REPRODUCTIVE ANATOMY

José Adán Amaya Duarte and
Kareling Alexandra Lopez Sandoval

ALLIED
HEALTH
PRESS

Reproductive Anatomy

Authors: **José Adán Amaya Duarte and Kareling Alexandra Lopez Sandoval**

Allied Health Press
4164 Lakeshore Road
Burlington ON L7L 1A4
Canada
www.alliedhealthpress.com
Email: orders@arclereducation.com

ISBN: 978-1-77956-262-3

ABOUT THE AUTHORS

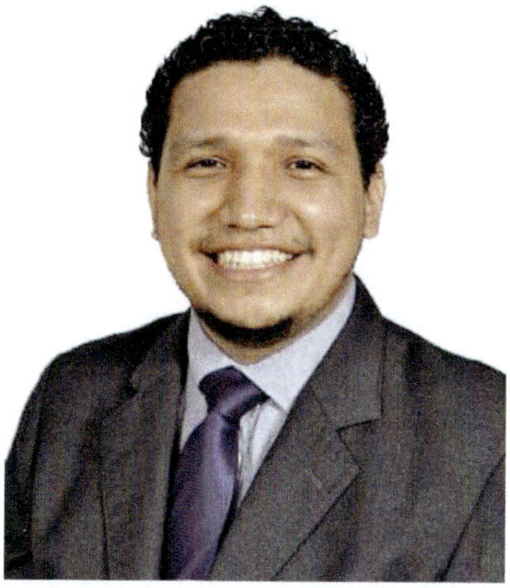

José Adan Amaya Duarte is a distinguished professional from León, Nicaragua, with a robust background in management, education, and public health. He currently serves as the General Manager and CEO of INVALA S.A., where he strategically oversees all operational aspects of the company to align with the board's objectives and ensure sustainable growth. José's career is also marked by significant contributions to education, specifically within the Pan American Health Organization, where he has held various roles such as Art Designer for Audiovisual Media, Virtual Learning Coach, and Content Creator. His work primarily involves creating educational content for public health, enhancing learning experiences through digital platforms. Educationally, José is a Doctor of Medicine and Surgery from UNAN-León, enriched by further training in areas such as 3D Printing and Biofabrication, Radiological Anatomy, and Medical Informatics. His proficiency in English and basic knowledge of German complements his extensive digital skills. José's commitment to continuous learning and professional development is evident through his active participation in various courses and workshops, including those on managing medical informatics and the effects of endocrine disruptors on health. His accolades include several honors for his educational contributions and innovations in mobile application development.

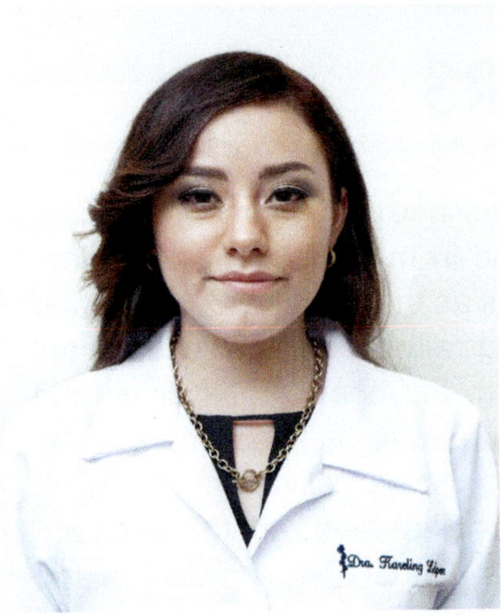

Kareling Alexandra Lopez Sandoval has made significant strides in the intersecting fields of medicine, management, and communication. Kareling currently excels as a Supervisor at OCLINICALS-GI Alliance, where she leads a team dedicated to enhancing patient engagement and practice performance in gastroenterology across the United States. Her role involves monitoring agent performance, providing training, and ensuring compliance with healthcare regulations, which she manages with a keen eye for detail and commitment to excellence. Before her current role, Kareling served as a Medical Scheduler at the same organization, where she coordinated patient appointments and ensured seamless communication between patients and healthcare providers. Her ability to handle complex cases and maintain high customer satisfaction has been a hallmark of her career. Kareling's expertise also extends to medical writing, where she contributed insightful articles on diseases and lab tests for C-MATER DEI Clinical Laboratory's website. This role allowed her to merge her clinical knowledge with her skill in communication, making complex medical information accessible to a broad audience. Kareling's academic background is as robust as her professional journey. She earned her Doctor of Medicine and Surgery from the National Autonomous University of Nicaragua, León, equipping her with a profound understanding of medical science, which she has applied throughout her career in health management and education.

ABOUT THE AUTHORS

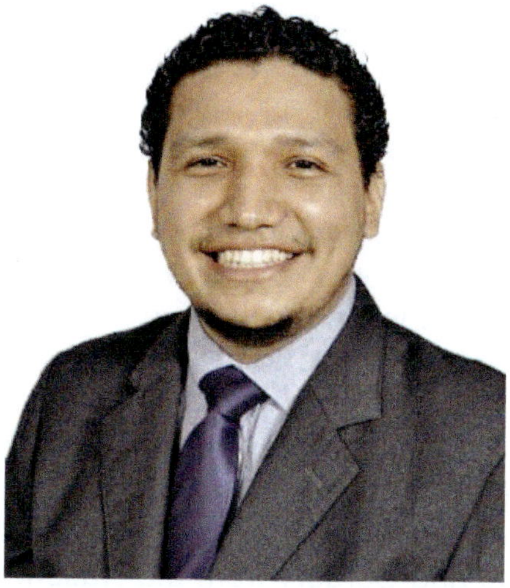

José Adan Amaya Duarte is a distinguished professional from León, Nicaragua, with a robust background in management, education, and public health. He currently serves as the General Manager and CEO of INVALA S.A., where he strategically oversees all operational aspects of the company to align with the board's objectives and ensure sustainable growth. José's career is also marked by significant contributions to education, specifically within the Pan American Health Organization, where he has held various roles such as Art Designer for Audiovisual Media, Virtual Learning Coach, and Content Creator. His work primarily involves creating educational content for public health, enhancing learning experiences through digital platforms. Educationally, José is a Doctor of Medicine and Surgery from UNAN-León, enriched by further training in areas such as 3D Printing and Biofabrication, Radiological Anatomy, and Medical Informatics. His proficiency in English and basic knowledge of German complements his extensive digital skills. José's commitment to continuous learning and professional development is evident through his active participation in various courses and workshops, including those on managing medical informatics and the effects of endocrine disruptors on health. His accolades include several honors for his educational contributions and innovations in mobile application development.

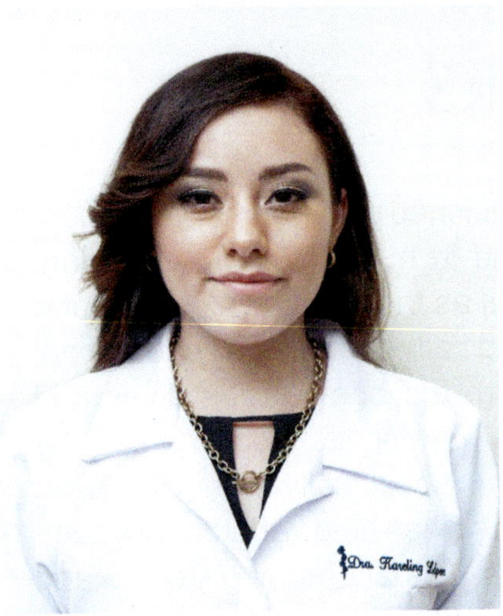

Kareling Alexandra Lopez Sandoval has made significant strides in the intersecting fields of medicine, management, and communication. Kareling currently excels as a Supervisor at OCLINICALS-GI Alliance, where she leads a team dedicated to enhancing patient engagement and practice performance in gastroenterology across the United States. Her role involves monitoring agent performance, providing training, and ensuring compliance with healthcare regulations, which she manages with a keen eye for detail and commitment to excellence. Before her current role, Kareling served as a Medical Scheduler at the same organization, where she coordinated patient appointments and ensured seamless communication between patients and healthcare providers. Her ability to handle complex cases and maintain high customer satisfaction has been a hallmark of her career. Kareling's expertise also extends to medical writing, where she contributed insightful articles on diseases and lab tests for C-MATER DEI Clinical Laboratory's website. This role allowed her to merge her clinical knowledge with her skill in communication, making complex medical information accessible to a broad audience. Kareling's academic background is as robust as her professional journey. She earned her Doctor of Medicine and Surgery from the National Autonomous University of Nicaragua, León, equipping her with a profound understanding of medical science, which she has applied throughout her career in health management and education.

Word Roots, Prefixes, and Suffixes by Chapter

Chapter 1 Introduction to Reproductive Anatomy

Ante-: Before
Dys-: Painful, difficult
Endo-: Within
Hydro-: Water
Intra-: Within
Multi-: Many

Chapter 2 Male Reproductive Anatomy

Neo-: New
Nulli-: None
Peri-: Around
Primi-: First
Secundi-: Second

Chapter 3 Female Reproductive Anatomy

-algia: Pain
-arche: Beginning
-cyesis: Pregnancy
-ectomy: Surgical removal of
-itis: Inflammation

Chapter 4 Gametogenesis

-optosis: Sagging
-orrhaphy: Suture
-orrhea: Discharge, flow
-oscopy: Visual examination
-otomy: Incision into

Chapter 5 Reproductive Hormones

-plasty: Surgical repair
-rrhagia: Burst forth, excessive flow
-salpinx: Fallopian tube
-tocia: Labor

Chapter 6 Menstrual Cycle

Amni/o: Amnion
Cephal/o: Head
Cervic/o: Cervix/neck
Chori/o: Chorion
Colp/o: Vagina
Culd/o: Retrouterine pouch (cul-de-sac)

Chapter 7 Fertilization and Early Development

Cyes/o, cyes/i: Pregnancy
Embry/o: Embryo
Endometri/o: Endometrium
Episi/o: Vulva
Fet/o: Fetus
Fimbri/o: Fimbria

Chapter 8 Pregnancy and Parturition

Galact/o: Milk
Genit/o: Genitalia
Gonad/o: Ovaries
Gravida: Pregnancy
Gynec/o, gyn/o: Woman, female
Hyster/o: Uterus
Lact/o: Milk

Chapter 9 Reproductive Disorders and Diseases

Lapar/o: Abdomen
Mamm/o, mast/o: Breast
Men/o: Menstruation
Metr/o, metr/io: Uterus
Mult/i: Many
My/o: Muscle
Myometri/o: Myometrium

Chapter 10 Reproductive Health and Ethics

Nat/o, nat/i: Birth
Null/i: None
Olig/o: Scanty
Omphal/o, umbilic/o: Umbilicus, navel
Oophor/o: Ovary
Ov/o, ov/i, ovul/o: Egg, ovum

Table of Contents

Table of Contents

7 Fertilization and Early Development 173

8 Pregnancy and Parturition 199

9 Reproductive Disorders and Diseases 225

10 Reproductive Health and Ethics 247

LIST OF FIGURES

activate epithelial Na+ channel (ENaC) that induce genes involved in implantation and post-implantation [illegible]. Developmentally compromised embryos [illegible]

LIST OF TABLES

PREFACE

The male and female reproductive systems are intricate and dynamic, reflecting complex underlying physiological processes. Despite significant advancements in scientific understanding, our current knowledge is primarily based on simplified views of individual cells and tissues. Processes like gamete production and hormone synthesis in the gonads are not isolated events but are part of extensive networks that undergo dynamic changes throughout development, from embryo to adulthood and into old age.

While molecular science has made great strides in identifying components of the reproductive system, the interactions and functions of these components in the context of time and space remain largely unknown. Recent innovations in microfluidics, stem cell biology, and the integration of single-cell transcriptomics with tissue dynamics offer promising approaches to unraveling these complexities. Understanding the reproductive system's normal functioning is crucial not only for fertility, but also for comprehending how it is impacted by diseases, environmental factors like endocrine disruptors, and aging. Additionally, the reproductive system is intricately linked with other physiological systems, playing a crucial role in maintaining health and well-being throughout life, including during pregnancy, puberty, adulthood, and old age.

A deeper understanding of the male and female reproductive systems is essential not just for fertility, but also for overall health across the lifespan. This understanding can help us address reproductive health issues, age-related changes, and the impacts of external factors, ultimately contributing to improved health and well-being.

The objective of this book is to provide a comprehensive resource for readers interested in understanding the intricate workings of the human reproductive system. It presents the latest scientific knowledge clearly and engagingly, catering to a diverse audience, including students, healthcare professionals, and individuals seeking a deeper understanding of their bodies.

Through detailed explanations and illustrations, it will explore the anatomy of both male and female reproductive systems, highlighting the structures and functions essential for reproduction. It will cover topics such as the development of reproductive organs, the hormonal regulation of reproductive processes, and the mechanisms of fertilization and pregnancy.

Common reproductive health issues, their causes, and available treatments empowering readers to make informed decisions about their reproductive health, are also discussed.

The book will serve as a valuable educational tool for students studying anatomy, biology, or healthcare-related fields, providing a solid foundation in reproductive anatomy. Healthcare professionals, including doctors, nurses, and midwives, will find it to be a useful reference guide, enhancing their understanding of reproductive health and enabling them to provide better care to their patients.

Chapter

INTRODUCTION TO REPRODUCTIVE ANATOMY

1

Contents

Unit Introduction

The biological system consisting of all the anatomical organs involved in sexual reproduction is called the reproductive system, or genital system, depending on the organism. Numerous inanimate materials, including hormones, pheromones, and fluids, are also crucial components of the reproductive system. In contrast to most organ systems, differentiated species frequently exhibit notable differences between the sexes. These variations enable the blending of genetic material between two individuals, potentially increasing the genetic fitness of the progeny.

Sexual activity typically results in internal fertilization of the human reproductive system. The male ejaculates sperm-containing semen into the female's vagina while inserting their erect penis there. After passing through the cervix and vagina, the sperm enters the uterus or uterine tubes to fertilize the ovum. When fertilization and implantation are successful, the fetus proceeds through a nine-month gestation period inside the female uterus; in humans, this is referred to as pregnancy. Childbirth marks the end of gestation, and delivery comes after labor. During labor, the cervix dilates, the uterine muscles contract and the baby passes out the vagina (the female genital organ). Human infants and kids are essentially defenseless and need intensive care from their parents for a long time. The use of a woman's mammary glands to nurse her infant is a significant form of parental care. The production of egg cells is the first purpose of the female reproductive system; the second is to safeguard and feed the fetus until it is born. The production and deposit of sperm is the sole purpose of the male reproductive system. Humans differ greatly in their sexual orientation. Apart from variations in almost all reproductive organs, multiple variations usually arise in secondary sexual traits.

The male reproductive system is a group of organs that are situated outside the body and in the male's pelvic area, and they are all involved in reproduction. The male reproductive system's main direct purpose is to supply male sperm for ovum fertilization. Three categories can be used to classify the major male reproductive organs. The creation and preservation of sperm is the first category. The temperature-regulating scrotum houses the testes, where production occurs. Immature sperm then move to the epididymis for development and storage. The second group consists of the glands that produce ejaculatory fluid, such as the vas deferens, prostate, and seminal vesicles. The last group consists of the organs that are utilized during copulation and spermatozoa (sperm) deposition within the male, such as Cowper's gland, the urethra, the penis, and the vas deferens.

Larger, more muscular stature, a deeper voice, facial and body hair, broad shoulders, and the emergence of Adam's apple are prominent secondary sex traits. Androgen, especially testosterone, is a key sexual hormone in men. The hormone that regulates sperm development is released by the testes. In addition, this hormone oversees the growth of physical traits in men like facial hair and a deep voice. The organs that are mostly found inside the body and in the vicinity of a woman's pelvic region and play a role in reproduction make up the human female reproductive system. The uterus, which houses the growing fetus, the vulva, which leads to the vagina and the vaginal opening, and the ovaries, which produce the female's ova, make up the human female reproductive system. Although the breasts participate in reproduction during the parenting stage, they are not regarded as a component of the female reproductive system in most classifications.

The vulva is where the vagina connects with the outside world, encompassing the labia, clitoris, and urethra. During intercourse, this area is lubricated by mucus from the greater vestibular glands. The vagina is linked to the uterus through the cervix, and the uterus is connected to the ovaries by the uterine tubes. Each ovary holds numerous ova, also known as ovum.

The pituitary gland secretes a hormone that encourages some ova to grow and develop once every 28 days. After release, a single ovum enters the uterus through the uterine tube. The ovaries secrete hormones that prime the uterus to receive the ovum. The ovum will pass through her uterine tubes and wait for fertilization to happen with the sperm. When this doesn't take place, i.e., the lining of the uterus or the endometrium, and unfertilized eggs are shed during each cycle during menstruation; no sperms are needed for fertilization. The process of embryonic development starts when the ovum attaches to the endometrium after being fertilized by sperm (Bradley, 2000; Marieb, 2000; Bergsjø, 2001; Cooper, 2001; Drake et al., 2004).

Orientation and Directional Terms

Terms	Definition	Illustration
Biological system	A biological system is a complex network which connects several biologically relevant entities.	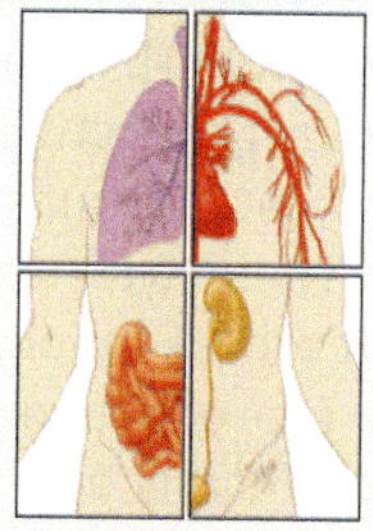
Reproductive system	The reproductive system of an organism, also known as the genital system, is the biological system made up of all the anatomical organs involved in sexual reproduction. Many non-living substances such as fluids, hormones, and pheromones are also important accessories to the reproductive system.	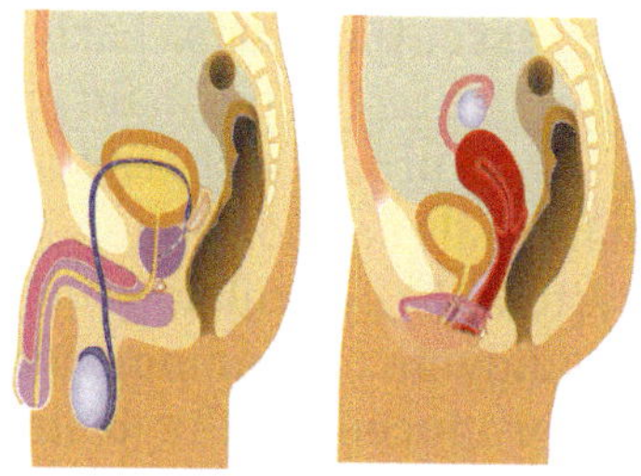
Vagina	The vagina is the elastic, muscular reproductive organ of the female genital tract. In humans, it extends from the vestibule to the cervix.	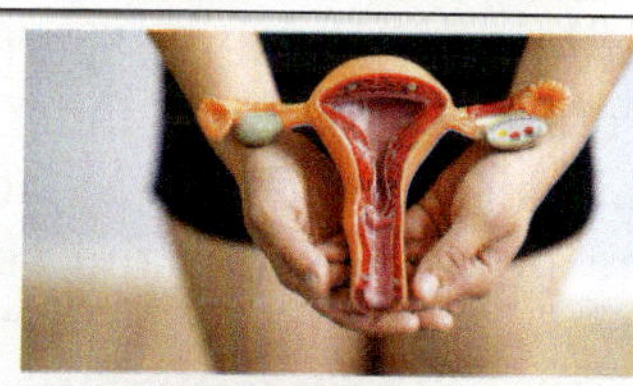
Menstruation	Menstruation is the regular discharge of blood and mucosal tissue from the inner lining of the uterus through the vagina.	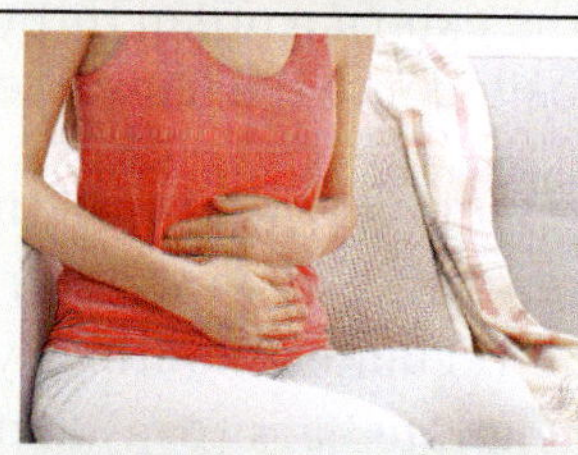
Epididymis	The epididymis is an elongated tubular structure attached to the posterior side of each one of the two male reproductive glands, the testicles.	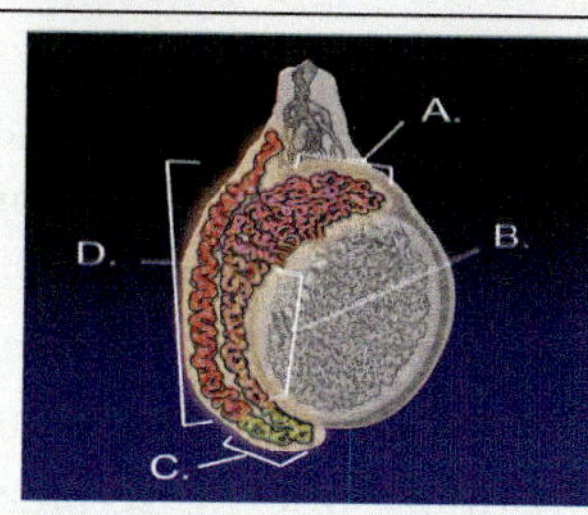

1.1. Overview of the Male and Female Reproductive Systems

The complex networks of organs and tissues that make up the reproductive systems of men and women are created to make reproduction easier for humans. Their structures and functions show notable differences tailored to their respective roles in the reproductive process, even though they both ultimately aim to produce offspring. The male reproductive system is made up of various essential parts, each with a distinct purpose. The testes, the main male reproductive organs that produce sperm, and testosterone, the main male sex hormone, are at the center of this system. The ejaculatory ducts, vas deferens, and epididymis are among the ducts that the sperm produced in the testes pass through before being released from the body through the urethra during ejaculation. Sperm are nourished and protected by seminal fluid, which includes semen, which is secreted by accessory glands like the prostate gland and seminal vesicles. Furthermore, during sexual activity, the penis acts as the external organ through which sperm are deposited into the female reproductive tract.

The female reproductive system, on the other hand, is more intricate and has a hormone-regulated monthly cycle. The ovaries, which generate eggs (ova) and secrete the two primary female sex hormones, progesterone, and estrogen, are the main organs of the female reproductive system. Ovulation is the process by which one egg is released from an ovary during each menstrual cycle and is caught by the uterine tube's fimbriae. When an egg is fertilized by sperm, it passes through the uterine tube, enters the uterus, implants into the lining of the uterus, and grows into a fetus. During menstruation, the uterine lining sheds if fertilization is unsuccessful. The pear-shaped organ known as the uterus, or womb, is where fetal development occurs during pregnancy. The vulva, which is made up of the vaginal opening, clitoris, labia majora, and labia minora, surrounds the external genitalia. Hormones produced by the pituitary gland, gonads, and hypothalamus affect the reproductive systems of both sexes, coordinating the intricate processes of gamete production, hormone secretion, and sexual differentiation. Furthermore, lifestyle decisions, genetic predispositions, and environmental influences can influence reproductive health in both sexes, resulting in diseases like cancers of the reproductive system, STDs, and infertility.

The reproductive systems of men and women are marvels of biological engineering, with unique structures and roles to guarantee the survival of humanity in each case. Comprehending the complexities of these systems is essential for maintaining fertility and reproductive health, as well as for developing medical treatments and technological advancements targeted at improving reproductive results.

1.1.1. Human Reproductive System

The male and female reproductive systems of humans are responsible for producing and depositing sperm and egg cells, respectively, and for protecting and nourishing the fetus until it is born. Humans differ greatly in their sexual orientation. There are variations in almost every reproductive organ as well as in the characteristics of typical secondary sex.

Sexual activity usually results in internal fertilization during human reproduction. This involves the male penetrating the female's vagina with his penis and ejaculating sperm-containing semen. A tiny percentage of sperm enter the uterus through the cervix, travel through it, and eventually exit into the uterine tubes to fertilize the ovum. Fertilization of the ovum requires only one sperm. The fertilized ovum, or zygote, exits the uterine tube and enters the uterus after successful fertilization, where it implants in the uterine wall. This is the start of gestation, or pregnancy, which lasts for about nine months while the fetus grows. Childbirth, which involves labor, marks the end of pregnancy when the fetus has reached a specific developmental stage. The uterine muscles contract, the cervix dilates over several hours, and the baby emerges from the vagina during labor. Human babies need a lot of parental care because they are entirely dependent on their caregivers. Babies look to their caregivers for food, clean clothes, and comfort. Food can be given through formula feeding or nursing.

1.1.1.1. Structure

1. **Female:** The organs that are mostly found inside the body and in the vicinity of near a woman's pelvic region and play a role in reproduction make up the human female reproductive system. The uterus, which houses the growing fetus, the vulva, which leads to the vagina and the vaginal opening, and the ovaries, which produce the female's ova, make up the human female reproductive system. Although the breasts are involved in reproduction during the parenting stage, they are not regarded as a component of the female reproductive system in most classifications.

   The vulva, which also contains the clitoris, urethra, and labia, is where the vagina joins the outside world. During sexual activity, mucus secreted by the greater vestibular glands lubricates this area. The uterine tubes connect the uterus to the ovaries, while the cervix connects the uterus to the vagina. Hundreds of egg cells, or ova (singular ovum), are found in each ovary.

   The pituitary gland secretes a hormone that encourages some ova to grow and develop once every 28 days. After release, a single ovum enters the uterus through the uterine tube. The ovaries secrete hormones that prime the uterus to receive the ovum. Menstruation is the process through which unfertilized eggs and the endometrium, the lining of the uterus, are shed each cycle. The ovum attaches to the endometrium and develops into a fetus if sperms fertilize it.

2. **Male:** The organs that surround a man's pelvic area and are external to the body make up the male reproductive system, which aids in reproduction. The male reproductive system's main direct purpose is to supply male sperm for ovum fertilization. Penile shrinkage brought on by chilly conditions. To control testicular temperatures, the scrotum is tense.

   Three categories can be used to classify the major male reproductive organs. Sperm (spermatozoa) are produced and stored by the first category. The temperature-regulating scrotum houses the testes, which produce these. Immature sperm then move to the epididymis for development and storage. The second group consists of glands that produce ejaculatory fluid, such as the vas deferens, seminal vesicles, prostate, and Cowper's gland (also known as the bulb-urethral gland).

The penis, urethra, and vas deferens are among the last group; these are used for copulation and sperm deposition inside the female.

The development of Adam's apple, a deeper voice, facial and body hair, larger, more muscular stature, and broad shoulders are some of the main secondary sexual traits. Androgen, especially testosterone, is a key sexual hormone in men. The hormone that regulates sperm development is released by the testes. In addition, this hormone oversees the growth of physical traits in men like facial hair and a deep voice.

1.1.1.2. Development

The development of the human fetus is intimately related to the development of the reproductive and urinary systems. The intermediate mesoderm is the source of both adult female and male differences. The mesonephric duct (Müllerian ducts), paramesonephric ducts (Wolffian ducts), and gonads are the three primary fetal precursors of the reproductive organs. One well-known and important controlling factor in the proper differentiation of the reproductive system is endocrine hormones.

In the male reproductive system, the mesonephric duct forms the vas deferens, ductus deferens, ejaculatory duct, and seminal vesicle; in the female reproductive system, it virtually vanishes. The paramesonephric ducts duct does the opposite in the male and female reproductive systems, essentially disappearing in the former and forming the uterus, uterine tubes, and vagina in the latter. The gonads develop into the testes and ovaries in both sexes; these organs are regarded as homologous because they originate from the same undeveloped structure. The reproductive systems of men and women share several other homologous structures. The male epididymis and vas deferens, as well as the female uterine tubes, have similar functions, but they are not homologous structures; rather, they are analogs because they develop from distinct fetal structures (Bradley, 2000; Marieb, 2000; Bergsjø, 2001; Cooper, 2001; Drake et al., 2004).

1.1.2. Reproduction

1.1.2.1. Production of Gametes

Gametogenesis is the process by which gametes are created inside the gonads. This happens when specific types of germ cells divide into haploid cells with only 23 chromosomes and normal diploid cells with 46 chromosomes during the meiotic process. This process, called spermatogenesis in males, occurs in the seminiferous tubules of the testes only after puberty. After entering the epididymis, the immature spermatozoa or sperm acquire a tail that allows for motility. Each of the four functional gametes that are produced by the initial diploid germ cells, also known as primary spermatocytes, is eternally young. Sperm production and viability depend on a temperature lower than the average body temperature. The temperature in the scrotum, which houses the testes, is around 3°C lower than the rest of the body because it is located outside the cavity.

Gametogenesis also referred to as oogenesis in females takes place in the ovarian follicles of the ovaries. It takes puberty for this process to produce a mature ovum. Unlike males, each of the initial diploid germ cells, also known as primary oocytes, will develop into three polar bodies that cannot be fertilized and one mature ovum. It has long been known that all a female's primary oocytes are produced before birth, in contrast to males, and that the last stages of ova production do not resume until puberty.

Recent scientific findings, however, have called into question that theory. According to this new research, female mammals in at least some species of mammals continue to produce new eggs long after giving birth.

1.1.2.2. Disease

Like all complex organ systems, the human reproductive system is affected by many diseases. There are four main categories of reproductive diseases in humans.

They are:

- Genetic or congenital abnormalities;
- Cancers;
- Infections, which are often sexually transmitted diseases;
- Varicocele;
- Functional problems are caused by environmental factors, physical damage, psychological issues, autoimmune disorders, or other causes. The best-known functional problems include sexual dysfunction and infertility, which are both broad terms relating to many disorders with many causes.

Certain reproductive diseases are challenging to categorize because they frequently exhibit symptoms of other illnesses or disorders or have multiple, unclear causes. For example, endometriosis in females and Peyronie's disease in males are examples of disorders that cannot be classified. Reproductive abnormalities are a common symptom of many congenital conditions, but their other symptoms are often more well-known.

1.1.3. Male Reproductive System

A variety of sex organs that are involved in human reproduction make up the male reproductive system. These organs are found inside the pelvis and on the exterior of the body. The primary male sex organs are the penis and the testicles, which secrete semen and sperm. During a sexual encounter, these substances fertilize an ovum in the female's body, which then grows into a fetus that is eventually born as an infant. The female reproductive system in females is the analogous system (Figure 1.1).

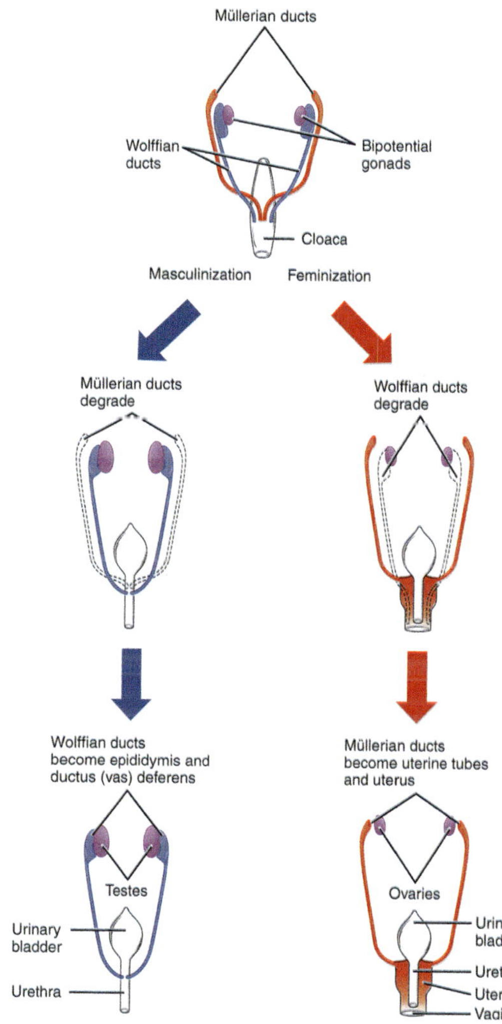

Figure 1.1. *Sexual differentiation in males and females.*

Source: By OpenStax College - Anatomy & Physiology, Connections Web site. http://cnx.org/content/col11496/1.6/, Jun 19, 2013., CC BY 3.0, https://commons.wikimedia.org/w/index.php?curid=30148605.

By the six weeks of development in both sexes, the primordial germ cells have moved from their previous extra embryonic position to the gonadal ridges, where they are encircled by the sex cords to form a pair of primitive gonads. Whether chromosomally XX or XY, the forming gonad has potential up until this moment. According to current theory, the coordinated action of several genes that support ovarian development in the absence of a Y chromosome or Y testicular development controls the development of an ovary or testis. Unless a gene called TDF (testis defined factor), located on the Y's shooting arm, functions as a switch, the ovarian pathway is followed, causing development to diverge into the male pathway.

One of the main focuses in medical genetics is currently finding the key gene that determines testis development. In the presence of the Y chromosome, medullary tissue forms traditional testes with seminiferous tubules and interstitial cells that can produce androgens when stimulated by human chorionic gonadotropin (HCG) from the placenta. Spermatogonia, derived from primordial germ cells through around 200 mitoses, line the walls of the seminiferous tubules with support from sustentacular cells. In the absence of a Y chromosome, the gonad defaults to developing into an ovary, with the cortex developing, the medulla regressing, and oogonia starting to develop within follicles. Oogonia are created from primitive germ cells through approximately 30 mitoses, fewer than needed for spermatogenesis.

At approximately the end of the third month, oogonia begins meiosis 1, but this process is halted at a stage known as dictyotene, during which the cell survives until ovulation occurs several years later. Just 400 of the oogonia mature into ova during the 30 years or so that a female reaches sexual maturity; the majority of oogonia degenerate before birth. As the primordial germ cells migrate to the genital ridges, thickenings in the ridges indicate the developing genital ducts, the mesonephric (formerly called Wolffian) and paramesonephric (formerly called Mullerian) ducts. The male genital ducts form when the mesonephric ducts are stimulated to form by the release of androgen by the Leydig cells of the fetal testes, and the paramesonephric duct formation is suppressed by a hormone produced by the sustentacular cells. In the female (or non-gonadic embryo), the paramesonephric ducts grow into the female duct system, while the mesonephric ducts regress. A genital tubercle, paired labioscrotal swellings, and paired urethra folds make up the outer genitals in an early embryo. Male external genitals develop from this undifferentiated state under the influence of androgens, while female external genitals are produced whether or not an ovary is present in the absence of a testis.

1.1.3.1. Male Phenotype

- To raise blood concentrations to the same level as those observed in adult males, fetal testicular cells secrete an adequate amount of testosterone. The TDF gene, also known as the SRY (sex-determining region of the Y chromosome), exerts an additional influence on testosterone accumulation by suppressing the production of aromatase and preventing the conversion of testosterone to estrogens. The development of the mesonephric ducts, which give rise to the internal male genital tracts, is stimulated by testosterone.
- Sertoli cells in the newly differentiated seminiferous tubule secrete a glycoprotein called anti-mullerian hormone (AMH) under the influence of the SRY gene product and various transcription factors, inducing

apoptosis of tubular epithelial cells and atrophy or reabsorption of the Mullerian ducts (which would have become the female internal genital tract).

- The urogenital sinus and genital tubercle are the primitive structures that give rise to the external genitalia in both sexes. The scrotum, prostate gland, and penis are formed by the fetal testis secreting testosterone, which is necessary for the masculinization of these structures. If androgen is not stimulated, those structures develop into the female external genitalia. When there is too much androgen in female embryos or insufficient androgen in male embryos, and the external genitalia are unclear, differentiation is not complete. Dihydrotestosterone, not testosterone, is what distinguishes male external genitalia.

1.1.3.2. Female Phenotype

- Estrogen is secreted by the ovaries in gonadal females but not by testosterone anti-mullerian hormone.
- Mesonephric ducts cannot distinguish without testosterone.
- Mullerian is not suppressed without anti-mullerian ducts and thus develops into the female internal genital tract.

1.1.3.3. External Genital Organs

1. **Penis:** The male intromittent organ is the penis. Its glans penis, an enlarged bulbous tip that supports and shields the foreskin, is situated at the end of its long shaft. The penis becomes erect and prepared for sexual activity when the male is aroused sexually. Blood fills the sinuses located in the penis' erectile tissue during an erection. Blood enters the erectile cartilage under pressure when the penis's arteries dilate, and its veins constrict. The pudendal artery supplies blood to the penis.
2. **Scrotum:** It is a pouch located behind the penis that houses and shields the testicles. Filled with nerves and blood vessels, it adapts to temperature changes by contracting the Cremaster muscle, which pulls the scrotum closer to the body, and the Dartos muscle, which gives it a wrinkled look. As temperatures rise, both muscles relax to lower the scrotum and smooth out any wrinkles.

   The inguinal canal keeps the scrotum attached to the abdomen or pelvic cavity. The spermatic cord enters the testis through the inguinal canal after being formed from the spermatic artery, vein, and nerve joined together with connective tissue (Figure 1.2).

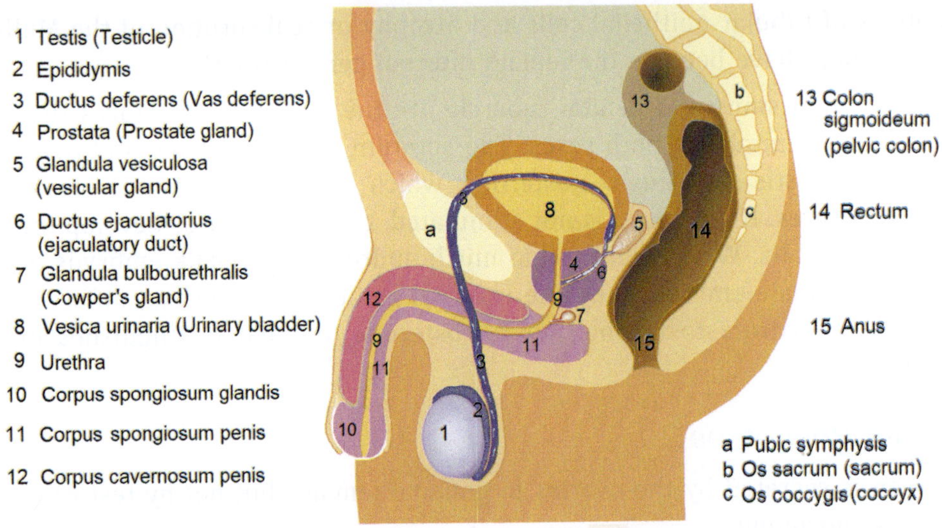

Figure 1.2. *Diagram showing the external and internal parts of the male reproductive system.*

Source: By The old versions were from Tsaitgaist. This new image is reworked, changed, and improved by Sciencia58 so that there is no problem anymore. File: Male and female anatomy.svg, CC BY-SA 4.0, https://commons.wikimedia.org/w/index.php?curid=140554261.

1.1.3.4. Internal Genital Organs

The production of sperm through the meiotic division of germ cells within seminiferous tubules and the synthesis and secretion of androgens, which control male reproductive functions, are the two main purposes of the testis. The interstitial cells found in the space between seminiferous tubules are where androgens are produced.

1. **Epididymis:** The epididymis is a long, white, tube that is tightly wound. The epididymis receives the sperm produced in the seminiferous tubules. Ion channels on the apical membrane of the epididymis act to concentrate the sperm during their maturation during passage through the epididymis.
2. **Vas Deferens:** The vas deferens, which is also known as the sperm duct, is a thin tube approximately 30 centimeters (0.98 ft) long that starts from the epididymis to the pelvic cavity. It carries the spermatozoa from the epididymis to the ejaculatory duct.
3. **Accessory Glands:** Three accessory glands provide fluids that lubricate the duct system and nourish the sperm cells. They are the seminal vesicles, the prostate gland, and the bulbourethral glands (Cowper glands).

1.1.3.5. Development

The process by which the reproductive organs develop mature, and become established in the male reproductive system occurs during the embryonic and prenatal stages. A single fertilized egg starts the process, which ends 38 weeks later with the birth of a male child. It's a phase of the sexual differentiation process. The male reproductive system and the urinary system develop at the same time. Together, their development can also be referred to as the development of the reproductive and urinary systems.

1.1.3.5.1. Sexual Determination

When a sperm cell with either an X or Y chromosome initiates the genetic sex of the zygote during fertilization, the zygote's sexual identity is established. A female child will develop if this sperm cell has an X chromosome, which matches the X chromosome of the ovum. An XY combination produced by a sperm cell with a Y chromosome leads to the development of a male offspring. Whether the gonads become the ovaries, or the testes is determined by genetic sex. If the testes are developed in the developing embryo, they will secrete and produce male sex hormones in the late stages of embryonic development, which will cause the development of the male's secondary sex organs.

1.1.3.6. Other Embryonic Reproductive Structures

The structures are masculinized by secretions of the testes:

- Urogenital sinus;
- Genital tubercle;
- Urogenital folds;
- Cloacal membrane;
- Labioscrotal folds.

The prostate gland derives from the urogenital sinus, and the other embryonic structures differentiate into the external genitalia. In the absence of testicular secretions, the female genitalia is formed.

1.1.3.7. External Structures

The external genitalia of the male and female have not yet differentiated at six weeks after conception. During the indifferent stage, a distinct phallus is visible at eight weeks. By the tenth or twelfth week, the genitalia, which are derived from their homologous structures, are identifiable as male or female. The genitalia is developed and distinct at 16 weeks after conception.

Testosterone secreted by the developing testes causes the masculinization of the developing reproductive structures. However, the active ingredient in these organs is not testosterone. Once within the target cells, testosterone is transformed into dihydrotestosterone (DHT) by an enzyme known as 5α-reductase. In these organs, the androgen effect is mediated by DHT.

1.1.3.8. Testes

Male gonad and testicular differentiation are well advanced at nine weeks. One of the internal changes is the formation of tubular seminar Chris tubules from the primary sex cord in the Rete testis. The gubernaculum, a Fibromuscular cord, develops on the exterior of each testis. A section of the embryonic mesonephric duct adjacent to the testis becomes attached and convoluted, informing the epididymis, at the same time as this structure attaches to the inferior portion of the testis and extends to the labial sacral fold of the same side. As the ductus deferens, another section of the mesonephric duct develops. The prostate gland arises from an Indo dermal outgrowth of the urogenital sinus; the bulbourethral glands develop from outgrowths in the membrane-like portion of the urethra; the seminal vesicles form from lateral outgrowths of the caudal and of each mesonephric duct.

The testes descend to their ultimate position at the anterior abdominal wall, and then the gubernaculum develops, pulling and translocating the testis into the growing scrotum. The passageway eventually shuts behind the testis. An infantile hydrocoele or an indirect inguinal hernia may result from a breakdown in this process. Between the sixth and the tenth week, the testes descend into the scrotal sac. Contrary to what is known, dissent into this does not happen until roughly the 28th week, and the abdominal wall forms canals that provide openings from the pelvic cavity to the scrotal sac. The mechanism by which a testis descends is poorly understood, but it appears to be linked to the shortening of the gubernaculum, which is attached to the testis and extends to the inguinal canal to the wall of the scrotum. It carries with it lymph vessels, a section of the abdominal muscle, and the ductus deference, or testicular vessels and nerves. By the time the testis reaches the scrotal sac, the gubernaculum has reduced to a scar-like remnant of tissue. All the structures continue to attach to the testis, forming what is known as the spermatic cord (Bradley, 2000; Marieb, 2000; Bergsjø, 2001; Cooper, 2001; Drake et al., 2004).

1.1.4. Female Reproductive System

The female reproductive system is made to do multiple tasks. It creates the ova, also known as oocytes, which are female egg cells required for reproduction. Its function is to deliver the eggs to the location of fertilization. The uterine tubes are where conception—the fertilization of an egg by a sperm—usually takes place. The fertilized egg will then proceed to implant into the uterine walls, initiating the first phases of pregnancy. The mechanism is intended to undergo menstruation, or the monthly shedding of the uterine lining if fertilization and/or implantation are unsuccessful. The female reproductive system also generates female sex hormones, which are necessary to keep the reproductive cycle going.

1.1.4.1. What Is the Female Reproductive System?

The word "vulva," which means "covering," refers to the external portion of the female reproductive organs. The vulva, which is situated between the legs, protects the opening to the vagina and other internal reproductive organs. The mons pubis is the term for the fleshy region that is situated just above the top of the vaginal opening. The vaginal opening is surrounded by two pairs of skin flaps known as the labia, or lips. The point where the labia folds converge in front of the vulva is home to the clitoris, a tiny sensory organ. The urethra, the canal that transports urine from the bladder to the outside of the body, and the vagina are accessible through the openings between the labia. Pubic hair covers the mons pubis and the outer labia in girls who reach sexual maturity.

A woman's uterus, uterine tubes, ovaries, and vagina are her internal reproductive organs. The muscular, hollow vagina tube connects the uterus to the vaginal opening. The vagina can expand and contract due to the muscle walls that support it. The vagina can fit something as thin as a tampon and as wide as a baby thanks to its ability to expand and contract. Mucous membranes line the muscular walls of the vagina, keeping it moist and protected.

The vagina serves three purposes:

- It's where the penis is inserted during sexual intercourse;
- It's the pathway (the birth canal) through which a baby leaves a woman's body during childbirth;
- It's the route through which menstrual blood leaves the body during periods.

The hymen is a thin piece of skin-like tissue that partially covers the opening of the vagina and can vary in appearance from woman to woman. Many women find that their hymens have stretched or torn after their first sexual encounter, often resulting in slight bleeding without much pain. However, some women may not experience any changes to their hymens after sex, while others may find that their hymens have already stretched before engaging in sexual activity. The uterus has a muscular wall and an inverted pear-like shape. In fact, the uterus has some of the strongest muscles in the female body. These muscles can contract and expand to meet the needs of a developing fetus and then assist in pushing the baby out during labor. The uterus is only about 3 inches (7.5 cm) long and 2 inches (5 centimeters) wide when a woman is not pregnant.

The uterine tubes connect the uterus to the ovaries at the upper corners of the uterus. Located above and to the right of the uterus are two oval-shaped organs called the ovaries. Ovulation is the process by which they create, store, and release eggs into the uterine tubes (pronounced: av-yoo-LAY-shun). Each of the two uterine tubes, which are connected to either side of the uterus, is pronounced fuh-LO-pee-un. There is a tiny opening no bigger than a sewing needle inside each tube. Each uterine tube has a fringed region that resembles a funnel at the other end. The ovary is encircled by this fringed region, which is not entirely attached to it. An egg enters the uterine tube after emerging from an ovary. Tiny hairs in the lining of the uterine tube assist in pushing the egg down the tiny passageway and toward the uterus once it is inside.

The ovaries (pronounced: OH-vuh-reez) are also part of the endocrine system because they produce female sex hormones such as estrogen (pronounced: ESS-truh-jun) and progesterone (pronounced: pro-JESS-tuh-rone) (Figure 1.3).

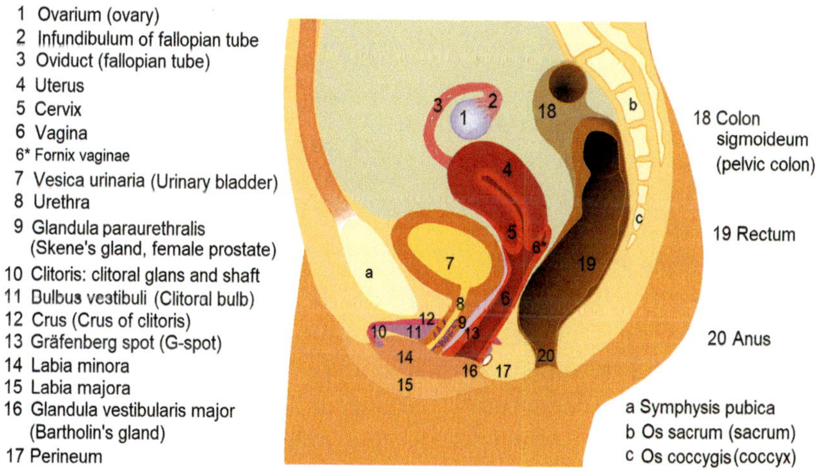

Figure 1.3. *Organs of the female reproductive system.*

Source: By The old versions were from Tsaitgaist. This new image is reworked, changed, and improved by Sciencia58 so that there is no problem anymore. File: Male and female anatomy.svg, CC BY-SA 4.0, https://commons.wikimedia.org/w/index.php?curid=140544867.

1.1.4.2. Organs of the Female Reproductive System

The female reproductive system's organs create and maintain the female sex cells, also known as ova or egg cells, move these cells to a location where sperm may fertilize them, give the developing fetus a good environment, remove the fetus from the mother when its development is complete, and produce the female sex hormones. The ovaries, uterine tubes, uterus, vagina, accessory glands, and external genital organs make up the female reproductive system.

- Ovaries;
- Genital tract;
- External genitalia;
- Female sexual response and hormonal control;
- Mammary glands.

1.1.4.3. Ovaries

The primary female reproductive organs, or gonads, are the two ovaries. Each ovary is a solid, ovoid structure about the size and shape of an almond (about 3.5 cm in length, 2 cm wide, and 1 cm thick). The ovaries are in shallow depressions, called ovarian fossae, one on each side of the uterus, in the lateral walls of the pelvic cavity. They are held loosely in place by peritoneal ligaments.

1.1.4.3.1. Structure

A layer of basic cuboidal epithelium known as germinal (ovarian) epithelium covers the outside of the ovaries. The tunica albuginea, a dense capsule of connective tissue, lies beneath this layer. There is a clear separation between the inner medulla and the outer cortex within the ovarian substance. Because there are many ovarian follicles in the cortex at different stages of development, the cortex appears denser and more granular. A female germ cell known as an oocyte is present in each follicle. There are many blood vessels, lymphatic vessels, and nerve fibers in the medulla, which is a loose connective tissue structure.

1.1.4.3.2. Oogenesis

Oogenesis is a type of meiosis that occurs in the ovaries to produce gametes or female sex cells. Though the timing and outcome are different, the events in oogenesis follow a similar sequence to those in spermatogenesis. Primitive germ cells in the ovaries differentiate into oogonia early in fetal development. These quickly divide to produce thousands of cells with a complete complement of 46 (23 pairs) chromosomes, which are still referred to as oogonia. After that, oogonia grow larger and go through a growth phase to become primary oocytes. The first meiotic division is initiated by the diploid (46 chromosomes) primary oocytes, but the process ends in prophase, leaving the cells in a suspended state that lasts until puberty. The two ovaries together contain about 7,00,000 oocytes at birth, although many of the primary oocytes degenerate before birth. There will never be another supply; this is the lifetime supply. This is significantly different from the male, where primary spermatocytes and spermatogonia are continuously produced during the reproductive lifetime. The quantity of primary oocytes has further decreased to roughly 4,00,000 by puberty.

The follicle-stimulating hormone causes a few primary oocytes to begin growing again every month starting during puberty. Meiosis I is resumed by one primary oocyte that appears to outgrow the others. The remaining cells deteriorate. The big cell divides unevenly, resulting in one cell that becomes a secondary oocyte and contains almost all the cytoplasm, organelles, and half of the chromosomes. The first polar body, a smaller cell, receives the other half of the chromosomes. The second meiotic division of the secondary oocyte starts, but it ends in metaphase. This is when ovulation takes place. In the event of fertilization, meiosis II proceeds. With all the cytoplasm going to the ovum, which contains 23 single-stranded chromosomes, this division is also unequal. A second polar body is produced by this division's smaller cell. During meiosis I, the first polar body typically divides again to create two even smaller polar bodies. The secondary oocyte degenerates and the second meiotic division is never finished in the event that fertilization is unsuccessful. Again, there are clear distinctions between the male and female in this instance. Each primary spermatocyte produces four viable sperm during spermatogenesis. During oogenesis, a primary oocyte gives rise to a single fertile cell. The remaining three cells undergo degeneracy and are polar bodies.

1.1.4.3.3. Ovarian Follicle Development

An oocyte in development is encased in one or more layers of cells known as follicular cells to form an ovarian follicle. The follicular cells undergo corresponding alterations while the oocyte advances through meiosis. At birth and throughout childhood, the ovaries contain primordial follicles, which are developed in the fetus and comprise a primary oocyte encircled by a single layer of flattened cells (Figure 1.4).

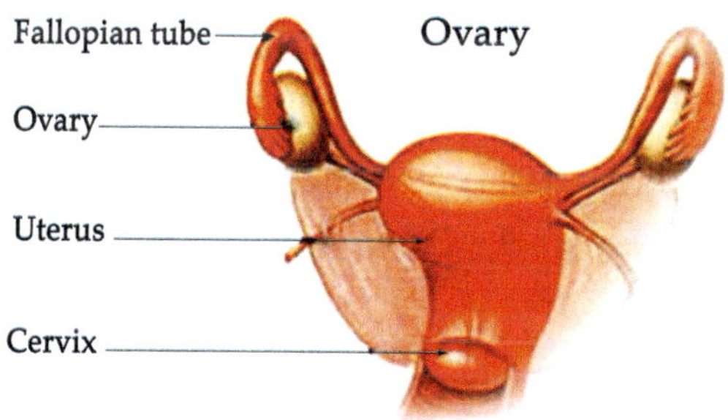

Figure 1.4. *Structure of the ovary.*

Source: Public Domain, https://commons.wikimedia.org/w/index.php?curid=10704998.

Follicle-stimulating hormone induces alterations in primordial follicles starting at puberty. The primary oocyte grows, the follicular cells take on a cuboidal shape, and it becomes a primary follicle. The follicle-stimulating hormone causes the follicles to keep growing, and as a result, the follicular cells multiply and surround the primary oocyte with multiple layers of granulose cells. One of these primary follicles usually develops each month, but most of them degenerate along with the primary oocytes inside of them. When the granulosa cells begin to secrete estrogen, the follicle develops an antrum or cavity. The follicle turns into a secondary follicle when the antrum begins to form. The zona pellucida, a transparent membrane that encircles the oocyte, is formed by a glycoprotein material secreted by the granulose cells. The follicle matures into a vesicular (graafian) follicle after roughly 10 days of growth. This follicle forms a swelling on the ovary's surface and contains a secondary oocyte that is ready for ovulation.

1.1.4.3.4. Ovulation

Ovulation is triggered by luteinizing hormone from the anterior pituitary, causing the mature follicle on the surface of the ovary to rupture. This releases the secondary oocyte into the peritoneal cavity. The ovulated secondary oocyte, prepared for fertilization, remains surrounded by the zona pellucida and a few layers of cells known as the corona radiata. If fertilization does not occur, the secondary oocyte will degrade in a matter of days. However, if a sperm breaches the corona radiata and zona pellucida and enters the cytoplasm of the secondary oocyte, the second meiotic division restarts, resulting in the formation of a polar body and a mature ovum.

The portion of the follicle that is still in the ovary enlarges and becomes a corpus luteum after ovulation in response to luteinizing hormone. Progesterone and a small amount of estrogen are secreted by the corpus luteum, a glandular structure. Its future is determined by the outcome of fertilization. The corpus luteum continues to produce hormones for approximately 10 days if fertilization is unsuccessful. After that, it starts to degenerate into a corpus albicans, which is essentially scar tissue. In the event of fertilization, the corpus luteum endures and keeps on secreting hormones until the placenta grows to the point where it can do so. Once more, the corpus luteum eventually gives way to corpus albicans, but this time it stays active for a longer amount of time.

1.1.4.4. Genital Tract

1.1.4.4.1. Uterine Tubes (Fallopian Tubes)

There are two uterine tubes, sometimes known as oviducts or uterine tubes. Every ovary has a single tube associated with it. The tube near the ovary expands to form an infundibulum that resembles a funnel and is encircled by fimbriae, which are projections that resemble fingers. The ovum enters the peritoneal cavity before the uterine tube due to the lack of a direct connection between the ovary and the infundibulum. The fimbriae become more active during ovulation, causing currents in the peritoneal fluid to assist in pushing the oocyte into the uterine tube. The oocyte is propelled through the uterine tube by the peristaltic action of the smooth muscle in the tube wall as well as the regular beating of cilia on the epithelial lining. The uterine tube travels for roughly seven days. Fertilization typically takes place in the uterine tube since the oocyte is only fertile for 24 to 48 hours.

1.1.4.4.2. Uterus

The uterus is a muscular organ that takes in the fertilized oocyte and gives the growing fetus a suitable environment. The uterus resembles a pear in size and shape before the first pregnancy, with the narrow end pointing inferiorly. The uterus typically grows after childbirth and then shrinks after menopause (Figure 1.5).

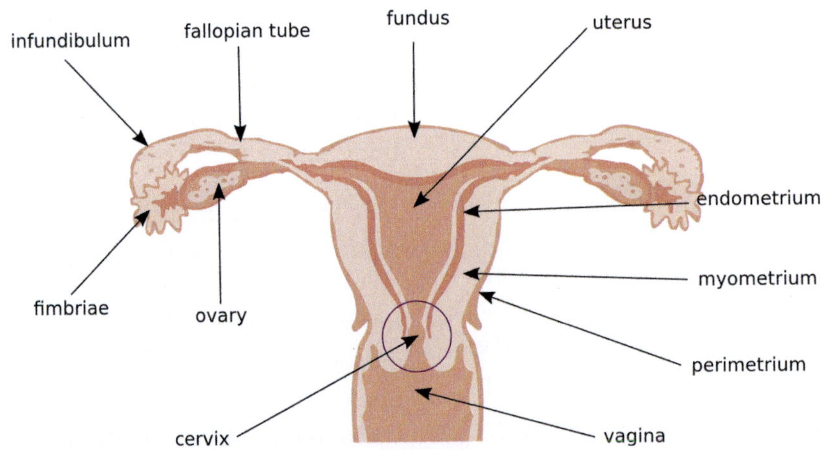

Figure 1.5. *Uterus and uterine tubes.*

Source: http By Original: US Government Vector: Pixel squid⍰ – Own work based on: Illu cervix. jpg: Public Domain, https://commons.wikimedia.org/w/index.php?curid=103131877.

The endometrium lines the inside of the uterus. During menstruation, the endometrial stratum functionale sheds. Rebuilding the stratum functionale is based on the deeper stratum basale.

1.1.4.4.3. Vagina

The vagina is a fibromuscular tube that connects the uterus's cervix to the outside. It is roughly 10 cm long. It is situated between the bladder and the rectum. The cervix projects into the vagina at almost a right angle because the vagina is tilted posteriorly as it ascends, and the cervix is tilted anteriorly. In addition to being the birth canal during childbirth, the vagina receives the erect penis during sexual activity and acts as a conduit for menstrual flow.

1.1.4.5. External Genitalia

The accessory structures of the female reproductive system that are located outside of the vagina are known as the external genitalia. They go by the name's pudendum and vulva as well. The labia majora, mons pubis, labia minora, clitoris, and vestibule glands are examples of external genitalia. Like the male penis, the clitoris is an erectile organ that reacts to sexual stimulation. The urethra, vagina, paraurethral glands, and greater vestibular glands (Bartholin's glands) open into the vestibule posterior to the clitoris (Figure 1.6).

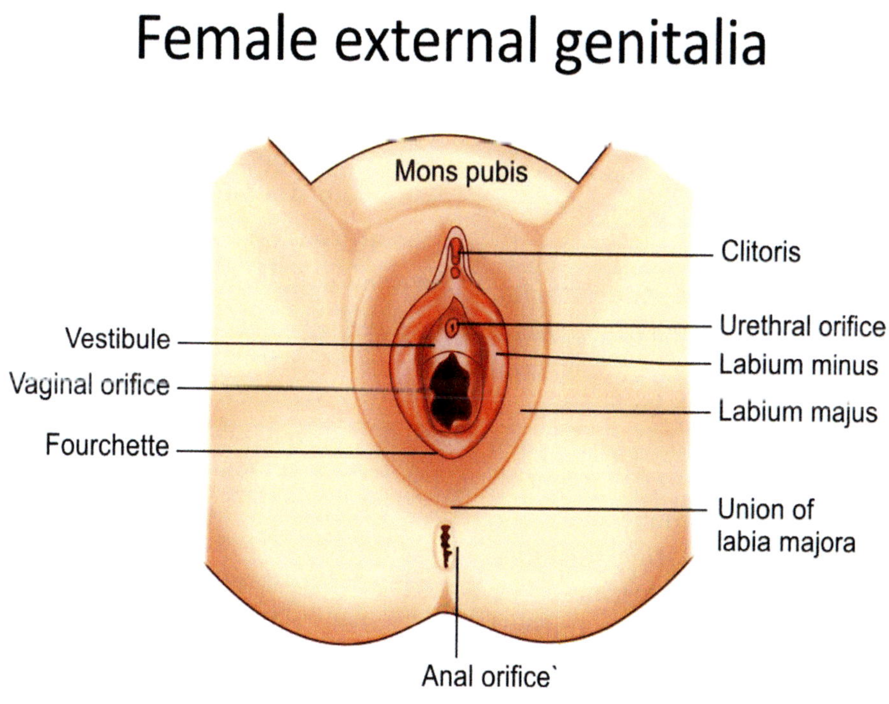

Figure 1.6. *Female external genitalia.*

Source: https://sp-uploads.s3.amazonaws.com/uploads/services/1616991/20220914155938_6321fa6ac8af1_female_reproductive_systempage2.jpg.

1.1.4.6. Female Sexual Response and Hormone Control

Arousal and orgasm are part of the female sexual response, but ejaculation is not present. Pregnancy can occur in women who do not experience an orgasm. Progesterone, estrogen, luteinizing hormone, and follicle-stimulating hormone all play important roles in controlling the activities of the female reproductive system.

Gonadotropin-releasing hormone is secreted by the hypothalamus in response to specific stimuli during puberty when the ovaries and uterus are developed enough to react to hormonal stimulation. After entering the bloodstream, this hormone travels to the anterior pituitary gland, where it stimulates the release of luteinizing hormone and follicle-stimulating hormone. The monthly cycles start because of these hormones' effects on the uterus and ovaries. The menstrual cycle of a woman lasts from menarche to menopause.

The development of follicles during the follicular phase, ovulation during the ovulatory phase, and the growth and regression of the corpus luteum during the luteal phase mark the beginning, middle, and end of the monthly ovarian cycle. The ovarian and uterine cycles happen at the same time.

The menstrual phase of the uterine cycle commences with menstruation, while the proliferative phase involves endometrial repair, and the secretory phase culminates in the growth of blood vessels and glands. When a woman's reproductive cycles end, she enters menopause. Lower ovarian hormone levels and higher pituitary follicle-stimulating hormone and luteinizing hormone levels are indicative of this phase. The symptoms of menopause are brought on by fluctuating hormone levels.

1.1.4.7. Mammary Glands

The mammary glands function to produce milk and are structurally modified sweat glands. Located in the breast overlying the pectoralis major muscles, mammary glands are present in both sexes but typically only functional in females. Each breast externally has a raised nipple surrounded by a pigmented area called the areola. The nipples are sensitive to touch and contain smooth muscle that contracts, causing them to become erect when stimulated.

Within the adult female breast, there are 15 to 20 lobes of glandular tissue arranged in a circular pattern around the nipple. These lobes are separated by connective tissue and adipose tissue, with the connective tissue providing support. Suspensory ligaments known as Cooper's ligaments run through the breast from the skin to the underlying muscles. The size and shape of the breast are determined by the amount and distribution of adipose tissue. Each lobe is made up of lobules containing glandular units that produce milk. Milk is collected from the lobules by lactiferous ducts, which carry it to the nipple. Before reaching the nipple, the ducts widen to form a reservoir called the lactiferous sinus. After the sinus, the duct narrows again, with each duct opening independently on the surface of the nipple.

Hormones control the function of the mammary glands. Increasing estrogen levels during puberty encourages the growth of glandular tissue in the female breast. Adipose tissue accumulation in the breast is another way that estrogen increases breast size. The duct system develops in response to progesterone. These hormones promote the mammary glands' continued development during pregnancy. The anterior pituitary's prolactin stimulates the glandular tissue's ability to produce milk, and oxytocin causes the glands to expel milk (Bradley, 2000; Marieb, 2000; Bergsjø, 2001; Cooper, 2001; Drake et al., 2004).

1.1.4.8. How Does the Female Reproductive System Work?

The female reproductive system enables a woman to:

- Produce eggs (ova);

- Have sexual intercourse;
- Protect and nourish a fertilized egg until it is fully developed;
- Give birth.

The gonads, or sexual organs, are necessary for sexual reproduction to occur. For most people, the male testicles are thought to be the gonads. However, gonads are present in both sexes. In females, gonads are the ovaries, which produce female gametes (eggs). Male gametes (sperm) are produced by male gonads. Upon birth, a girl's ovaries hold hundreds of thousands of eggs, which are dormant until the onset of puberty. The pituitary gland, located in the brain's central region, begins producing hormones during puberty that encourage the ovaries to produce estrogen and other female sex hormones. These hormones cause a girl to become a sexually mature woman by secreting them.

Girls start releasing eggs at the end of puberty as part of the menstrual cycle, which is a monthly event. An ovary releases a tiny egg into one of the uterine tubes once a month during ovulation. Menstruation occurs when an egg exits the body through the uterus approximately two weeks after it is laid, barring fertilization by a sperm while the egg is still in the uterine tube.

Menstrual flow is made up of blood and tissues from the uterus's inner lining. It typically lasts three to five days for girls. Menarche is the term for a girl's first menstrual cycle (pronounced MEH-nar-kee).

It's common for women and girls to have some discomfort in the days leading to their periods. Premenstrual syndrome (PMS) includes both physical and emotional symptoms that many girls and women get right before their periods, such as:

- Acne;
- Bloating;
- Tiredness;
- Backaches;
- Sore breasts;
- Headaches;
- Constipation;
- Diarrhea;
- Food cravings;
- Depression;
- Irritability;
- Trouble concentrating or handling stress.

PMS typically peaks seven days before the onset of a girl's menstrual cycle and subsides thereafter. Prostaglandins, which are bodily chemicals that cause the smooth muscle in the uterus to contract, are also responsible for many girls' stomach cramps during the first few days of their menstrual cycle. These uncontrollably occurring spasms can be mild or severe and powerful.

A girl's body may not develop a regular menstrual cycle for up to two years after menarche. Her body is acclimating to the hormones that come with puberty during that period. An adult woman's monthly cycle lasts 28 days on average, although it can vary from 23 to 35 days.

1.1.4.9. What Happens If an Egg Is Fertilized?

Fertilization can occur if a female and male have sex a few days after the female ovulates. A tiny quantity of semen is deposited into the vagina by the male during ejaculation, which is the release of semen from the penis. This tiny amount of semen contains millions of sperm, which swim up from the vagina, through the cervix and uterus, and meet the egg in the uterine tube. One sperm is all that is needed to fertilize an egg.

A multicellular blastocyst is formed from the fertilized egg (pronounced "zygote") approximately five to six days after the sperm fertilizes the egg. Pronounced BLAS-tuh-sist, a blastocyst is a hollow ball of cells with fluid inside that is roughly the size of a pinhead. The endometrium, the lining of the uterus, is where the blastocyst burrows itself. The endometrium (pronounced "en-doh-MEE-tree-um") thickens and becomes more blood-rich because of the hormone estrogen. For the blastocyst to adhere to the uterus and take up nutrients from it, progesterone, another hormone secreted by the ovaries, maintains the endometrial blood thinning. We refer to this procedure as implantation.

The embryo is roughly the size of a raspberry after eight weeks, but nearly every component has developed, including the heart and blood, the stomach and intestines, the brain and nerves, the muscles, and the skin. The nine weeks following fertilization until delivery, or the fetal stage, are a time of continued development as cells divide, move, and undergo transformation. Inside the amniotic sac, the fetus (pronounced FEE-tis) floats in amniotic fluid (pronounced am-nee-AH-tik). The placenta (pronounced pluh-SEN-tuh) carries nutrients and oxygen from the mother's blood to the developing fetus. The umbilical (pronounced um-BIL-ih-kul) cord connects this disk-shaped structure to the fetus and adheres to the uterine lining. The fetus is protected from bumps and shocks to the mother's body by the amniotic fluid and membrane.

An average pregnancy lasts 280 days, or roughly nine months. The cervix widens and relaxes in preparation for the baby's passage into and through the vagina when the baby is ready to be born, pressing on it with its head. The cervix has a plug made of mucus that is now loosening. It emerges through the vagina when the mother's water breaks, along with amniotic fluid. The pituitary hormone oxytocin (pronounced: ahk-see-TOE-sin) stimulates the uterine walls to contract when labor contractions start. The cervix opens up and widens as a result of the contractions. The cervix becomes sufficiently dilated (opened) to allow the baby to pass through after several hours of this widening. The baby is forced through the cervix, out of the uterus, and down the birth canal. Usually, the head of the baby comes first. The baby comes out with the umbilical cord. After delivery, it is clamped and sliced near the navel.

The placenta, also known as the afterbirth at that point, is delivered during the final stage of childbirth. The uterus contracts to push it out along with its fluids and membranes after it has detached from the inner lining (Bradley, 2000; Marieb, 2000; Bergsjø, 2001; Cooper, 2001; Drake et al., 2004).

A Closer Look

Human Reproductive

The human reproductive system is a marvel of biological engineering, ensuring the continuation of the species through the complex interplay of organs, hormones, and processes. In males, the journey begins with the testes, which produce sperm and testosterone. Sperm mature in the epididymis and travel via the vas deferens to mix with fluids from seminal vesicles and the prostate, forming semen ejaculated through the penis during intercourse.

Females possess ovaries that cyclically release eggs into the fallopian tubes, where fertilization typically occurs. The uterus, or womb, prepares each month to receive a fertilized egg, supported by hormones like estrogen and progesterone. If fertilization occurs, the embryo implants in the uterus for development into a fetus. The cervix connects the uterus to the vagina, allowing sperm entry during intercourse and serving as a passage for childbirth.

Hormonal regulation guides these processes, orchestrating menstrual cycles in females and maintaining reproductive function in both sexes, ensuring the perpetuation of human life.

Summary

- The reproductive system of an organism, also known as the genital system, is the biological system made up of all the anatomical organs involved in sexual reproduction.
- The male and female reproductive systems are intricate networks of organs and tissues designed to facilitate the process of human reproduction. While they share the ultimate goal of producing offspring, their structures and functions exhibit significant differences tailored to their respective roles in the reproductive process.
- The female reproductive system is designed to carry out several functions. It produces the female egg cells necessary for reproduction, called the ova or oocytes. The system is designed to transport the ova to the site of fertilization.
- Anatomical terminology is a form of scientific terminology used by anatomists, zoologists, and health professionals such as doctors, physicians, and pharmacists. Anatomical terminology uses many unique terms, suffixes, and prefixes deriving from Ancient Greek and Latin.
- The organs of the female reproductive system produce and sustain the female sex cells (egg cells or ova), transport these cells to a site where they may be fertilized by sperm, provide a favorable environment for the developing fetus, move the fetus to the outside at the end of the development period, and produce the female sex hormones.
- A serous membrane is one of the thin membranes that cover the walls and organs in the thoracic and abdominopelvic cavities. The parietal layers of the membranes line the walls of the body cavity (pariet- refers to a cavity wall).

References

1. Al-Agha OM, Axiotis CA. An in-depth look at Leydig cell tumor of the testis. Arch Pathol Lab Med. 2007 Feb;131(2):311-7.
2. Anderson DJ, Marathe J, Pudney J. The structure of the human vaginal stratum corneum and its role in immune defense. Am J Reprod Immunol. 2014 Jun;71(6):618-23.
3. Bonomi M, Rochira V, Pasquali D, Balercia G, Jannini EA, Ferlin A., Klinefelter ItaliaN Group (KING). Klinefelter syndrome (KS): genetics, clinical phenotype and hypogonadism. J Endocrinol Invest. 2017 Feb;40(2):123-134.
4. Chen WN, Yeong KY. Scopolamine, a toxin-induced experimental model, used for research in Alzheimer's disease. CNS Neurol Disord Drug Targets. 2020;19:85–93.
5. de Ziegler D, Pirtea P, Galliano D, Cicinelli E, Meldrum D. Optimal uterine anatomy and physiology necessary for normal implantation and placentation. Fertil Steril. 2016 Apr;105(4):844-54.
6. Dimitriadis F, Tsiampali C, Chaliasos N, Tsounapi P, Takenaka A, Sofikitis N. The Sertoli cell as the orchestra conductor of spermatogenesis: spermatogenic cells dance to the tune of testosterone. Hormones (Athens). 2015 Oct-Dec;14(4):479-503.
7. Esteves SC. Clinical relevance of routine semen analysis and controversies surrounding the 2010 World Health Organization criteria for semen examination. Int Braz J Urol. 2014 Jul-Aug;40(4):443-53.

8. Gacci M, Coppi M, Baldi E, Sebastianelli A, Zaccaro C, Morselli S, et al. Semen impairment and occurrence of SARS-CoV-2 virus in semen after recovery from COVID-19. Hum Reprod. 2021;36:1520–1529.
9. Gibbons T, Reavey J, Georgiou EX, Becker CM. Timed intercourse for couples trying to conceive. Cochrane Database Syst Rev. 2023 Sep 15;9(9):CD011345.
10. Kelleher AM, DeMayo FJ, Spencer TE. Uterine Glands: Developmental Biology and Functional Roles in Pregnancy. Endocr Rev. 2019 Oct 01;40(5):1424-1445.
11. Khare S, Azevedo M, Parajuli P, Gokulan K. Conformational changes of the receptor binding domain of SARS-CoV-2 spike protein and prediction of a B-cell antigenic epitope using structural data. Front Artif Intell. 2021;4:630955.
12. Lin Y, Wu Y, Zhong P, Hou B, Liu J, Chen Y, et al. A clinical staging proposal of the disease course over time in non-severe patients with coronavirus disease 2019. Sci Rep. 2021;11:10681.
13. Mawhinney M, Mariotti A. Physiology, pathology and pharmacology of the male reproductive system. Periodontol 2000. 2013 Feb;61(1):232-51.
14. Plant TM, Marshall GR. The functional significance of FSH in spermatogenesis and the control of its secretion in male primates. Endocr Rev. 2001 Dec;22(6):764-86.
15. Shan D, Johnson JM, Fernandes SC, Suib H, Hwang S, Wuelfing D, et al. N-protein presents early in blood, dried blood and saliva during asymptomatic and symptomatic SARS-CoV-2 infection. Nat Commun. 2021;12:1931.
16. Stocco C, Telleria C, Gibori G. The molecular control of corpus luteum formation, function, and regression. Endocr Rev. 2007 Feb;28(1):117-49.
17. Trevisan CM, Montagna E, de Oliveira R, Christofolini DM, Barbosa CP, Crandall KA, Bianco B. Kisspeptin/GPR54 System: What Do We Know About Its Role in Human Reproduction? Cell Physiol Biochem. 2018;49(4):1259-1276.
18. Xu H, Wang Z, Feng C, Yu W, Chen Y, Zeng X, et al. Effects of SARS-CoV-2 infection on male sex-related hormones in recovering patients. Andrology. 2021;9:107–114.
19. Yoon JY, Cheon CK. Evaluation and management of amenorrhea related to congenital sex hormonal disorders. Ann Pediatr Endocrinol Metab. 2019 Sep;24(3):149-157.
20. Zhou L, Ayeh SK, Chidambaram V, Karakousis PC. Modes of transmission of SARS-CoV-2 and evidence for preventive behavioral interventions. BMC Infect Dis. 2021;21:496.

Chapter

MALE REPRODUCTIVE ANATOMY

2

Contents

Unit Introduction

The male reproductive system is a sophisticated network of tissues and organs that oversee secreting hormones necessary for sexual development and function in addition to producing and delivering sperm. Various important parts make up this system, and each one plays a specific role in the reproduction process. The testes, the main organs in charge of producing sperm and testosterone, are at the center of the male reproductive system. The testes are housed outside the body in the scrotum to maintain a temperature that is favorable to produce sperm. Seminiferous tubules, which are found inside the testes, are the site of spermatogenesis, or the process of producing sperm. Within these tubules, sperm cells are continuously produced through a convoluted series of cellular divisions and maturation processes.

Sperm are produced and then mature in the coiled tube called the epididymis, which is behind each testis. Before sperm are ejaculated, the epididymis is where they mature and store, gaining motility and the ability to fertilize. Sperm are released from the body through the ejaculatory ducts, which join the urethra and epididymis when a person is sexually aroused. In men, the urethra has two purposes: it transports urine from the bladder and facilitates the movement of sperm during ejaculation. Fluids from the prostate gland, ejaculatory ducts, seminal vesicles, and bulbourethral glands are added to semen, which feeds and shields sperm cells as they pass through the female reproductive system.

To supply energy for sperm motility, the seminal vesicles, which are found behind the bladder, secrete a fluid that is high in fructose and other nutrients. The milky alkaline fluid secreted by the prostate gland, which is located beneath the bladder and encircles the urethra, balances the acidic pH of the vagina and improves sperm viability and motility. Furthermore, the urethra is lubricated, and any residual acidic urine is neutralized by the clear, viscous fluid secreted by the bulbourethral glands, which are situated beneath the prostate gland. This creates an environment that is more favorable for sperm (Guyton & Hall, 2006; Sembulingam & Sembulingam, 2006; Mescher, 2010; Rhoades & Bell, 2012).

Orientation and Directional Terms:

Terms	Definition	Illustration
Cellular divisions	There are two types of cell division: mitosis and meiosis. Most of the time when people refer to "cell division," they mean mitosis, the process of making new body cells.	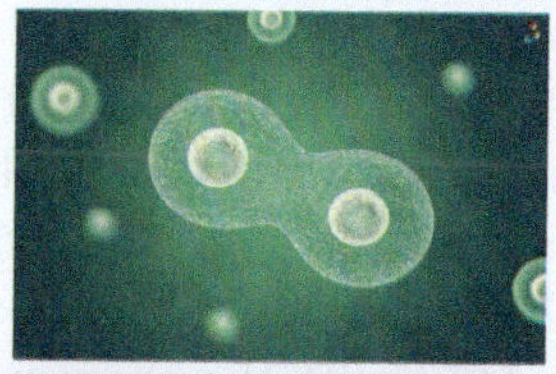
Sperm	Sperm is the male reproductive cell, or gamete, in anisogamous forms of sexual reproduction.	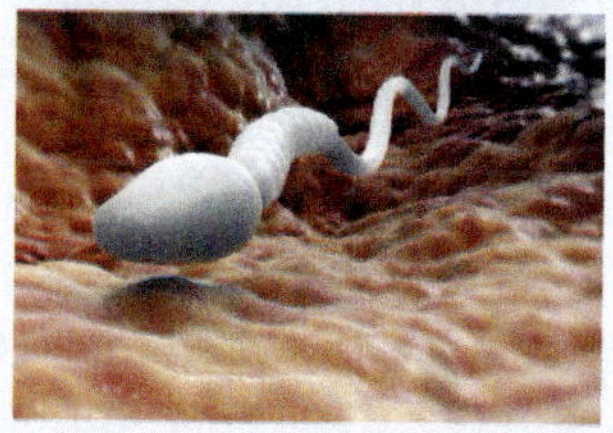
Urethra	The urethra is the tube that lets urine leave your bladder and your body. If you were assigned male at birth, your urethra passes through your prostate and into your penis.	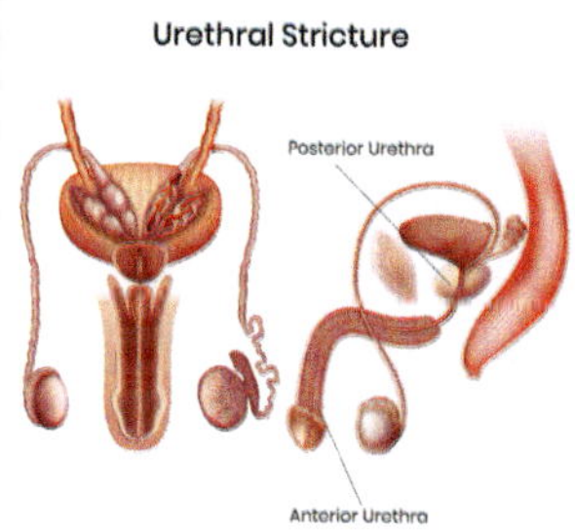
Scrotum	The scrotum is a part of a male's body that is located below the penis. The scrotum is the sac (pouch) that contains the testes, epididymis, and the lower part of the spermatic cord (blood vessels and vas deferens).	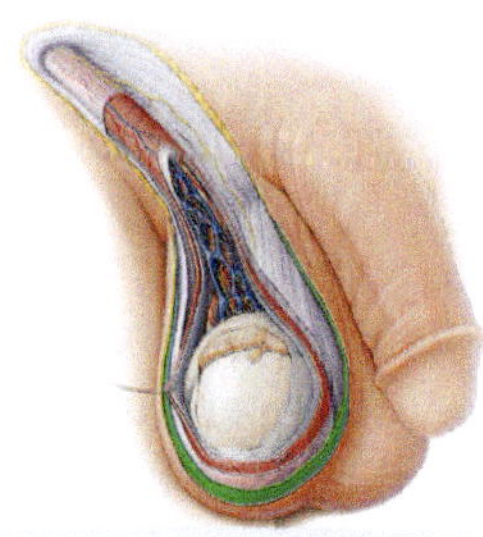

2.1. The Concept of Male Reproductive Anatomy

Reproduction is the process of creating new offspring; it is also referred to as breeding. Ensure the birth of the next generation of domestic, wild, and laboratory vertebrate organisms, involves a set of physiological processes that typically occur in the female reproductive system along with the corresponding behaviors and anatomical structures. While these occur within the female's system, in vertebrates, fertilization is the process by which haploid gametes from the male (sperm cell) and female (ovum) fuse. Male reproductive system: testes, ductus deferens, epididymis, accessory glands, penis. The primary role of the male reproductive system is spermatogenesis, which produces male gametes (spermatozoa), which are then produced, maintained, and temporarily stored. Through the process of steroidogenesis, it generates both estrogen and androgens. Crucially, it is linked to the penis, the organ of copulation, which facilitates the introduction of spermatozoa-containing semen into the female genital system through mating.

2.1.1. Functional Anatomy of Male Reproductive System

Most of the male reproductive system is external to the body. The scrotum, testicles, and penis are examples of these external organs. The urethra, prostate, and vas deferens are examples of internal organs. The male reproductive system oversees both urination and sexual function. A man's reproductive and urinary systems are composed of a collection of organs known as the male reproductive system.

These organs do the following jobs within your body:

- They produce, maintain, and transport sperm (the male reproductive cells) and semen (the protective fluid around sperm).
- They discharge sperm into the female reproductive tract.
- They produce and secrete male sex hormones.

The internal (found inside your body) and external (found outside your body) components comprise the male reproductive system. These organs work together to enable you to urinate (get rid of liquid waste products from your body), engage in sexual activity, and become pregnant (Guyton & Hall, 2006; Sembulingam & Sembulingam, 2006; Mescher, 2010; Rhoades & Bell, 2012).

2.1.2. Male Reproductive System Function

The internal (found inside your body) and external (found outside your body) components comprise the male reproductive system. These organs work together to enable you to urinate (get rid of liquid waste products from your body), engage in sexual activity, and become pregnant.

The pituitary gland produces both LH and FSH. It is housed at the base of the brain and oversees numerous bodily processes. Spermatogenesis, the process of producing sperm, requires FSH. To keep the spermatogenesis process going, testosterone must be produced, which is stimulated by LH. The development of masculine traits like bone mass, sex drive, fat distribution, and muscle mass and strength are also influenced by testosterone (Figure 2.1).

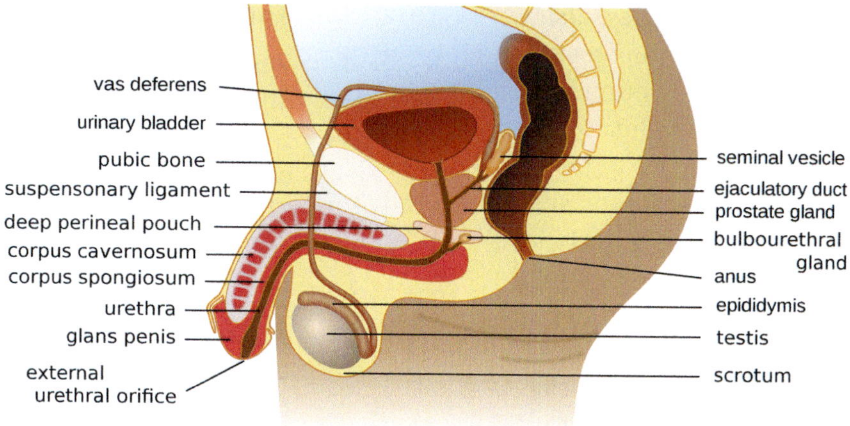

Figure 2.1. *Male reproductive system*

Source: By Wumingbai – Own work, CC BY-SA 4.0, https://commons.wikimedia.org/w/index.php?curid=102958455.

2.1.3. Anatomy: External Male Reproductive Structures

Most of the male reproductive system is situated outside the pelvis and abdominal cavity. The penis, scrotum, and testicles are the external components of the male reproductive system.

1. **Penis:** The penis is the male organ for sexual intercourse. It has three parts:
   - i. **The Root:** This is the part of the penis that attaches to the wall of your abdomen.
   - ii. **The Body or Shaft:** The penis body has three internal chambers and is shaped like a tube or cylinder. There is a unique, sponge-like erectile tissue inside these chambers that has thousands of large spaces that fill with blood when you become sexually aroused. The penis gets stiff and erect as it fills with blood, allowing for penetration during intercourse. Because the penis' skin is elastic and loose, it can change size during an erection.
   - iii. **The Glans:** This is the cone-shaped end of the penis. The glans, which are also called the head of the penis, are covered with a loose layer of skin called the foreskin. This skin is sometimes removed in a procedure called circumcision.

   The tip of the glans penis is where the urethra, the tube that carries urine and semen out of the body, opens. There are a lot of delicate nerve endings in the penis as well. When a man reaches his sexual climax, sperm-containing semen is released (ejaculated) through the tip of the penis (orgasm). The urethra cannot flow urine when the penis is erect, so the only substance that can be ejaculated during an orgasm is semen.

2. **Scrotum:** The loose sac-like sac of skin that dangles behind the penis is called the scrotum. It contains numerous blood vessels and nerves

in addition to the testicles, also known as the testes. Your testicles are shielded by the scrotum, which also acts as a kind of climate control system. The testes need to be just below body temperature for sperm to develop normally. The testicles can move closer to the body for warmth and protection or farther away to lower body temperature thanks to special muscles in the scrotal wall that contract and relax.

3. **Testicles (Testes):** The spermatic cord secures the testes at both ends, which are oval organs the size of large olives that are in the scrotum. Men typically have two testes. The testes are the organs that produce sperm and testosterone, the main hormone involved in male sex. Seminiferous tubules are coiled masses of tubes found inside the testes. Through a process known as spermatogenesis, these tubules oversee producing the sperm cells.
4. **Epididymis:** Located behind each testicle, the epididymis is a lengthy, twisted tube responsible for carrying and storing sperm cells produced in the testes. Furthermore, it plays a crucial role in allowing the sperm to reach maturity, as the sperm initially produced in the testes are immature and cannot fertilize. When sexually aroused, contractions help propel the sperm into the vas deferens.

2.1.3.1. Internal Male Reproductive Organs

You have several internal organs also called accessory organs that play a big part in the male reproductive system. These organs include:

1. **Vas Deferens:** The vas deferens is a long, muscular tube that travels from the epididymis into the pelvic cavity, to just behind the bladder. The vas deferens transports mature sperm to the urethra in preparation for ejaculation.
2. **Ejaculatory Ducts:** These ducts are formed by the fusion of the vas deferens and the seminal vesicles. The ejaculatory ducts empty into the urethra.
3. **Urethra:** The urethra is the tube that carries urine from the bladder to the outside of your body. In males, it has the additional function of expelling (ejaculating) semen when you reach orgasm. When the penis is erect during sex, the flow of urine is blocked from the urethra, allowing only semen to be ejaculated at orgasm.
4. **Seminal Vesicles:** The seminal vesicles are sac-like pouches that attach to the vas deferens near the base of the bladder. The seminal vesicles make a sugar-rich fluid (fructose) that provides sperm with a source of energy and helps with the sperm's ability to move (motility). The fluid of the seminal vesicles makes up most of the volume of your ejaculatory fluid, or ejaculate.
5. **Prostate Gland:** The prostate gland is a walnut-sized structure that's located below the urinary bladder in front of the rectum. The prostate gland contributes additional fluid to the ejaculate. Prostate fluids also help to nourish the sperm. The

urethra, which carries the ejaculate to be expelled during orgasm, runs through the center of the prostate gland.

6. **Bulbourethral Glands:** The bulbourethral glands, or Cowper's glands, are pea-sized structures located on the sides of the urethra, just below the prostate gland. These glands produce a clear, slippery fluid that empties directly into the urethra. This fluid serves to lubricate the urethra and to neutralize any acidity that may be present due to residual drops of urine in the urethra (Guyton & Hall, 2006; Sembulingam & Sembulingam, 2006; Mescher, 2010; Rhoades & Bell, 2012).

2.1.4. Primary and Secondary Sexual Characteristics

The external and internal genitalia (e.g., sperm and eggs) are the primary sexual characteristics that are present from birth. The vagina and ovaries in females, and the penis and testes in males). The traits that surface during the prepubescent and postpubescent stages are known as secondary sexual characteristics (e.g., breasts in women and facial hair color in men). Physical changes during puberty fall into two categories: (i) changes to primary sex characteristics; and (ii) changes to secondary sex characteristics. Changes to the sexual organs themselves—the uterus, vagina, penis, and testes—are referred to as primary sex characteristics. The term "secondary sex characteristics" refers to additional outward manifestations of adult maturation, like height and body shape changes.

For boys, the enlargement of the testes, penis, prostate gland, and seminal vesicles are primary sex characteristic changes. Between the ages of 9 and 14 is usually when these changes start to happen. They typically reach their full growth potential between the ages of 12 and 16. For young men, the most notable and significant change associated with puberty is spermarche or the first ejaculation. In most cases, spermarche happens between the ages of 12 and 16. The spermarche shows that a boy is now generating sperm, which may fertilize a female egg through intercourse and cause a pregnancy in the female. This initial ejaculation frequently takes place while you're asleep; it's also known as a "wet dream." While they are awake, young men may also get spontaneous erections. This could happen for no apparent reason at all or when they experience emotional stimulation. These unplanned erections may cause discomfort or embarrassment to young men.

For girls, the main changes in sex characteristics are the uterus beginning to form a lining that will eventually be shed during menstruation and the vagina starting to secrete a substance that resembles mucus. This mucus-like discharge is an early stage of vaginal lubrication, not the actual menstrual flow. When the young woman reaches adulthood, she will be able to produce this lubricant in different amounts even when she isn't feeling sexually aroused. A girl may go through these changes weeks or months before she experiences her first menstrual period or menarche. Every young person's experience is a little bit unique.

The onset of the first menstrual period, or menarche, is the most notable and significant primary sex change for young women. This happens when the uterus sheds its initial layer of tissue and blood. The uterus is the organ that will eventually carry and nourish a baby. This lining sheds once a month, or roughly every 28 days, in adult women. The lining serves to prepare the uterus for the first stage of pregnancy, during which the fertilized egg must adhere to the lining of the uterus. Every month, the lining sheds when the body recognizes it is not pregnant. When a woman has her menstrual period, there is no open wound and no bleeding. Rather, the bloody lining tissue that has developed inside their uterus over the past month is just being shed and released by it.

A girl is not guaranteed to be able to conceive after menarche. Pregnancy can happen before menarche in certain situations, but it can also wait months after menarche in other situations. Some girls may wait up to 12 to 18 months after the onset of their periods before their ovaries start producing eggs. Before their first menstruation, other girls will have started to release mature eggs. For this reason, if young women are to engage in sexual activity, they should be taught that getting pregnant before the onset of their first period is possible, if not common. The primary characteristics of sexuality (penises vs. vaginas). During puberty, secondary sexual traits (such as high voices and no facial hair in human females, and low voices and beards in human males) appear.

2.1.4.1. Primary Sexual Characteristics

Other than the gonads, primary sexual characteristics are those that are directly necessary for reproduction. The scrotum and penis are the main somatic sexual organs of men, and they are all necessary for producing and releasing sperm. The clitoris, cervix, uterine tubes, vagina, and the capacity to procreate are the main sexual features of women.

The primary sexual traits are those that exist from birth. The sex of mammals is decided by hormonal processes that occur in utero and are normally regulated by the X and Y chromosomes together. The gonads should develop into ovaries and the offspring will be female if an egg is fertilized by a sperm carrying the X chromosome; the gonads should develop into testes and the offspring will be male if the egg is fertilized by a sperm carrying the Y chromosome. Although there are numerous exceptions to this rule, they are regarded as anomalies.

Certain reptile species, such as turtles and alligators, use temperature-dependent sex determination to regulate the gender ratios of their young. When eggs are kept at a low temperature, they tend to produce one gender, while eggs kept at a higher temperature will result in the opposite gender.

2.1.4.2. Secondary Sexual Characteristics

The sexually dimorphic traits that are not directly related to reproduction are known as secondary sexual traits. Secondary features of males include more hair on their faces and chests, more hair overall, a pelvic build (without rounded hips), a muscular upper body, and the capacity to build muscle mass more quickly than a female. Secondary sex characteristics in females include a menstrual cycle, increased body fat composition, round hips and figures, breasts, a decreased ability to generate muscle mass quickly, a decrease in upper body strength, and, in some cases, thicker hair on the head. Any attempt to categorize individuals into the various traditionally defined sex categories using a list of features is not without its exceptions, of course. For example, not all women who otherwise meet the traditional definition of female are successful in nursing their babies.

Secondary sexual traits that are traditionally associated with either gender are developed by hormones secreted through the hypothalamus. Most sexually dimorphic species—species with two forms that are determined by their sex—have these secondary sexual traits, which are not utilized in reproduction. The mane on a male lion, the bright, showy plumage of many male birds and fish, human female breasts, and human male facial hair are examples of secondary sexual characteristics.

2.1.4.3. Female Mate Choice

Male-male competition and/or female mate preference are thought to be the main factors behind the persistence of male ornamentation in animal populations. According to the choosy female theory, females select males with larger, brighter, and better ornamentation to select a mate with better genes and increase the viability of her offspring. Two mechanisms can lead to this increase in viability.

According to the "sexy sons" theory, the female selects the handsome male because her sons will inherit his ornamentation, increasing the likelihood that they will reproduce and carry on her genes. According to the good genes hypothesis, the female selects the showier male because his ornamentation might indicate greater resistance to disease or other fitness advantages that she might pass on to her progeny.

2.1.4.4. Male-Male Competition

A dominant male has an advantage due to certain secondary sexual traits. For example, if he can outfight his rivals in combat, he may be granted the opportunity to mate with a female and contribute more genetic material to the population. Due to superior features like tusks and antlers that can be used as weapons when fighting other males, this dominant male will be able to mate with more females than less dominant males. The genes for the superior fighting trait will proliferate in the population because of his increased ability to mate with females; in other words, that trait will be selected naturally (Guyton & Hall, 2006; Sembulingam & Sembulingam, 2006; Mescher, 2010; Rhoades & Bell, 2012).

2.2. Fundamental Component of Male Reproductive Anatomy

The male reproductive anatomy is divided into five components which are very fundamental to human reproductive health. These include.

1. **Gonadal Development:** At eight weeks of gestation (period of pregnancy), Y chromosomal synthesis of H-Y antigen occurs. In males, this H-Y antigen causes undifferentiated sex glands to develop into testes while in females, lack of the H-Y antigen causes undifferentiated sex glands to develop into ovaries.
2. **Duct Development:** The Mullerian duct, which develops into the uterine tubes, uterus, and inner vagina, and the mesonephric duct, which develops into the epididymis, vas deferens, and seminal vesicles, are similar in both sexes at birth. During development, the male fetal interstitial cells secrete enough testosterone to match that of adult men, while the sustentacular cells secrete the anti-mullerian hormone (AMH). The testes determining factor (TDF) gene or the sex-determining region of the Y chromosome (SRY) gene product, which inhibits the expression of aromatase and thereby prevents the conversion of testosterone to estrogen, also contributes to the accumulation of testosterone (androgen), which is responsible for male sex differentiation during embryogenesis (9th and 13th weeks of pregnancy). As a

result, testosterone promotes the development and differentiation of the Wolffian ducts into the male internal genital tracts. However, a glycoprotein known as anti-mullerian hormone (AMH) is secreted by sustentacular cells in newly differentiated seminiferous tubules under the influence of specific transcription factors and the SRY gene product. This results in the death of tubular epithelial cells and the atrophy or reabsorption of the Mullerian ducts 9, which would have formed the female internal genital tract. Nevertheless, the SOX9 and steroidogenesis factor (SF1) are among the genes downstream of those that make up the SRY gene product. These categorized products promote the development of tunica albuginea as well as the differentiation of sustentacular cells and interstitial cells in the testes.

3. **External Genital Development:** The external genitalia in both sexes are derived from two primitive reproductive anatomy structures. This covers the urogenital sinus and genital tubercle. These structures develop into the female external genitalia (clitoris, labia, vaginal opening, etc.), but the masculinization of these structures to form the penis, scrotum, and prostate gland depends on the testosterone secreted by the fetal testes unless stimulated by androgens. The external genitalia are unclear, and differentiation is incomplete in male embryos with insufficient androgen or female embryos with excessive androgen. Rather than testosterone, dihydrotestosterone is what differentiates the masculine external genitalia. The process by which this happens is when an enzyme known as 5α-reductase converts testosterone into dihydrotestosterone (DHT).

$$\text{testosterone} \xrightarrow{\text{5?alpha reductase}} \text{dihydrotestosterone} \quad (1)$$

4. **Brain Development:** Sex hormones such as testosterone and estradiol exert their influence during the development of the fetus. Testosterone secreted into the blood reaches the brain and gets converted into estradiol by an enzyme called Aromatase. The estradiol is what helps in the masculinization of the human brain. In the female, the estradiol secreted by the ovaries binds to a particular protein called α-fetoprotein and therefore prevents its entering into the brain to protect the female brain from being masculinized by estradiol.

$$\text{testosterone} \xrightarrow{\text{Aromatase}} \text{estradiol} \quad (2)$$

5. **Neural Development:** One of the first systems to start and the last to finish after birth is neural development. The most complex structure within the embryo is produced by this development, and because it takes so long, an in-utero injury during pregnancy may have an impact on the nervous system's development. The basic neural plate that gives rise to the neural groove and subsequently the neural tube is the earliest form of the central nervous system. The

neuropores are formed when this early neural is initially open at both ends. One of the main classes of neural abnormalities (neural tube defects) is caused by these openings failing to close. The two main cell classes that comprise the bulk of the nervous system, neurons, and glia, are produced by neural tube stem cells. These two classes of cells can differentiate into a wide variety of types with highly specialized forms and functions.

2.2.1. The Physio-Anatomy of the Testes

The testis is a powerful, oval-shaped male gonad that measures approximately 4 cm in length and 2.5 cm in width in adult males. The scrotum contains the testes, which control its temperature to roughly 23°C, which is lower than the average body temperature. The right testis is typically slightly larger and heavier than the left, weighing approximately 963 ı 0 grams. Normally, there are two testes, each weighing approximately 11–17 grams. A saccular extension of the peritoneum inside the scrotum known as the tunica vaginalis envelops a testis (singular). Under the tunica vaginalis, the white, fibrous capsule that surrounds the testis is formed by the confined tunica albuginea. The testis mediastinum, from which the fibrous septa enter the testis and split into roughly 200–300 wedge-shaped lobules, is subsequently assembled by thickening the tunica albuginea.

Each testicular lobule contains one to four tightly coiled seminiferous tubules that produce sperm. The germ cells and the supporting cells, also known as sustentacular cells, are the two main cell types found in testis seminiferous tubules. The sustentacular cells are uniformly distributed in the seminiferous epithelium alongside developing germ cells, providing nourishment to the germ cells as they grow. The seminiferous tubule is lined by peritubular myoid cells, which are part of the basal lamina. Because they keep big molecules out of the germinal epithelium, myoid cells form a barrier with partial permeability. It is the close and gap junctions between neighboring sustentacular cells that serve as the primary barrier to exclusion, though. These inter-Sertoli cell junctions, also known as the blood testis barrier, split the seminiferous epithelium into two separate compartments: the basal and the adluminal compartments. Living in the basal compartment, spermatogonia, and early spermatocytes are easily accessible for systemic circulation. Meiotic and post-meiotic spermatocytes are found in the adluminal compartment, which is isolated from the systemic circulation and only comes into contact with substances carried by sustentacular cells. During the process of spermatogenesis, the undifferentiated spermatogonia that live in the basal compartment of the seminiferous epithelium go through many mitotic divisions to form primary spermatocytes (Figure 2.2).

The inter-Sertoli closed junctions must be completely restructured to transfer the primary spermatocyte to the adluminal compartment. In the adluminal compartment, the spermatocytes go through two successive rounds of meiosis to become mature haploid spermatids. Sustentacular cells provide a unique environment in the adluminal compartment, which oversees moving sperm from the testis to the epididymis by creating a specialized testis, in addition to providing physical support for germ cells. Important functions of the testis include the provision of nutrients and development factors necessary for the survival of germ cells. On the other hand, Sertoli cell behavior is also significantly regulated by germ cell variables. The interactions between germ cells and sustentacular cells are critical for successful spermatogenesis. Interstitial cells, which secrete steroids, blood and lymphatic vessels, nerves, macrophages, fibroblasts, and loose connective tissues comprise the interstitial compartment of the testis. The interstitial cells of the interstitial matrix, however, are the main cells in this compartment.

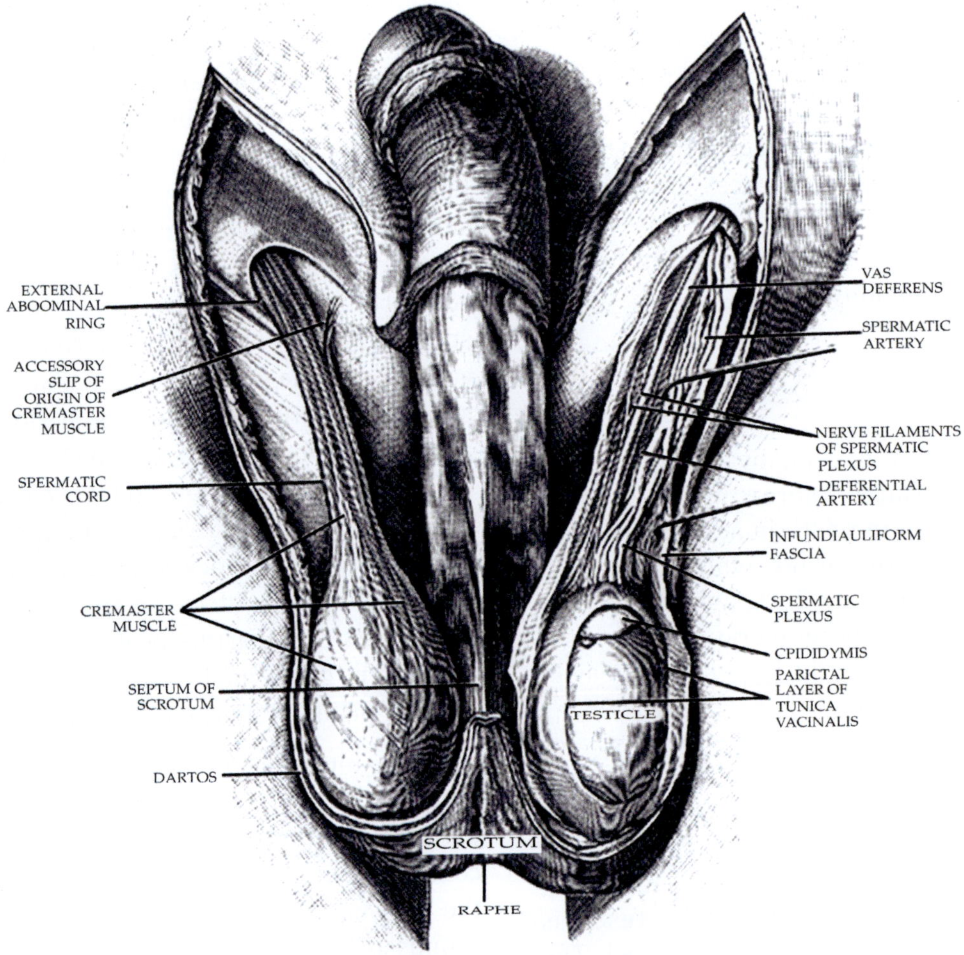

Figure 2.2. *The testis is a strong oval-shaped male gonad.*

Source: By Henry, G., (1918); Anatomy of the Human Body (See "Book" section below) Bartleby.com: Gray's Anatomy, Plate 1144, Public Domain, https://commons.wikimedia.org/w/index.php?curid=35171279.

2.2.2. Epithelial Cells of the Testes

2.2.2.1. Sertoli Cells (Also Called Substantial Cells)

Large, asymmetrical somatic cells are called sustentacular cells. Tight junctions bind sustentacular cells to one another at the base. Their intimate contact demonstrates the importance of sustentacular cells in the development of germ cells. Up to 6 or 12 spermatids can be connected to a single Sertoli cell. Sustentacular cells support the process of spermiation, which is the process by which mature spermatozoa finally separate and enter the lumen of the seminiferous tubule. Sustentacular cells also target and phagocytize damaged germ cells and excess cytoplasm left over from the transformation of spermatids into spermatozoa. Additionally, the sustentacular cells secrete fluid and offer structural support and nutrition to germ cells. The columnar cells that extend from the basal to the luminal compartment of the seminiferous epithelium of adult rats are found to occupy a volume of roughly 17–19%. Inhibin is a nonsteroidal pituitary receptor of gonadal origin secreted by sustentacular cells. Non-germinal sustentacular cells formed a continuous layer around the circumference of each tubule, creating the tight junctions that lead to the blood testis barrier.

Blood molecules attach themselves to germinal cells through the cytoplasm of sustentacular cells. Sustentacular cells secrete a protein known as androgen-binding protein into the lumen of the seminiferous tubules. The growing germ cells are enveloped by the Sertoli cell cytoplasm, which travels from the tubule lumen to the periphery. It assists in defending the seminiferous tubules against immune damage; the FAS ligand is produced by sustentacular cells on the surface of T lymphocytes, which bind to the FAS receptor. In this manner, it prevents the developing sperm's immune attack by causing T lymphocytes to undergo apoptosis. The somatic cells of the testes are referred to as sustentacular cells, and they are crucial for both spermatogenesis and testicular development. These cells (Sertoli) influence the environment inside the seminiferous tubules directly and regulate them to facilitate the development of germ cells into spermatozoa. As a "gatekeeper," the blood testes barrier (BTB), which is created by nearby sustentacular cells close to the basement membrane, keeps dangerous materials from getting to germ cells, particularly during post-mediotic spermatids. To facilitate the growth of post-meiotic spermatids, or spermiogenesis, in the apical compartment behind the BTB in a unique microenvironment, the BTB additionally divides the seminiferous epithelium into the basal and luminal (apical) compartments. In addition, the BTB plays a role in the immune privilege status of the testis, at least partially, preventing the production of anti-sperm antibodies against antigens that are momentarily expressed during spermatogenesis. Because of their constantly changing, three-dimensional relationship with growing germ cells throughout the 14 phases of the epithelial cycle, sustentacular cells have become extremely difficult to remain morphologically stable.

2.2.2.2. Leydig Cells

Leydig cells are the predominant cell type found in the interstitial tissue next to the seminiferous tubules and blood vessels. In addition to interstitial cells, other cell types such as fibroblasts, macrophages, and a few mast cells are also present in this space. Interstitial cells are responsible for producing testosterone, the main hormone found in the male bloodstream. These cells contain a high number of mitochondria, granular endoplasmic reticulum, lipid droplets, and occasionally protein crystals in their cytoplasm. While interstitial cells do not have receptors for follicle-stimulating hormone (FSH), their growth is indirectly influenced by FSH through stimulation of Sertoli cell development. Leydig cell growth can also be stimulated by androgens. However, estrogen receptors in interstitial cells can reduce their proliferation and activity. Luteinizing hormone (LH) binds to receptors on interstitial cells, leading to the secretion of androgens through a cAMP-dependent mechanism. While testosterone is the primary hormone produced by interstitial cells, it also produces dehydroepiandrosterone (DHEA) and androstenedione, which are androgens with lower biological activity. The human testes have adapted to the cooler temperature of the scrotum and are unable to generate sperm at the core body temperature of 37°C.

There are three mechanisms in the scrotum to control test temperature:

1. **Cremaster Muscle:** The spermatic cord of the internal abdominal oblique muscle is entangled by strips that make up the cremaster muscle. To keep the testicles warm in the winter, the cremaster contracts and draws them closer to the body. Warmness causes the cremaster to relax and the testicles to hang farther from the body.
2. **Darto Muscle:** The darto muscle (tunica dartos) is a smooth muscle layer found beneath the skin. It contracts as well in cold weather, causing the scrotum to stiffen and wrinkle. The teaching of the scrotum reduces the scrotal surface area, which in turn reduces heat loss and helps to keep the testes snugly against the warm body.
3. **The Pampiniform Plexus:** It is an extensive network of veins in the spermatic cord from the testes that surround the testicular artery. These converge as they pass through the inguinal canal to form the testicular vein, which emerges into the pelvic cavity from the canal. Warm arterial blood will heat the testicles and prevent spermatogenesis without the pampiniform plexus. However, by serving as a countercurrent heat exchanger, the pampiniform plexus avoids this. Such a process in the spermatic cord eliminates heat from the descending arterial blood, so this blood is 1.5°C to 2.5°C cooler than the core body temperature by the time it enters the testicles.

Most amphibians and fish lack seminiferous tubules. Instead, the sperm form spherical structures called sperm ampullae. These are seasonal structures that release their material during the breeding season and then the body absorbs it again. The ampullae of fresh sperm start to grow and mature before the next breeding season. Other than that, the ampullae of higher vertebrates are almost exactly like the seminiferous tubules, sharing the same range of cell types (Guyton & Hall, 2006; Sembulingam & Sembulingam, 2006; Mescher, 2010; Rhoades & Bell, 2012).

2.2.3. Testicular Temperature Regulation of Testes

The ideal temperature for the testes is just below the body's core temperature. Spermatogenesis is less successful at both higher and lower temperatures. The testicles may be external to the body for this reason. There are several methods to maintain the tests at the ideal temperature.

2.2.3.1. Testicular Development

In the third week following fertilization, the germ cells move from the yolk sac to the genital ridge. In male embryos, primordial germ cells move from the yolk sac wall to the gonads, and testes emerge from the genital ridges between the fourth and eighth week of development. Human chorionic gonadotropin is influencing the beginning of the evolution of the interstitial cells in the developing testis. It secretes testosterone. Around week nine, the labioscrotal swellings unite to form the scrotum. To form the seminal vesicles, vas deferens, and epididymis, testosterone also stimulates the production of mesonephric (Wolfian) ducts. Between the 7th and the 12th week, the gubernaculum shortens and pushes the testes, the deferent duct, and its vessels downward. Between the third and seventh months, the testes stay near the inguinal canal to enter it. They enter the scrotum around the time of birth, controlled by the androgen hormone. At approximately 13 weeks of development, the vaginal process emerges as an outpouching of the parietal peritoneum. The internal inguinal ring, where the vaginal process begins, is where the testis remains for 10 to 12 weeks. To generate an increased intra-abdominal input, the abdominal wall musculature is at least partially responsible for this patent herniation mechanism. If the abdominal muscles are not able to increase intra-abdominal pressure, the testis may not descend into the scrotum and the patent processus vaginalis does not advance through the inguinal canal. Every testis originates from one of three sources: first, teste production is visible during the seventh week of intrauterine life.

The base of each testis is the medulla of the undifferentiated genital ridge, the cortex of which regresses. The genital ridge is formed by the proliferation of coelomic mesothelium covering the mesonephric ridge's medial surface. Primitive sex cells, or gonocytes, are generated from the proliferation of the endoderm of the hind intestine's dorsal wall and emerge in the genital ridge because of active migration between the gut's primitive dorsal mesentery layers on the dorsal and cephalic sides. Multiple solid cellular testis cords protrude into the interior of the genital ridge from its surface. Primitive sex cells are inserted into the testis cords. The inner ends of the testis cords form a cellular plexus that is connected to the rete cord, which is situated close to the blind ends of the mesonephric tubules. The mesenchymal cells from the mesonephric ridge invaded the genital ridge and spread beneath the surface, eventually severing the peripheral ends of the testis cords from the surface. This part of the infected cells is composed of Tunica albuginea. During intrauterine development, some mesenchymal cells form septa testis while others detach to create interstitial cells. The testis cords and rete cords become canalized, forming seminiferous tubules and rete testis by the 7th month of gestation. Efferent testis ductules are then formed and connect with the rete testis. The epididymis and vas deferens develop from the mesonephric duct in the third trimester, with the epididymis entering the processus vaginalis before descending into the scrotum. The closure of the vaginal process at full term prevents contact between the peritoneum and the inguinal canal or scrotum. A remnant of tissue known as the appendix epididymis may persist, often attaching to the caput epididymis. The paramesonephric structures regress due to the Müllerian inhibiting substance secreted by sustentacular cells in the developing testis (Guyton & Hall, 2006; Sembulingam & Sembulingam, 2006; Mescher, 2010; Rhoades & Bell, 2012).

2.2.4. Blood Neurovascular Supply of the Testes

The delivery of oxygenated, nutrient-rich blood and the elimination of metabolic waste products are essential for the survival of cells in their target organs. Furthermore, most organs depend on neural signaling to carry out specific functions. Regarding the testes, a simple bilateral neurovascular network supplies each of the spherical reproductive organs. The testes' extensive vascular supply performs many tasks in addition to bringing in nutrients and waste products and removing them from the body. This is because the organs have dual functions as reproductive organs and endocrine glands, both of which are temperature-sensitive.

2.2.4.1. Arterial Supply

The two arteries that emerge directly from the abdominal aorta on either side are known as the testicular arteries. They emerge from the anterolateral surface of the massive artery caudal to the renal vessels at the level of the base of the L1–L2 vertebra. After crossing the inferior vena cava anteriorly, the right testicular artery proceeds inferolaterally, medially to the right testicular vein and the proximal portion of the right ureter. The artery continues its inferior course on the psoas major body after crossing the ureter anteriorly. On the left side, the testicular vein and left testicular artery run medially.

Its proximal path is more vertical than that of the right testicular artery. Additionally, it goes through the left ureter anteriorly. Both the left and right testicular arteries supply blood to the common and external iliac vessels. They do not cross the external iliac vessels until they enter the inguinal canal through the deep inguinal ring, at which point they transform into the femoral vessels. They extend laterally to the vas (ductus) deferens and its artery. After entering the scrotum, the testicular artery branches off into the epididymis and then divides into medial and lateral branches. These two branches are further divided to directly puncture the organ's material. Additionally, three significant vascular anastomotic connections with the testicular artery have been formed. The anteromedial side of each corresponding inferior epigastric artery (a branch of the external iliac artery) is where the cremasteric arteries begin. As they pass through the spermatic cord (in the inguinal canal), they anastomose with the testicular artery. The ductus deferens artery is born out of the inferior vesical artery, which is supplied by the anterior segment of the internal iliac artery. Additionally, anastomosis joins it to the testicular artery.

2.2.4.2. Venous Drainage

A dense network of connected veins forms a venous plexus around the testicular artery. A network known as the pampiniform plexus transports colder, less oxygenated, and less nutrient-rich blood cranially. As the plexus emerges from the scrotum and moves into the spermatic cord, its branches continue to converge, eventually forming four branches. On either side of the testicular artery, two branches come together at the deep inguinal ring. Consequently, two valvular testicular veins run parallel to each testicular artery until they reach their drainage sites. The two veins then combine to form the testicular vein, which crosses the anterior surface of the psoas muscle and flows laterally beside the testicular artery. Although the neurovascular supply to the testes is a difficult subject to study, interactive anatomy can make it more bearable. On the front surface of the psoas muscles, each testicular vein crosses the corresponding ureter approximately at the level of the L3 vertebra. After that, the left testicular vein passes between the ureter on the lateral side and the testicular artery on the medial side before almost vertically piercing the left renal vein. The right testicular vein, on the other hand, drains directly into the inferior vena cava after traveling almost vertically on the left, then obliquely on the right (along with the ureter lateral and the testicular artery medial).

2.2.4.3. Innervation

The T10 spinal segment is the source of the sympathetic nerve fibers that innervate the testes. They travel to the celiac ganglion via the lesser splanchnic nerves, where they synapse. The post-ganglionic fibers subsequently follow the testicular artery to its site of innervation. Similar sensory root fibers carry information to the dorsal root ganglion cells of the T10 segment. Specifically, the genital branch (L2) of the genitofemoral nerve (L1, L2) of the lumbar plexus innervates the tunica vaginalis of the testes.

2.2.4.4. Lymphatic Drainage

The only parts of the male genitalia that do not leak into the inguinal lymph nodes are the testes. Its lymphatics travel alongside the testicular veins until they arrive at the para-aortic lymph nodes located at the level of the L2 vertebrae (Guyton & Hall, 2006; Sembulingam & Sembulingam, 2006; Mescher, 2010; Rhoades & Bell, 2012).

2.3. Spermatogenesis: Process of Sperm Production

A carefully planned biological process called spermatogenesis is necessary for male organisms, including humans, to reproduce sexually. This complex process starts in the testes' seminiferous tubules, where specialized cells go through many transformational phases before producing mature spermatozoa that can fertilize an egg. Spermatogonia, undifferentiated diploid cells, are found around the periphery of seminiferous tubules at the beginning of spermatogenesis. These progenitor cells multiply through a process known as mitosis, guaranteeing a consistent supply of precursor cells to produce sperm. Setting the stage for the amazing journey ahead, some spermatogonia commit to the path of differentiation, while others stay reserve cells.

During the following stage, which is defined by growth and maturation, some spermatogonia develop into primary spermatocytes. These initial spermatocytes go through a crucial process called meiosis I while still having a diploid chromosome complement. Haploid secondary spermatocytes are created because of the alignment and genetic material exchange between the chromosome pairs during this process. Meiosis II proceeds quickly after, with secondary spermatocytes dividing once more to produce haploid round spermatids. The spermatozoa that result from this reduction in chromosome number will only carry one set of chromosomes, which is essential for successful fertilization upon fusion with an egg.

Spermiogenesis is the next stage on the path to spermatozoa, during which there are significant structural changes. Round spermatids acquire the characteristic characteristics of mature sperm cells through a series of morphological changes that are coordinated by complex molecular mechanisms. The formation of the acrosome, a specialized organelle that houses enzymes necessary for piercing the egg's protective layers, the condensation of the nucleus to support genetic integrity, and the elongation of the cell to form a tail-like flagellum, which is essential for sperm motility, are a few of the noteworthy events that occur during spermiogenesis.

Excess cytoplasm is shed during spermiogenesis, which streamlines the spermatozoa for ideal performance. Cellular remodeling guarantees that developed sperm cells have the form and capacity to go through the female reproductive system and fertilize an egg that is waiting to be fertilized. Spermiation, or the release of mature spermatozoa from the seminiferous tubules into the convoluted duct known as the epididymis, signifies the end of spermatogenesis. Here, sperm undergo additional maturation and acquire motility. Spermatozoa experience physiological changes in the epididymis, such as modifications to their membranes and the activation of flagellar movement to give them motility. Sperm cells are primed for their eventual journey through the male reproductive tract and eventual interaction with an ovum by this maturation process. The process of spermatogenesis is tightly controlled by a complex interaction between hormonal signals and molecular cues. Follicle-stimulating hormone (FSH) and testosterone are two important hormones that regulate different phases of sperm production and maintain male fertility.

Male infertility can result from spermatogenesis abnormalities or disruptions, underscoring the crucial role that this process plays in reproductive health. To address male infertility, extensive research and clinical interventions are required because spermatogenesis can be negatively impacted by a variety of factors, including genetic mutations, hormonal imbalances, environmental toxins, and lifestyle decisions. The intricate and well-coordinated process of producing sperm, known as spermatogenesis, is necessary for sexual reproduction. Spermatogonia differentiate into mature spermatozoa capable of fertilizing an egg through a sequence of precisely regulated cellular events, demonstrating the astounding complexity of biological reproduction.

The male reproductive organs are specialized for the following functions:

- Spermatogenic function; for sperm production;
- Maintenance and transport of sperm (the male reproductive cells and protective fluid semen);
- Sperm Discharge function; for discharging sperm inside the female reproductive tract;
- Hormonal function; for producing and secreting male sex hormones like testosterone.

2.3.1. Spermatogenic Functions

Spermatogenesis is the process by which spermatogonia, the primitive germ cells in the testes, undergo mitotic divisions and differentiate into mature sperm cells (spermatozoa). This complex process involves several stages, each with distinct cellular changes and functions:

1. ***Spermatogonial proliferation***: The process begins with spermatogonial stem cells undergoing mitotic divisions to produce more spermatogonia. These cells are located on the basement membrane of the seminiferous tubules in the testes.
2. **Meiosis:** Spermatogonia undergoes two consecutive divisions to produce haploid cells called spermatids. This process occurs in the adluminal compartment of the seminiferous tubules. Meiosis I reduces the chromosome number from diploid to haploid, while meiosis II further divides the haploid cells to generate spermatids.
3. **Spermiogenesis:** Spermatids undergo extensive morphological changes to become mature spermatozoa. This involves the formation of the acrosome, condensation of the nucleus, development of the flagellum, and removal of excess cytoplasm.
4. **Spermiation:** Mature spermatozoa are released from the sustentacular cells into the lumen of the seminiferous tubules. They then move to the epididymis, where they undergo further maturation and acquire motility.

Functions of spermatogenesis include:

i. **Production of Sperm:** The primary function of spermatogenesis is to produce mature sperm cells capable of fertilizing an egg. This ensures the continuation of the species through sexual reproduction.

ii. **Genetic Diversity:** During meiosis, genetic recombination occurs, leading to the shuffling and exchange of genetic material between homologous chromosomes. This process introduces genetic variation among sperm cells, contributing to genetic diversity within a population.

iii. **Hormonal Regulation:** Spermatogenesis is tightly regulated by hormones, including follicle-stimulating hormone (FSH) and testosterone. FSH stimulates the proliferation and maturation of germ cells, while testosterone is essential for the maintenance of spermatogenesis and the development of secondary sexual characteristics.

iv. **Sperm Quality Control:** Spermatogenesis involves quality control mechanisms to ensure the production of functionally competent spermatozoa. Defects in spermatogenesis can lead to infertility or genetic abnormalities in offspring.

Overall, spermatogenesis is a critical process for male fertility and reproductive success. It involves precise cellular and molecular events that ensure the production of mature and functional sperm cells (Guyton & Hall, 2006; Sembulingam & Sembulingam, 2006; Mescher, 2010; Rhoades & Bell, 2012).

2.3.2. Spermatogenesis

Spermatogenesis, which has two main components, is the term used to describe the cellular divisions and developmental changes that take place within the seminiferous tubules of the testes (Figure 2.3). In the first section, spermatocytogenesis takes place.

It begins with spermatogonia, which is the early stage of mitotic stem cell division into spermatocytes and is followed by meiosis, which reduces the number of chromosomes to form spermatids. The process of spermiogenesis, in which spermatids undergo metamorphic changes to become sperm, takes place in part 2. Spermatogenesis is a highly structured, intricate process that typically lasts a lifetime. According to the description given above, spermatogenesis is divided into three main divisions: spermatocytogenesis, meiosis, and spermiogenesis.

The process starts with spermatogonial stem cells, which are located on the seminiferous tubules' basement membrane. These cells typically multiply for self-renewal and give rise to progeny that are differentiating spermatogenic cells, including primary, secondary, spermatid, and spermatozoa. The spermatogonia divides by mitosis, and one of the duplicate members—referred to as the primary spermatocyte—goes through meiosis to produce secondary spermatocytes. Two daughter haploid cells, referred to as secondary spermatocytes, are created when the diploid primary spermatocytes, or spermatogonia, finish the first round of meiosis. Each of the two secondary spermatocytes produced two haploid spermatids by the end of the second (2nd) meiotic cell division. The spermatids initially exhibit the typical traits of epithelioid cells, but they eventually differentiate and lengthen into mature spermatozoa.

A fully developed spermatozoon consists of a head, a tail, and a thin layer of surrounding membranous material as well as condensed nuclear material. The creation of the acrosome, which is derived from the Golgi apparatus, condensation, nucleus elongation, flagellum formation, and extensive cytoplasmic shedding of the spermiated spermatozoa—which are composed of a head, middle piece, and tail—are among the main characteristics of spermiogenesis (Figure 2.4).

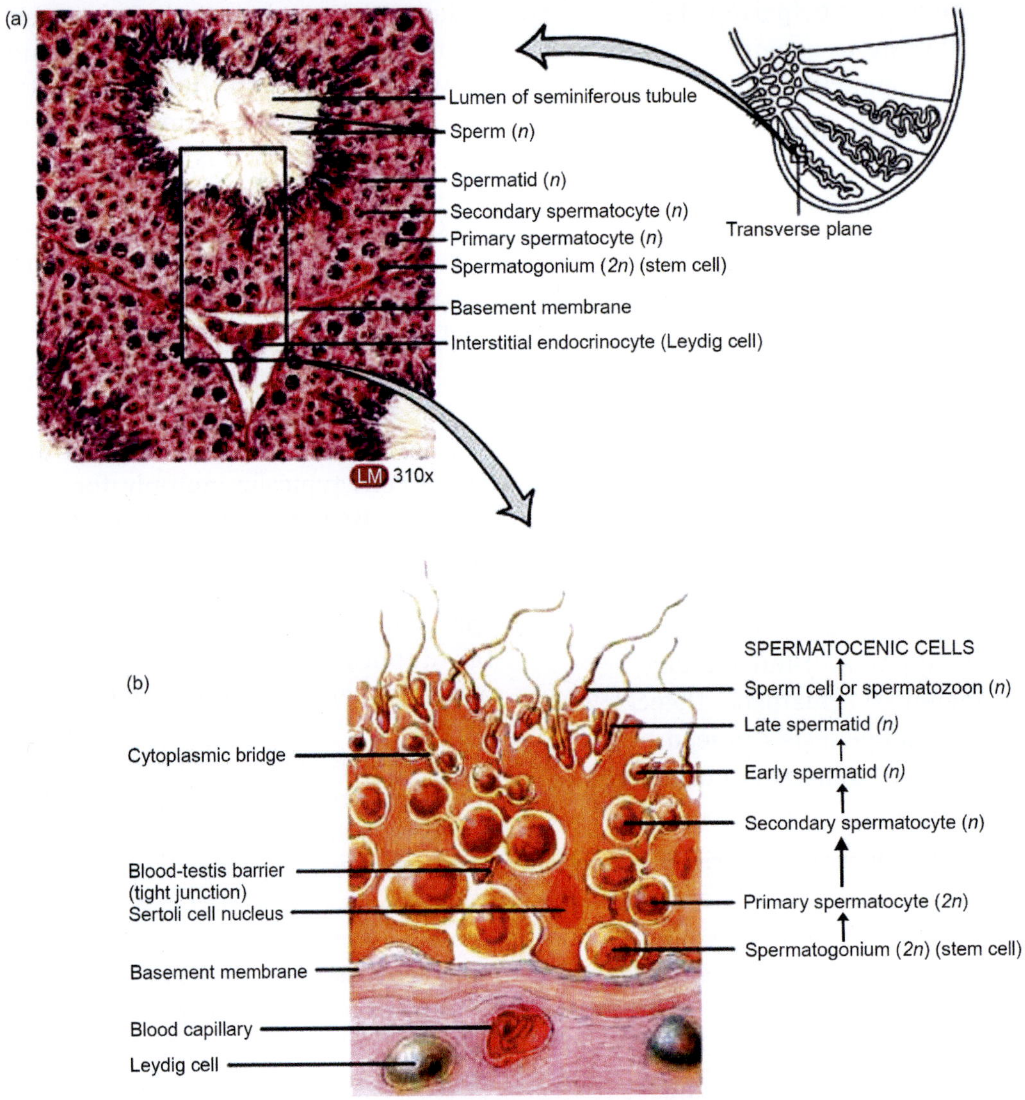

Figure 2.3. *The microscopic anatomy of the seminiferous tubules.*

Source: Mega, O. O., Eze, K. N., Arientare, R. R., & Victor, E., (2022). The concept of male reproductive anatomy. IntechOpen. doi: 10.5772/intechopen.99742.

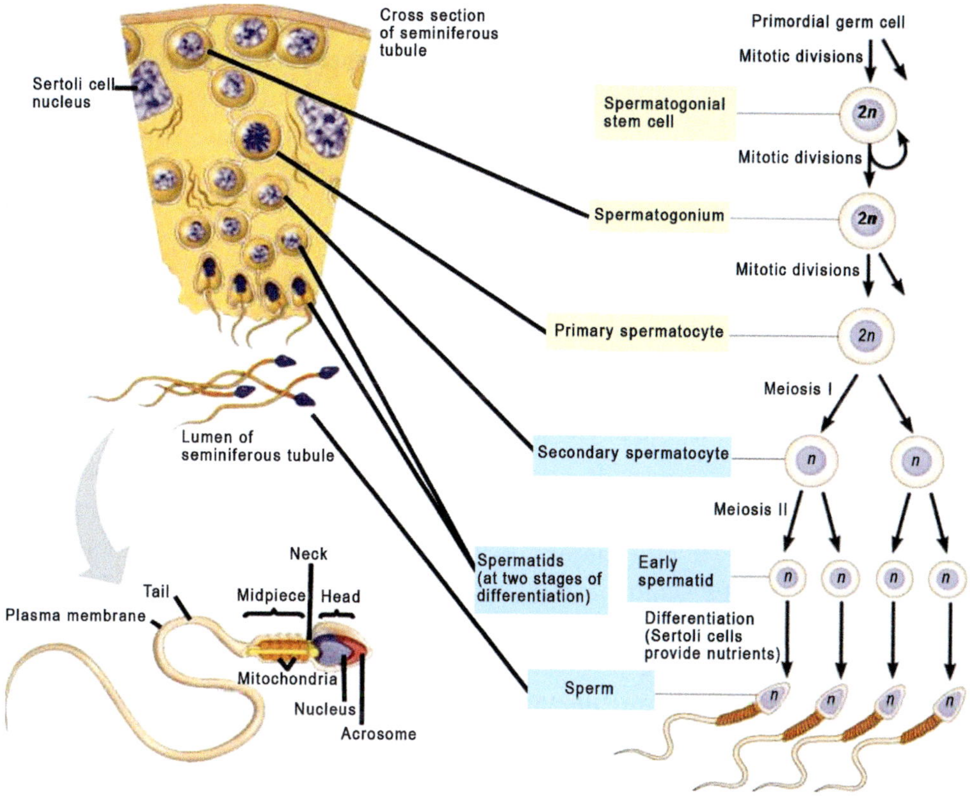

Figure 2.4. *An overview of spermatogenesis.*

Source: Mega, O. O., Eze, K. N., Arientare, R. R., & Victor, E., (2022). The concept of male reproductive anatomy. IntechOpen. doi: 10.5772/intechopen.99742. Adapted from: bio1151.nicerweb.com.

2.3.2.1. Structure of Mature Spermatozoa and Its Membrane

The head, center, and tail make up the sperm. The head is made up of nuclei encircled by an acrosome of chromatin that is closely packed. Enzymes for oocyte penetration are present in the acrosome. To produce ATP necessary for the sperm to pass through the female reproductive tract, a unique arrangement of mitochondria spirals around the center of the sperm. The spermatozoa's flagellum, or tail, is what propels them forward. The microtubule and associated protein bundle known as the axoneme is in the center of the flagellum of eukaryotic sperm and oversees movement. Sperm cells are found in the fluid expelled during an organism's ejaculation, along with secretions from the prostate, seminal vesicles, Cowper's gland, and possibly the urethral glands.

It has a fixed gravity (1.028), a bright, opalescent fluid, and a pH of 7.35–7.50. For each ejaculation, the approximate volume of semen is 2.5 to 3.5 ml after several days of consistency. The seminal vesicles contain the bulk of this secretion or fluid (about 60%), and the prostate gland contributes the remainder (about 40%). Components of seminal vesicle secretion include fructose, phosphorylcholine, ergothioneine, ascorbic acid, flavins, and prostaglandins, while spermine, citric acid, cholesterol phospholipids, fibrinolysis, fibrinogenase, zinc, and acid phosphate are components of prostate secretion. Hyaluronidase and buffers (phosphate and bicarbonate) are also known to be present in semen. With repeated ejaculations, the volume of the sperm-containing semen rapidly decreases. Even though it only takes one sperm to fertilize the ovum, male humans have between 60 and 150 million sperm per millimeter in their ejaculated semen, which makes up around 20% of the total volume of semen. After copulation or sexual contact, human sperm travels through the female genital tract at a speed of roughly 3 nm/min and enters the uterine tubes 30 to 60 minutes later.

Oligospemia is the term for a sperm concentration below roughly 10 millimeters, and it is linked to lower fertility. Oligospermia can be brought on by several things, such as heat from a hot tub or sauna, different prescription drugs, lead and arsenic poisoning, and illegal substances like cocaine, marijuana, and anabolic steroids. Some men and women experience infertility due to antibodies against sperm antigens, which is a common cause in men who have had a vasectomy, in addition to low sperm counts. These antibodies lower fertility but generally have no effect on well-being. Only 1% of the semen or seminal fluid sperm is composed of sperm composition and secretions from the prostate, bulbourethral, seminal vesicles, and epididymis; the remaining 1% is composed of accessory gland fluids. Although semen is more than 90% water, it also contains a variety of substances, including fructose, which is high in energy, vitamins like C and Inositol, and trace minerals like calcium, zinc, magnesium, copper, and sulfur. Prostaglandin is likewise found in the highest concentration of semen. Semen ranges in consistency from a thick, viscous liquid to a nearly watery one. The first cells that will develop into semen are called primordial germ cells. They are created in the yolk sac, a membrane that is attached to the developing embryo. In the fifth or sixth week of development, they invade the embryo itself, moving past the blood testis barrier (BTB) and into the seminiferous tubule. Spermatogonia reproduces by mitosis, giving rise to two kinds of type A daughter cells and type B spermatogonia. Beyond the blood test barrier, type A cells proliferate starting at puberty and continue to do so until death. Men therefore never run out of gametes and usually continue to be fertile into old age. Spermatogonia type B migrates inward toward the tubule lumen, where it differentiates into primary spermatocytes, which are slightly larger cells. These cells have to enter the tubule lumen after passing through the blood testicular membrane.

Before the primary spermatocyte, the tight junction between two sustentacular cells is typically broken down, and a new tight junction forms on the other side. After undergoing mitosis 1, the primary spermatocyte divides into two haploid secondary spermatocytes of the same size. Every one of these goes through meiosis II and splits into two spermatids, or four in total, depending on the spermatogonia. Every stage approaches the tubule a little bit more closely than the ones before it. All stages on the luminal side of the blood-testicular barrier are tightly encased in the tendrils of the sustentacular cells and connected to them by gap junctions and tight junctions. The daughter cells do not fully separate during this meiotic division; instead, they stay joined by tiny cytoplasmic bridges. Thus, spermiogenesis refers to the remaining stages of spermatogenesis. Instead of additional cell division, each spermatid (immature sperm) gradually changes into a mature spermatozoon (Figure 2.5).

As sperm travel through the epididymis, they undergo maturation processes that result in the development of progressive motility and the ability to fertilize an egg. These changes, known as sperm maturation, involve dynamic morphological and metabolic alterations. One important aspect of sperm maturation is the completion of nuclear condensation and modifications to the distribution and expression of surface molecules. Phospholipid hydroperoxide glutathione peroxidase (GPx4) plays a role in this process by helping to oxidize proteins in the sperm nucleus and protect against oxidative DNA damage. Additionally, reactive oxygen species may play a role in initiating sperm motility by enhancing cAMP synthesis and protein phosphorylation at the time of ejaculation.

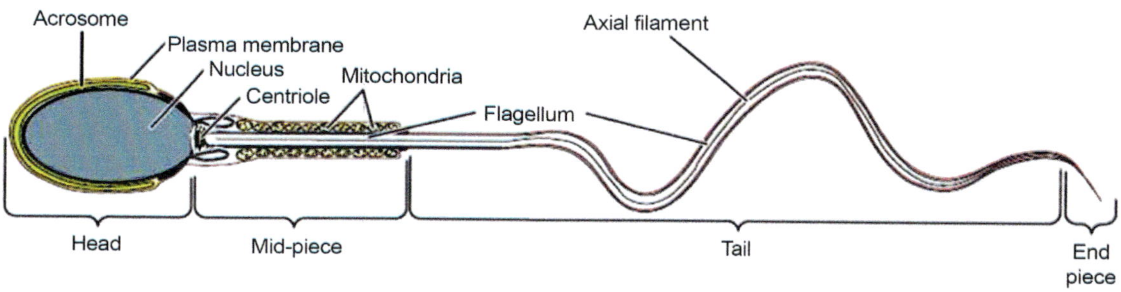

Figure 2.5. *Structure of a mature spermatozoon.*

Source: Mega, O. O., Eze, K. N., Arientare, R. R., & Victor, E., (2022). The concept of male reproductive anatomy. IntechOpen. doi: 10.5772/intechopen.99742.

Since the acrosome reaction and sperm-oocyte fusion are membrane-associated processes, the membrane structure is crucial for successful fertilization. In fact, the lipids in the spermatozoal membrane are what give the spermatozoa their fluidity and flexibility. However, these lipids are also the main substrates for peroxidation, which can result in severe disorders related to sperm function, along with membrane proteins. Excessive levels of oxidants have been demonstrated to cause sperm pathology, including ATP depletion, which results in insufficient axonemal phosphorylation, lipid peroxidation, and a reduction in motility and viability. The peroxidative damage of the sperm plasma membrane is the cause of the harmful effects of reactive oxygen species (ROS). Furthermore, oxidative stress-mediated sperm plasma membrane damage can explain observed defective sperm function in a significant number of infertile patients. The ionic environment and ionic fluxes across the membrane play a critical role in spermatozoa maturation, capacitation, and the start of the gamete interaction process. Different types of ion channels are present in the plasma membrane of mammalian sperm, suggesting a variety of roles in sperm physiology and gamete interaction.

The plasma membrane integral enzymes in most animal cells are Na^+/K^+-ATPase (E.C. 3.6.1.9) and Ca^{2+}-ATPase (E.C. 3.6.1.3) and are important components involved in ionic homeostasis. Changes in the surrounding of the sperm membrane and thus in fluidity change the activities of these enzymes, requiring the existence of phospholipids closely linked to their structure. The Na + pump is a heteromeric protein consisting of several isozymes and is not only responsible for maintaining cell osmotic equilibrium, volume, and pH, but also for maintaining the capacity of the cell resting membrane and supplying chemical energy across the cell membrane for the secondary Na^+–coupled transport of other ions, solutes, and water. The Ca^{2+} pump, on the other hand, is responsible for the homeostasis of calcium which is central to normal cell function. A distinctive Na^+/K^+-ATPase isoform expression profile has been found in the mammalian testis regarding the Na^+ pump. The human Na^+/K^+-ATPase 4 isoform has different functional properties and plays a primary role in the motility of sperm. Enzymes that contain sulfhydryl (SH) are thought to be ATPases, and nitric oxide (NO) and its byproducts, like peroxynitrite (ONOO-), may target their thiol groups. It has actually been demonstrated unequivocally that NO and NO-derived reactive nitrogen species modify the activity of various enzymes and can, as a result, damage cells, resulting in sperm dysfunction.

This can be achieved through raising lipid peroxidation, completely depleting the sulfhydryl group, and forming nitrotyrosine, or by inactivating proteins and damaging nucleic acids, which can then modify or disturb the structure and function of membranes. The accumulation of oxidative damage leads to the development of various disease states in humans. Specifically, the gradual conversion of sperm thiols to disulfides is responsible for sperm chromatin condensation and stabilization of the tail structure, which is necessary for the subsequent initiation of motility. Specifically, it has been discovered that a decrease in the quantity of protein thiol groups and a change in the substrate dependency curve of the enzyme occurs when peroxynitrite inhibits the activity of Na+/K+-ATPase. This indicates that its inhibition is caused by the blockade of Na+/K+-ATPase SH-groups. The pattern of this inhibition is consistent either with the oxidation of SH groups that are outside the active site of the enzyme but necessary for the enzyme's activity or with the oxidation of thiol groups directly involved in the binding of ATP but in a way that cannot be resolved by raising the concentration of the substrate.

2.3.2.2. Capacitation and Acrosome Reaction

Capacitation is a process where sperm undergo morphological changes through hyperactivation and acrosome reaction to be able to fuse with an egg. Hyperactivation involves strong, asymmetric movements of the sperm tail, allowing it to penetrate the outer layers of the egg. The acrosome reaction then takes place, releasing enzymes that help the sperm break through the protective barriers surrounding the egg. Research has shown that the presence of O_2 is crucial for both hyperactivation and acrosome reaction. Other characteristics of capacitation include increased membrane fluidity, tyrosine phosphorylation, pH levels, cAMP levels, and calcium influx. Certain substances in semen and secretions from the egg can also influence capacitation, but it can also occur spontaneously under the right conditions. Additionally, reactive oxygen species produced by sperm can play a role in regulating capacitation.

The redox effect on protein tyrosine phosphorylation is supported by various signal transduction pathways, such as sarcoma and extracellular kinase-regulated pathways, as well as the inhibition of tyrosine phosphatase activity through cAMP generation. Capacitation involves increasing membrane fluidity, cholesterol efflux, ion fluxes altering sperm membrane potential, increased tyrosine protein phosphorylation, hyperactivation induction, and acrosome reaction. Reactive oxygen species, along with factors like bicarbonate and membrane cholesterol loss, and increased intracellular Ca^{2+} levels, activate adenyl cyclase (AC), leading to cAMP production and activation of protein kinase A (PKA) for tyrosine protein phosphorylation. Adenyl cyclase can be activated by superoxides or hydrogen peroxides, acting as a bicarbonate substitute. Increased cAMP activates PKA, which in turn activates tyrosine kinases and inhibits tyrosine phosphatase (TP).

The involvement of PKA and its inhibitor H89 was confirmed. Hydrogen peroxide can stimulate tyrosine kinases directly and inhibit TP. Tyrosine phosphorylation plays a key role in capacitation, leading to hyperactivation, binding to the zona, and acrosome reaction. *In vitro* studies on mouse sperm showed a 50% increase in fertilization rates through mild lipid peroxidation induced by a ferrous ion and ascorbic acid mixture. Hydrogen peroxide-induced oxidative stress enhances sperm activity and fertilization rates. Superoxide anion induces capacitation in incubation conditions by acting as an oxidase. Further stimulation of ROS development – superoxide anion, hydrogen peroxide – leads to the release of unesterified fatty acids from the plasma of these cells.

2.3.2.3. Sperm Abnormalities

Sperm anomalies include oligospermia (sperm concentration less than 20 million/ml), which are typically based on sperm concentration, motility, and morphology which revealed a low rate of conception when the concentration of human sperm was less than 20 million/ml. A total absence of spermatozoa in an ejaculate is known as azoospermia, and it is estimated that this causes 10–15% of cases of male infertility. Sperm concentration was also affected by partial sperm duct obstruction. A disorder known as asthenospermia, or poor sperm motility, occurs when spermatozoa move too slowly and are unable to fertilize an egg or move in a straight line through the cervical mucus in the female reproductive system. Sperm motility is considered normal when 60% or more of the sperm actively travel in a straight line, and the quality is at least average. When the sperm motility percentage is less than 40%, the condition is considered less qualitative. Sperm motility issues, whether genetic or not, may be the cause of their slow motion, which may prevent them from fertilizing the egg. DNA fragmentation-related poor sperm motility can raise the possibility of genetic illnesses being passed on to progeny. There are two methods to rate sperm motility: general motility, which is the percentage of total motility, and progressive motility, which is the rate of individual forward progressive sperm movement. The latter is a grade that is based on how most motile sperm behave. Its values range from null, which indicates no movement, to four, which indicates excellent forward progress. Notably, a minimum of 50% progressive motility is required for a sperm sample. Teratospermia, also known as morphologic abnormalities, are typically classified according to where a spermatozoon's deformity is located—on its head, neck (midpiece), or tail.

The two most significant classification scheme types are primary and secondary anomalies. Primary anomalies are structural defects that affect the head, midpiece, and tail in the location. A more serious primary defect is thought to have originated when the sperm was still inside the seminiferous epithelium of the testis. Less severe secondary defects are thought to have originated during the passage of the sperm through the epididymis or because of improper handling after ejaculation. Changes in the form of different sperm components are a part of the heterogeneous state of teratozoospermia. Morphological defects and the possibility of sperm fertilization are closely related because mature spermatozoa structures are best organized to fulfill specific roles. Therefore, teratozoospermia can be defined as a combination of morphological abnormalities and sperm function impairments.

2.3.2.4. Factors Influencing Spermatogenesis

Temperature and hormone changes have a significant impact on the spermatogenesis process. Large local concentrations of testosterone are required to maintain the process, which is carried out by bidding testosterone with androgen binding protein found in the seminiferous tubules. Ledig cells, or interstitial cells, are cells that live next to the seminiferous tubule and produce testosterone. The testes are located outside the body in a skin sac known as the scrotum because the seminiferous epithelium in humans and some other animals is sensitive to high temperatures and can be negatively impacted by temperatures as high as the average body temperature. The ideal temperature is maintained when the body temperature is 20°C (human) or 80°C (mouse) below. Controlling blood flow and orienting the dartos smooth muscle and cremasteric muscle with or away from the body's heat are two ways this is achieved. The rate of spermatogenesis may also be negatively impacted by anabolic steroids, metals (lead and cadmium), X-ray exposure, dioxin, alcohol, drug toxicants, and pathogen-related illnesses (Guyton & Hall, 2006; Sembulingam & Sembulingam, 2006; Mescher, 2010; Rhoades & Bell, 2012).

2.3.3. Testicular Steroidogenesis

Steroidogenesis, which involves the production of testosterone (T) and dihydrotestosterone (DHT) from cholesterol by a series of P450 enzymes in the Leydig testis cells, is crucial for both spermatogenesis and the development of secondary sex characteristics. T (produced locally by the interstitial cells regulated by LH) is responsible for the differentiation of the mesonephric ducts into the epididymides, vasa deferentia, seminal vesicles, and the development of the levatorani-muscle and bulbocavernosus gland (the LABC complex). DHT is the hormone that causes the nipple anlagen in male fetuses to recede and the genital tubercle to separate from the external genitalia and the urogenital sinus into the glands of the prostate and Cowper. It is produced locally in the testis through T conversion using the enzyme 5-alpha-reductase. Steroid hormones are categorized into five groups based on the receptors they bind to mineralocorticoids, glucocorticoids, androgens, estrogen, and progestogens. The primary building block for the biosynthesis of all steroid hormones, cholesterol, is either synthesized de novo from acetate within the cell or integrated into the Leydig cell by receptor-mediated endocytosis from low-density lipoproteins. The quantity of cytoplasmic lipid droplets in interstitial cells is thought to be inversely correlated with the rate of androgen synthesis. The droplets contain cholesterol in an ester form.

During steroidogenesis, cholesterol ester is hydrolyzed by LH-induced cholesterol ester hydrolase activation and then transferred into the mitochondria of interstitial cells. Cholesterol is transported from the exterior to the inner mitochondrial membrane by the StAR protein. However, it is still unknown how precisely the StAR protein transports cholesterol to the mitochondria. StAR protein expression is severely reliant on trophic hormone stimulation, which is acutely regulated, e.g., LH and ACTH). It becomes vulnerable to environmental toxins as a result, including various xenobiotics. It has been reported that 4-tert-octylphenyl and the pesticides Lindane (1,2,3,4,5,6-hexachlorocyclohexane) and glyphosate Roundup (2-(phosphonomethylamino) acetate) interfere with the steroidogenesis by inhibitor of StAR protein expression. Mutations in the StAR gene are thought to be the cause of the condition known as lipoid congenital adrenal hyperplasia, or lipoid CAH. In lipoid CAH, an autosomal recessive fatal condition, cholesterol and cholesterol esters build up and the newborn is unable to synthesize enough steroids. StAR knockout mice exhibit a phenotype strikingly like lipoid CAH in humans, offering a useful model for deciphering the mechanism underlying the significant role that StAR protein plays in steroidogenesis and endocrine production.

The monooxygenase enzyme cytochrome P450scc side chain cleavage converts cholesterol to pregnenolone inside the inner mitochondrial membrane. This step involves the following three consecutive monooxygenations: C20–C22 bond cleavage, 20-hydroxylation, and 22-hydroxylation. Following its diffusion across the mitochondrial membrane, pregnenolone is transferred to the endoplasmic reticulum, where it engages in a sequence of biochemical reactions that result in the formation of testosterone. In the Delta 5 pathway, pregnenolone is hydroxylated on carbon 17 times to produce 17 alpha-hydroxypregnenolone. This compound is subsequently split between carbon 17 and carbon 20 bonds to form DHEA. These reactions are catalyzed by the cytochrome P450 17 alpha-hydroxylase/C17, 20 lyase. 3β-HSD can convert DHEA to androstenedione, and 17β-HSD can convert DHEA to testosterone. The type and current activity of 17β-HSD determine the balance between these androgens. Leydig testis cells express types 3 and 5 of 17β-HSD, which catalyze the conversion of androstenedione to testosterone, whereas type 2 of the enzyme exhibits the opposite reaction (found among others in the prostate and placenta).

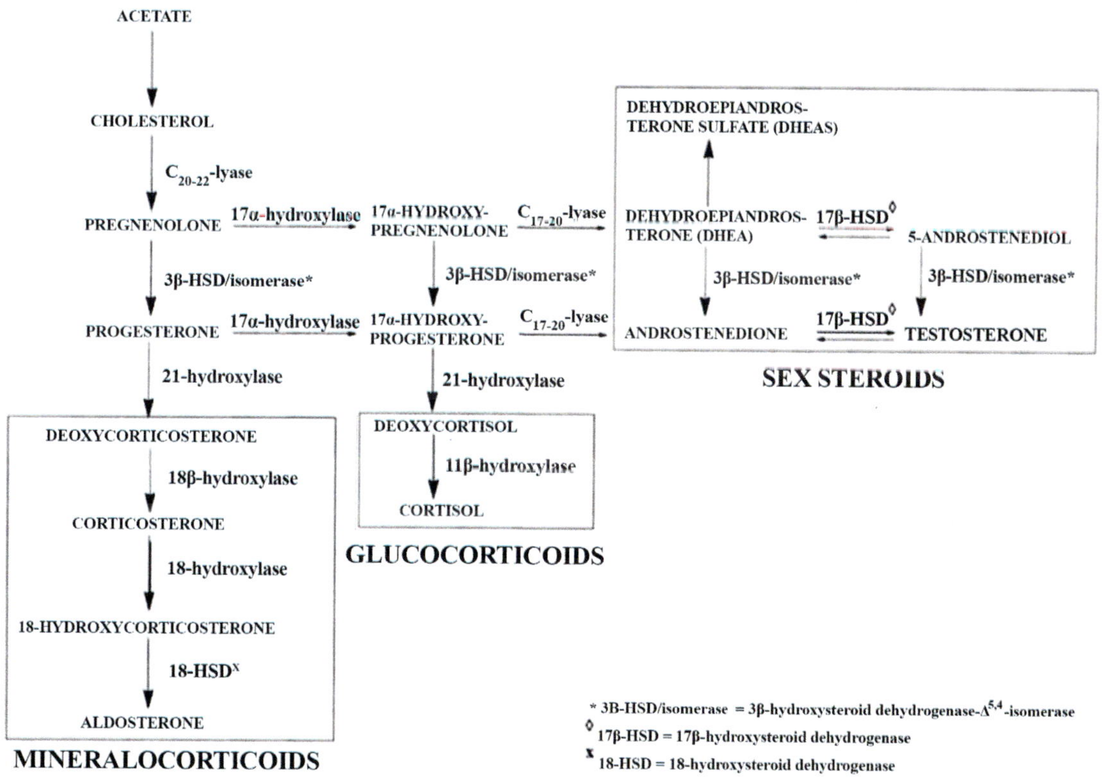

Figure 2.6. *The major pathways in steroid biosynthesis.*

Source: Mega, O. O., Eze, K. N., Arientare, R. R., & Victor, E., (2022). The concept of male reproductive anatomy. IntechOpen. doi: 10.5772/intechopen.99742.

The enzyme 3β-HSD is widely expressed in both steroidogenic and non-steroidogenic tissues, including the prostate, asthetes, skin, and brain. In the rat, four 3β-HSD isozymes with variable and tissue-specific expression were identified. Testosterone is released into the bloodstream through the spermatic vein. LH controls the synthesis of testosterone in interstitial cells. In addition, cytokines, insulin-like growth factor-1, and FSH all influence the biosynthesis of testosterone. FSH controls spermatogenesis through the paracrine regulation of testicular functions (Figure 2.6).

2.3.4. Sperm Discharge Function

The discharge of semen into the reproductive tract of a female has to do with the following steps:

1. **Libido:** This is the biological need (sexual drive) for sexual activity and is often expressed as conduct that seeks sex. Its strength is variable over a given time between people and within a person. In stable older but not younger men, higher serum testosterone tends to be associated with greater sexual action.
2. **Erection:** The penis is in an erect state when it is enlarged and firm. Some of the factors that influence it are the dynamic interplay of endocrine, neuronal, vascular, and psychological factors. A penile erection happens when venous blood enlarges the corpora cavernosa, two tubular structures that run the length of the penis. Any of the various physiological stimuli may cause this. Located directly below the cavernosa corpora, which is the urethra from which urine and semen pass during ejaculation, is a single tubular structure called the corpus spongiosum. This is frequently slightly engorged with blood, but not as much as the corpora canvernosa penile erection, which is typically brought on by sexual arousal and/or excitement. It can also happen spontaneously during the day or at night, frequently during romantic or wet dreams, or in response to triggers like a full bladder. An erection leads to penile swelling and enlargement. An erection facilitates sexual intercourse and other sexual activities, though it is not required for all of them (sexual functions).
3. **Ejaculation:** Sperm delivery into the female genital tract requires ejaculation and erection (without technical assistance). It is important to consider two things that happen during ejaculation: the first is the seminal emission or deposition of semen into the posterior urethra, and the second is the expulsion of semen from the urethra. The sympathetic nervous system regulates the release of sperm and their ejaculation. The vas, vas ampulla, seminal vesicles, prostate covering muscle, and myoid complexes are among the structures that emit. Closing the bladder neck is necessary during ejaculation to avoid or stop retrograde semen flow, along with contraction of the periurethral muscles, particularly the bulbocavernosus muscle.
4. **Orgasm:** An orgasm, is a powerfully pleasurable sensation that usually occurs at the peak of sexual arousal and is accompanied by a release of tension in the sexual area. An orgasm does not always follow sexual arousal because different people require different stimuli in different amounts and under different conditions to experience

one. An orgasm consists of a series of rhythmic contractions in the genital and pelvic regions. Blood pressure, heart rate, and breathing rate all sharply rise throughout the body. Muscle contractions in the back, buttocks, and extremities can result from a generalized contraction of the muscles. In men, the organism goes through two stages. First, seminal fluid is sent to the bulb by the contraction of the vas deferens, seminal vesicles, and prostate at the base of the urethral, and the man experiences an inevitability of ejaculation—a sensation that ejaculation is either about to occur or cannot be prevented. Second, ejaculation is a mechanism that involves the rhythmic contraction of the penis and urethra bulb to expel sperm; however, some men experience orgasms at a different time from ejaculation (Guyton & Hall, 2006; Sembulingam & Sembulingam, 2006; Mescher, 2010; Rhoades & Bell, 2012).

2.3.5. Endocrine and Neuroendocrine Factors Regulating Testicular Functions

The spermatogenic and steroidogenic activities of the testes are finely regulated by the brain (upon stimulation), the master endocrine gland, and local factors produced by the testes. During intrauterine life, testosterone—secreted by the Leydig cell upon activation by placenta-released human chorionic gonadotropin (HCG)—carefully regulates the growth of the testes and the proliferation of primitive germ cells. After birth, the testes no longer receive hormonal guidance, and they remain silent until the onset of puberty. During puberty, specific cells in the hypothalamus activate GnRH-secreting cells, which in turn triggers the testicular function setting (Figure 2.7). These cells, which are in the anteroventral periventricular nucleus (AVPV), periventricular nucleus (PVN), preoptic nucleus (PN), and arcuate nucleus (ARC), are known as kisspeptin-secreting cells.

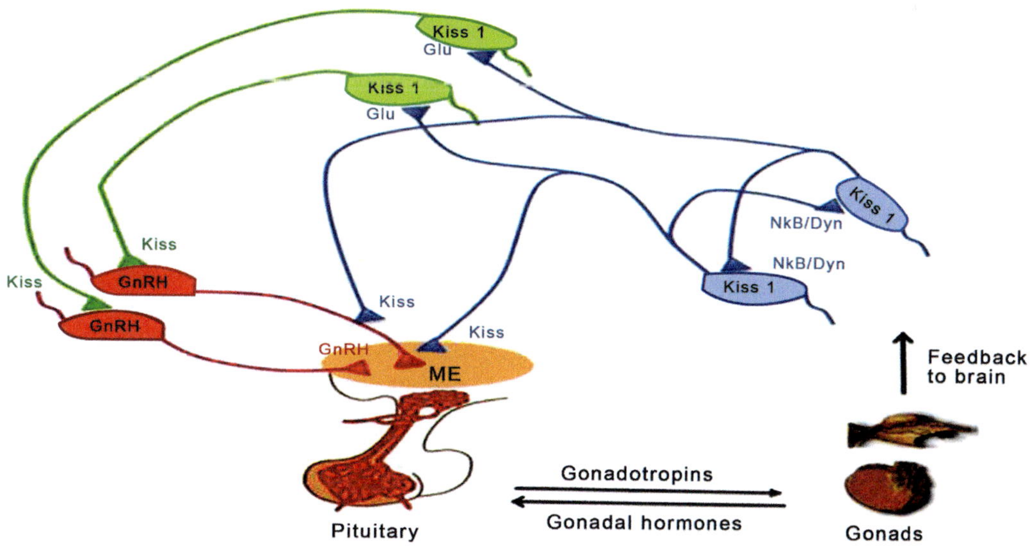

Figure 2.7. *The kisspeptin cell connections with GnRH cells.*

Source: Mega, O. O., Eze, K. N., Arientare, R. R., & Victor, E., (2022). The concept of male reproductive anatomy. IntechOpen. doi: 10.5772/intechopen.99742.

Testicular functions are thought to be impacted by the binding of steroids, leptin, and other systemic factors to receptors on these cells that secrete kisspeptin. Through the median eminence, kisspeptin induces GnRH cells to release gonadotropin-releasing hormone (Figure 2.8). Because they have the GPR54 receptor expressed on their cell membrane, which binds to kisspeptin released by kisspeptin-secreting cells, the cells that secrete GnRH are controlled by kisspeptin. This hormone travels via the hypothalamus-hypophyseal portal system to the anterior pituitary. There, luteinizing hormone (LH) and follicle-stimulating hormone (FSH), which are the tropics for interstitial and sustentacular cells, respectively, are released by the gonadotrophs when GnRH stimulates them. This is the testicular regulation neuroendocrine axis. Upon stimulation, the gonadotrophs in the adenohypophysis release growth hormone, LH, and FSH, which control testicular function. This is the testicular regulation endocrine axis. The development of spermatozoa is dependent on the release of LH and FSH by the pituitary in response to the pulsatile release of GnRH from the hypothalamus.

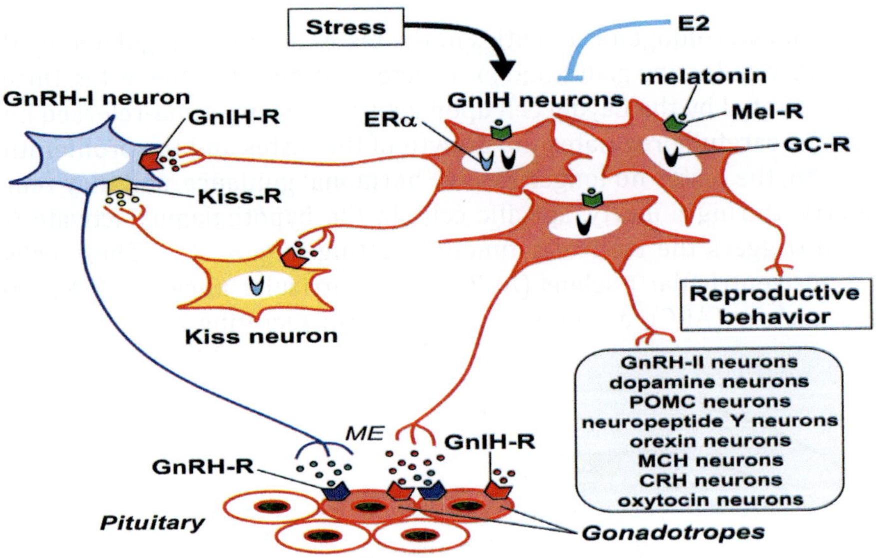

Figure 2.8. *Regulation of kisspeptin-GnRH axis (wikipedia.org.) It is through this kisspeptin-GnRH axis that factors such as steroid stress, leptin light and dark, etc., influence the functions of the testicles.*

Source: Mega, O. O., Eze, K. N., Arientare, R. R., & Victor, E., (2022). The concept of male reproductive anatomy. IntechOpen. doi: 10.5772/intechopen.99742.

As an endocrine gland, the testes secrete steroids and other regional substances that control their function by paracrine and autocrine means. Via a negative feedback mechanism, the steroids and inhibin produced by interstitial and sustentacular cells, respectively, regulate neuroendocrine and endocrine factors. Functionalities related to male reproduction arise from abnormalities in these testicular regulation levels. Due to a misdirection in GnRH cell migration from the olfactory cells during development, this is hypogonadotropin-hypogonadism.

GnRH works by interacting with a specific receptor that is present on gonadotrope cell membranes. These receptors interact with the hormone to form a hormone-receptor complex; they are G-protein coupled receptors. As a result, calcium is released from intracellular stores and enters the cell from extracellular sources through the interaction of phosphoinositide with Gp protein hydrolysis and the release of diacylglycerol and inositol triphosphate. This calcium influx triggers gonadotrophs to release gonadotropin into the bloodstream (Guyton & Hall, 2006; Sembulingam & Sembulingam, 2006; Mescher, 2010; Rhoades & Bell, 2012).

2.3.6. Clinical Implications of Gonadotropins and Steroidogenic Hormones

The release of pituitary and hypothalamic hormones may be negatively impacted by the induction of testosterone synthesis by LH through its binding to receptors on interstitial cells in the testis. The production of androgen-binding protein, which is induced by FSH and targets the receptors on sustentacular cells, aids in the transportation of testosterone through the tight junction complexes on sustentacular cells. FSH also triggers the release of inhibin and activin from sustentacular cells, which are antagonistic to the release of hormones from the pituitary and hypothalamus. FSH is the main hormone produced by the body that regulates testicular function. To control the number of germ cells moving through the mitotic and meiotic spermatogenesis phases, FSH is essential in controlling Sertoli cell populations. FSH controls or regulates DNA synthesis in mitotic and meiotic spermatogonia. In round spermatids, it also inhibits the induction of apoptosis. It has been demonstrated that FSH causes sustentacular cells to release a variety of products. It has been reported that Sertoli cell products are involved in the regulation of Leydig cell functions. The ability of LH to act on the LH receptors found on interstitial cells is crucial for the successful processes of spermatogenesis and steroidogenesis. Leydig cell growth, cell count, testosterone biosynthesis, and secretion are all regulated by LH. It has been demonstrated that spermatid separation from sustentacular cells and complete spermatogenesis stoppage are caused by the removal of testosterone. Testosterone and FSH collaborate to start, maintain, and finish spermatogenesis. Specifically, testosterone plays a role in the development of the blood testis barrier, the upkeep of the interactions between germ cells and Sertoli, and the release of mature sperm from sustentacular cells. In the absence of testosterone, the formation of the blood testis barrier is compromised, and germ cells are prematurely released from the sustentacular cells.

Spermatogenesis is regulated by estrogens, which are found in the epididymis, efferent ductules, and Leydig and Sertoli testis cells. There is evidence that germ cells secrete estrogen into the seminiferous tubular fluid, which may be necessary for the efferent ductules and epididymis to function properly. It is claimed that the growth and differentiation of germ cells are both stimulated and inhibited by estrogen. It has been demonstrated that giving male monkeys aromatase inhibitors causes a decrease in spermatogenesis and sperm concentrations, indicating the critical role estrogen plays in maintaining spermatogenesis. High levels of estrogen are found in sustentacular cells that are proliferating; these levels fall as sustentacular cells begin to avoid differentiation and begin to mature. Estrogens regulate the expression of neural cadherins, a molecule involved in maintaining the adhesion of germ cells, or sustentacular cells.

Male fertility is known to be negatively impacted by environmental estrogens, and research has demonstrated that newborn exposure to exogenous estrogens causes irreversible changes in the expression of certain genes in the reproductive system. It has been demonstrated that adult testicular steroidogenesis reduces a newborn's susceptibility to the synthetic estrogen diethylstilbestrol. It has been demonstrated that adult rats given 17β-estradiol have reduced basal and stimulated testosterone production by 33–48%. When treated with estradiol, adult male rats exhibited significant decreases in circulating concentrations of FSH and LH, which in turn led to reductions in serum and testicular testosterone levels. Testicular functions have been demonstrated to be impacted by many other factors besides hormones (Figure 2.9).

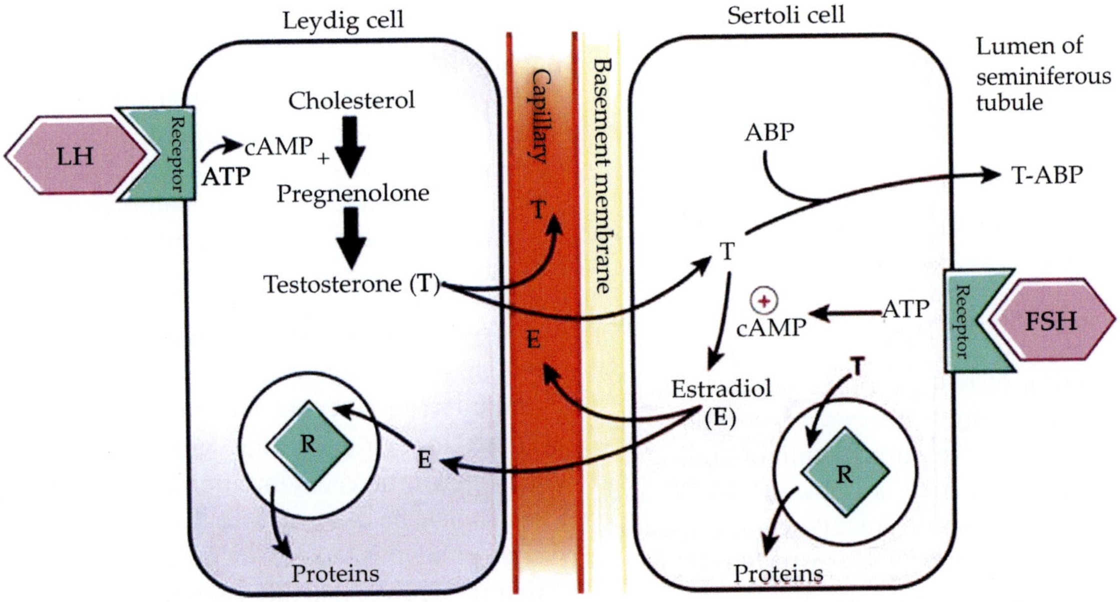

Figure 2.9. *The main product of interstitial cells (e.g., testosterone), regulation, hormonal products, Leydig, and sustentacular cells interaction. [AB: Androgen binding protein; ATP: adenosine triphosphate; cAMP: cyclic adenosine monophosphate; E: estradiol; FSH: follicle-stimulating hormone; LH: luteinizing hormone; and T: testosterone].*

Source: Mega, O. O., Eze, K. N., Arientare, R. R., & Victor, E., (2022). The concept of male reproductive anatomy. IntechOpen. doi: 10.5772/intechopen.99742.

2.3.7. Other Factors Necessary for Male Reproductive Functions

1. **Growth Hormone:** This hormone is usually synthesized by the anterior pituitary (AP) and influences virtually all tissues and organs of the body. It is essential for the general metabolic processes in the testes. It is also necessary for the proliferation of spermatogenesis and plays a key role in the proliferation, growth, and maturation of spermatids.
2. **Local Factors:** Some of the most important local factors produced in the testes by the interstitial cells are testosterone and insulin-like factors, while those of sustentacular cells are inhibin and growth factors. Stem cell factors, immunological factors, opioids, oxytocin, vasopressin, peritubular cell modifying factors, rennin, angiotensin, GnRH, CRH, ACTH, GHRH, calmodulin, plasminogen activator, metalloproteases, dynorphin, PACAP, etc., are some of the other local factors that are believed to have effects on

the functions of the testes. Apart from these factors, glucose has also been shown to be important for the proper functioning of the testis.

3. **Insulin Signaling and Glucose Transport:** In addition to these, glucose has been demonstrated to be crucial for the testes to function properly. For high-energy, difficult testicular spermatogenesis and steroidogenesis to be successfully completed, glucose is necessary. It has been demonstrated that the glucose transport inhibitor cytochalasin B competitively binds to proteins involved in the glucose absorption facilitated by interstitial cells and inhibits the LH-stimulated synthesis of testosterone. It has been demonstrated that there is no testosterone production in the absence of glucose, even though high testosterone production has been seen in the presence of glucose, indicating the need for this compound for testosterone production in addition to LH. Glucose is transferred across plasma membranes by the facilitative glucose transporter (GLUT) protein family. Thus far, 13 families of GLUT proteins have been identified. It has been shown that various types of rat testicular cells express glucose transporter-1 to -3. Because they need glucose for both essential cell functions like motility and fertilization ability as well as for specific functions like basic cell activity, mature spermatozoa also express glucose transporters. GLUT-8, a recently cloned member of the GLUT family, is recognized as the primary glucose transporter in the testis. GLUT-8 is expressed in the heart, skeletal muscles, brain, spleen, prostate, and intestine. However, testis expression of GLUT-8 is higher than that of any other tissue, suggesting that GLUT-8 is involved in glucose transport for Leydig cell steroidogenesis. Furthermore, it has been demonstrated that GLUT-2 is widely expressed in various testicular cell types.

The high expression of glucose transporters and insulin signaling molecules in the testis indicates that contractile testicular cells use a lot of energy and rely on glucose as a fuel source. The development of the gonads in the testis is another important function of the insulin receptor family. The expression of the sex determining region Y (SRY) in somatic progenitor cells that are destined to become sustentacular cells is what causes the differentiation of the testis. It has been demonstrated that Sertoli, Leydig, interstitial, and myoid cells express IRS-1 and IRS-2, indicating that these cell types depend on insulin. Insulin and leptin have been shown to improve the ability of human spermatozoa to fertilize by increasing sperm motility, progressive motility, and acrosome reaction. Furthermore, it has been demonstrated that human spermatozoa release autocrine-regulated pulsatile insulin, and it has been suggested that sperm-derived insulin may contribute to sperm capacitation. As a result, insulin is crucial for maintaining spermatozoa's ability to fertilize as well as the testis' normal operation. Numerous factors are known to impact the body's glucose transport and insulin signaling. As one of the primary regulators among the various variables (Guyton & Hall, 2006; Sembulingam & Sembulingam, 2006; Mescher, 2010; Rhoades & Bell, 2012).

A Closer Look

Hormones

Hormones are biochemical messengers that are produced by different endocrine system glands. They are essential for controlling a wide range of physiological processes. These chemicals are secreted straight into the bloodstream, where they find their way to target tissues and organs and cause particular reactions. The three primary types of hormones are peptide hormones, steroid hormones, and hormones derived from amino acids. Each type of hormone has a unique structure and function.

Peptide hormones are made up of chains of amino acids and are soluble in water, which makes them easy to pass through the bloodstream. Examples of peptide hormones are insulin and growth hormone. Usually, they attach themselves to target cell receptors to start a series of intracellular reactions. Lipid-soluble steroid hormones, such as cortisol, and sex hormones like estrogen and testosterone, can penetrate cell membranes and attach to intracellular receptors, thereby affecting protein synthesis and gene expression. Single amino acids are used to create hormones that are derived from them, such as thyroxine and adrenaline. These hormones have special qualities that enable them to act swiftly and widely.

In the endocrine system, the hypothalamus and pituitary gland are important regulators that control the release of different hormones. Hormones that regulate the pituitary gland, which secretes hormones that regulate other endocrine glands like the thyroid, adrenals, and gonads, are released and inhibited by the hypothalamus. The exact regulation of biological processes, such as metabolism, growth, reproduction, and stress responses, is ensured by this hierarchical control.

Numerous health problems, including diabetes, thyroid disorders, infertility, and growth deficiencies, can be brought on by hormonal imbalances. Hormone replacement therapy and other medications that aid in the management of these conditions have been developed because of advances in medical science. Comprehending the multifaceted functions of hormones remains essential for the diagnosis and treatment of endocrine disorders, as well as for appreciating the intricate interactions among the physiological processes they regulate (Guyton & Hall, 2006; Sembulingam & Sembulingam, 2006; Mescher, 2010; Rhoades & Bell, 2012).

Summary

- The male reproductive system is a complex network of organs and tissues responsible for the production and delivery of sperm, as well as the secretion of hormones essential for sexual development and function.
- Primary sexual characteristics are present at birth and comprise the external and internal genitalia (e.g., the penis and testes in males and the vagina and ovaries in females). Secondary sexual characteristics are those that emerge during the prepubescent through post pubescent phases (e.g., breasts in females and pigmented facial hair in males).
- In adult males, the testis is a strong oval-shaped male gonad, about 4 cm long and 2.5 cm wide in size. Testes are located in the scrotum that regulates its temperature below the normal body temperature to approximately 23°C.
- Sertoli cells are large, irregularly shaped somatic cells. Sertoli cells are bound by tight junctions to each other at their base. Sertoli cells, as shown by their close contact, are essential to the formation of germ cells.
- The survival of the cells in target organs depends on the delivery of nutrient-rich, oxygenated blood and the removal of metabolic waste. In addition, neural signaling is required for most organs to perform specific duties.
- LH binds to the receptors located on the Leydig cells in the testis and induces testosterone synthesis, which in turn could adversely affect the release of hypothalamic and pituitary hormones.

References

1. Agarwal, A., Gupta, S., & Sikka, S. (2006). The role of free radicals and antioxidants in reproduction. *Current Opinion in Obstetrics & Gynecology, 18*(3), 325–332.
2. Aitken, R. J., Ryan, A. L., Baker, M. A., & McLaughlin, E. A. (2004). Redox activity is associated with the maturation and capacitation of mammalian spermatozoa. *Free Radical Biology & Medicine, 36*(8), 994–1010.
3. Akinsola, A. R., Oluwaseun, H., Adewale, A., Olusegun, S., & Adesina, M. (2012). Effect of the methanolic extract of *Trichosanthes cucumerina* seed (snake gourd/tomato) on hormone-influenced seminal vesicle weight in adult Wistar rats. *Webmedcentral Anatomy, 3*(6), 1–8.
4. Aquila, S., Gentile, M., & Middea, E. (2005). Autocrine regulation of insulin secretion in human ejaculated spermatozoa. *Endocrinology, 146*(2), 552–557.
5. Breitbart, H. (2003). Signaling pathways in sperm capacitation and acrosome reaction. *Cellular and Molecular Biology (Noisy-le-Grand, France), 49*(3), 321–327.
6. Bucci, D., Rodriguez-Gil, J. E., Vallorani, C., Spinaci, M., Galeati, G., & Tamanini, C. (2010). GLUTs and mammalian sperm metabolism. *Journal of Andrology, 32*(4), 348–355.
7. Carreau, S., Bouraima-Lelong, H., & Delalande, C. (2012). Estrogen is a female hormone involved in spermatogenesis. *Advances in Medical Sciences, 57*(1), 31–36.
8. Chang, L., Xu, J., & Zhao, J. (2006). Taurine antagonized oxidative stress injury induced by homocysteine in rat vascular smooth muscle cells. *Acta Pharmacologica Sinica, 25*(3), 341–346.

9. Chen, Y., Nagpal, M. L., & Lin, T. (2003). Expression and regulation of glucose transporter 8 in rat Leydig cells. *Journal of Endocrinology, 179*, 63–72.

10. Clarke, I. J. (2011). Control of GnRH secretion: One step back. *Frontiers in Neuroendocrinology, 32*(3), 367–375. https://doi.org/10.1016/j.yfrne.2011.01.001.

11. Cooper, T. G. (2011). The epididymis, cytoplasmic droplets, and male fertility. *Asian Journal of Andrology, 13*, 130–138.

12. Dharia, S., Slane, A., Jian, M., Conner, M., Conley, A. J., & Parker, C. R., Jr. (2004). Colocalization of P450c17 and cytochrome b5 in androgen-synthesizing tissues of the human. *Biology of Reproduction, 71*(1), 83–88.

13. Ferramosca, A., & Zara, V. (2014). Bioenergetics of mammalian sperm capacitation. *BioMed Research International, 2014*, Article ID 902953, 1–8.

14. Gaboriau, D., Howes, E. A., Clark, J., & Jones, R. (2007). Binding of sperm proacrosin/βacrosin to zona pellucida glycoproteins is sulfate and stereo dependent: Synthesis of a novel fertilization inhibitor. *Developmental Biology, 306*, 646–657.

15. Gadella, B. M., Rathi, R., Brouwers, J. F. H. M., Stout, T. A. E., & Colenbrander, B. (2001). Capacitation and the acrosome reaction in equine sperm. *Animal Reproduction Science, 68*, 249–265.

16. Ganong, W. F. (2010). Review of medical physiology (23rd ed.). The McGraw-Hill Companies.

17. García-González, F. (2004). Infertile mating and sperm competition: The effect of "nonsperm representation" on intraspecific variation in sperm precedence patterns. *The American Naturalist, 164*(4), 457–472.

18. Gomez, O., Ballester, B., Romero, A., Arnal, E., Almansa, I., Miranda, M., & Terrado, J. (2009). Expression and regulation of insulin and the glucose transporter GLUT8 in the testes of diabetic rats. *Hormone and Metabolic Research, 41*, 343–349.

19. Gonzales, G. F. (2001). Function of seminal vesicles and their role on male fertility. *Asian Journal of Andrology, 3*(4), 251–258.

20. Gribbins, K. M., Happ, C. S., & Sever, D. M. (2005). Ultrastructure of the reproductive system of the Black Swamp Snake (*Seminatrix pygaea*). V. The temporal germ cell development strategy of the testis. *Acta Zoologica, 86*(4), 223–230.

21. Guyton, C. A., & Hall, J. E. (2006). *Textbook of Medical Physiology* (11th ed.). Philadelphia, PA: Saunders.

22. Hess, R. A., & Renato de Franca, L. (2008). Spermatogenesis and cycle of the seminiferous epithelium. *Advances in Experimental Medicine and Biology, 636*, 1–15.

23. Iammarrone, E., Balet, R., Lower, A. M., Gillott, C., & Grudzinskas, J. G. (2003). Male infertility. *Best Practice & Research Clinical Obstetrics & Gynaecology, 17*(2), 211–229.

24. Ibberson, M., Riederer, B. M., Uldry, M., Guhl, B., Roth, J., & Thorens, B. (2002). Immunolocalization of GLUTX1 in the testis and to specific brain areas and vasopressin-containing neurons. *Endocrinology, 143*, 276–284.

25. Ibberson, M., Uldry, M., & Thorens, B. (2000). GLUTX1: A novel mammalian glucose transporter expressed in the central nervous system and insulin-sensitive tissues. *Journal of Biological Chemistry, 275*, 4607–4612.

26. Kierszenbaum, A. (2002). Sperm axoneme: A tale of tubulin post-translation diversity. *Molecular Reproduction and Development, 62*(1), 1–3.

27. Kierszenbaum, A. L., & Tres, L. (2015). *Histology and cell biology: An introduction to pathology* (4th ed.). Elsevier Health Sciences.

28. Kim, H. H., Goldstein, M., & Marc, G. (2010). Chapter 53: Anatomy of the epididymis, vas deferens, and seminal vesicle. In S. D. Graham, T. E. Keane, & J. F. Glenn (Eds.), *Glenn's Urological Surgery* (7th ed., p. 356). Lippincott Williams & Wilkins.

29. Kishore, K. P., & Raju, A. B. (2011). A review on male fertility. *Hygeia Journal of Drugs and Medicines, 3*(1), 20–28.

30. Koçak-Toker, N., Aktan, G., & Aykaç-Toker, G. (2002). The role of Na, KATPase in human sperm motility. *International Journal of Andrology, 25*, 180–185.

31. Kunle-Alabi, O. T., Akindele, O. O., Mega, O., Oyovwi, D., Duro-Ladiipo, A. M., & Raji, Y. (2014). *Cocos nucifera L. water improves reproductive indices in Wistar rats. African Journal of Medical and Medical Sciences, 43*, 305–313.

32. McEntee, M. (2012). *Reproductive pathology of domestic mammals.* Elsevier Science.

33. Mescher, A. L. (2010). Chapter 21: The male reproductive system. In L. Junqueira & J. Carneiro (Eds.), *Junqueira's Basic Histology Text and Atlas* (12th ed., pp. 333). McGraw-Hill.

34. Mindnich, R., Moller, G., & Adamski, J. (2004). The role of 17 beta-hydroxysteroid dehydrogenases. *Molecular and Cellular Endocrinology, 218*(1–2), 7–20.

35. Moore, K. L., & Persaud, T. V. N. (2008). *Before we are born: Essentials of embryology and birth defects* (7th ed.). Saunders Elsevier.

36. Nakamoto, T., Shiratsuchi, A., Oda, H., Inoue, K., Matsumura, T., Ichikawa, M., & Hirai, H. (2004). Impaired spermatogenesis and male fertility defects in CIZ/Nmp4-disrupted mice. *Genes to Cells, 9*(6), 575–589.

37. Ohmura, M., Ogawa, T., Ono, M., Dezawa, M., Hosaka, M., Kubota, Y., & Sawada, H. (2003). The increment of murine spermatogonial cell number by gonadotropin-releasing hormone analog is independent of stem cell factor c-kit signal. *Biology of Reproduction, 68*(6), 2304–2313.

38. Oyovwi, M. O., Tesi, P. E., Rotu, R. A., Nwangwa, N. K., Emojevwe, V., Benneth Ben-Azu, & Ozegbe, Q. E. B. (2021). Ameliorative effects of lutein against cyclosporine-induced testicular oxidative stress, apoptotic and inflammatory flux in male Wistar rats. *Clinical and Experimental Obstetrics & Gynecology, 48*(3), 733–777. https://doi.org/10.31083/j.ceog.2021.03.0511.

39. Petersen, C., & Söder, O. (2006). The Sertoli cell - a hormonal target and 'super' nurse for germ cells that determines testicular size. *Hormone Research, 66*(4), 153–161.

40. Pfeifer, H. M., Conrad, D., Roethlein, A., Kyriakopoulos, M., & Brielmeier, G. W. (2001). Identification of a specific sperm nuclei selenoenzyme necessary for protamine thiol cross-linking during sperm maturation. *The FASEB Journal, 15*, 1236–1238.

41. Rhoades, R. A., & Bell, D. R. (Eds.). (2012). *Medical Physiology: Principles for Clinical Medicine* (4th ed.). Lippincott Williams & Wilkins.

42. Rhoades, R. A., & Tanner, G. A. (2004). *Medical Physiology: Part X, Reproductive Physiology: The Male Reproductive System* (2nd ed.). Lippincott Williams & Wilkins.

43. Ridge, I. L., Dubuque, I. A., & Madison, W. I. (2004). *Human Physiology* (8th ed.). McGraw-Hill Companies, Americas.

44. Rivlin, J., Mendel, J., Rubinstein, S., Ektovitz, N., & Breitbart, H. (2004). Role of hydrogen peroxide in sperm capacitation and acrosome reaction. *Biology of Reproduction, 70*(2), 518–522.

45. Saladin, K. S. (2008). Chapter 26: Reproductive system. In *Human Anatomy* (2nd ed., pp. 736–769). McGraw-Hill Companies.

46. Schurmann, A., Axer, H., Scheepers, A., Doege, H., & Joost, H. G. (2002). The glucose transport facilitator GLUT8 is predominantly associated with the acrosomal region of mature spermatozoa. *Cell and Tissue Research, 307*(2), 237–242.

47. Sofikitis, N., Giotitsas, N. T., Sounapi, P., Baltogiannis, D., Giannakis, D., & Pardalidis, N. (2008). Hormonal regulation of spermatogenesis and spermiogenesis. *Journal of Steroid Biochemistry and Molecular Biology, 109*(3–5), 323–330.

48. Stevens, A., & Lowe, J. (2005). Chapter 16: Male reproductive system. In *Human Histology* (3rd ed., pp. 327–343).

49. Vigier, M., Weiss, M., Perrard, M. H., Godet, M., & Durand, P. (2004). The effects of FSH and testosterone on the completion of meiosis and the very early steps of spermiogenesis of the rat: An in vitro study. *Journal of Molecular Endocrinology, 33*, 729–742.

50. Walsh, L. P., & Stocco, D. M. (2000). Effects of lindane on steroidogenesis and steroidogenic acute regulatory protein expression. *Biology of Reproduction, 63*(4), 1024–1033.

51. Walsh, L. P., McCormick, C., Martin, C., & Stocco, D. M. (2000). Roundup inhibits steroidogenesis by disrupting steroidogenic acute regulatory (Star) protein expression. *Environmental Health Perspectives, 108*(8), 769–776.

52. Weinbauer, G. F., Luetjens, C. M., Simoni, M., & Nieschlag, E. (2010). Physiology of testicular function. In E. Nieschlag, H. M. Behre, & S. Nieschlag (Eds.), *Andrology-Male Reproductive Health and Dysfunction* (pp. 11–59). Springer-Verlag.

Chapter 3

FEMALE REPRODUCTIVE ANATOMY

Contents

Unit Introduction

The intricate and multifaceted female reproductive anatomy, which consists of multiple structures that cooperate to support reproduction and childrearing, is a marvel of design. The uterus, uterine tubes, cervix, vagina, and ovaries are central to this anatomy, and each is essential to the reproductive process. The ovaries are two almond-sized organs that are situated on either side of the pelvis and form the center of the female reproductive system. Ovaries perform two tasks: they secrete hormones, such as progesterone and estrogen, which control the menstrual cycle and preserve reproductive health, and they produce eggs (ova) through the process of oogenesis.

The oviducts, or uterine tubes, are thin tubes that connect the ovaries and uterus. Their main responsibility is to catch the eggs that the ovaries release during ovulation and act as a conduit to deliver them to the uterus. Usually, the uterine tubes are where sperm and egg meet to fertilize. The uterus, also known as the womb, is a muscular, hollow organ that is located between the rectum and bladder in the pelvic cavity. Its main purpose during pregnancy is to give a developing fetus a loving environment. In response to hormonal fluctuations, the endometrium, or inner lining of the uterus, undergoes cyclic changes that either prepare it for the implantation of a fertilized egg or, in the absence of pregnancy, cause it to shed during menstruation. The cervix, a cylindrical structure made of dense connective tissue, connects the uterus to the vagina. The cervix acts as a passageway between the vagina and the uterus, supporting the latter structurally and enabling the flow of menstrual blood during the menstrual cycle. Additionally, it is essential for reproduction because it produces mucus, which alters in consistency during the menstrual cycle to either aid or hinder sperm passage.

Finally, the vagina is a muscular canal that connects the external genitalia to the cervix. It accommodates the penis during sexual activity and acts as the birth canal during childbirth. Mucous membranes that create lubrication and keep the pH of the vaginal walls slightly acidic to ward against infections line the walls of the vagina. The female reproductive anatomy is made up of interconnected structures, which work together to facilitate ovulation, fertilization, implantation, gestation, and childbirth. Comprehending the complexities of this structure is crucial for maintaining reproductive health, promoting fertility, and treating a range of gynecological disorders (Jaffe et al., 2017; Richards et al., 2018; Sikandar & Ali, 2020).

Orientation and Directional Terms:

Terms	Definition	Illustration
Oviducts	The oviduct in vertebrates is the passageway from an ovary. In human females, this is more usually known as the fallopian tube. The eggs travel along the oviduct.	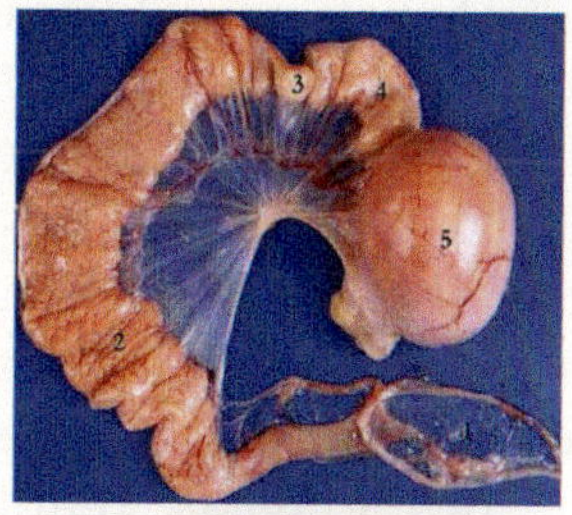
Embryo	An embryo is the initial stage of development for a multicellular organism.	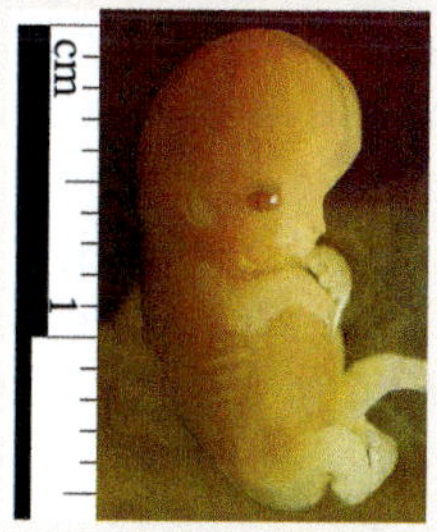
Progestogens	The progestogens are one of three types of sex hormones, the others being estrogens like estradiol and androgens/ anabolic steroids like testosterone.	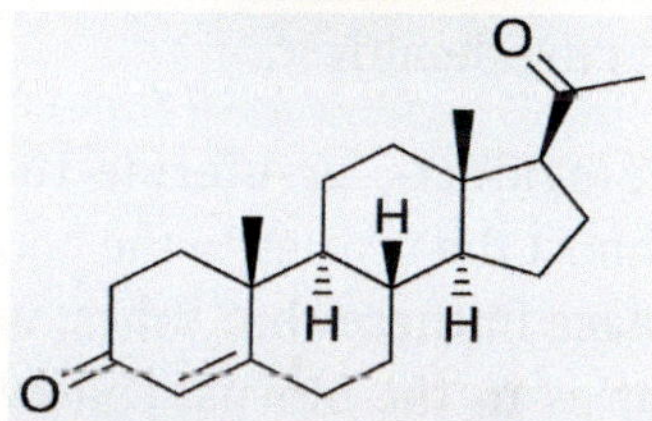
Estrogens	Estrogens act on many tissues and functions in the body, from our skin, blood clotting, electrolyte balance, cholesterol mobilization, bone and brain, to the uterus, vagina, breast, ovaries, and likely other sites not yet identified.	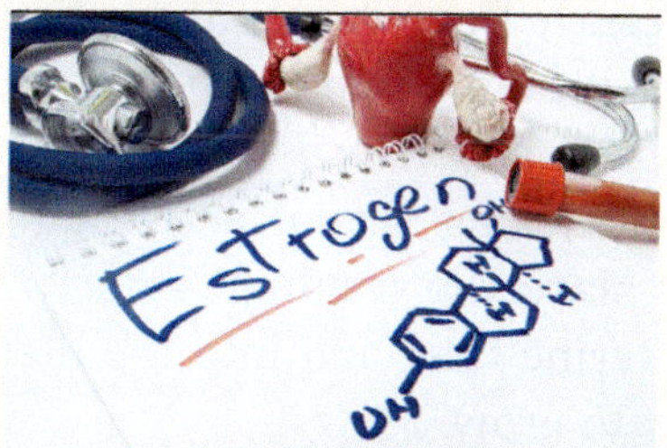
External Genitalia	The external genitalia are the accessory structures of the female reproductive system that are external to the vagina.	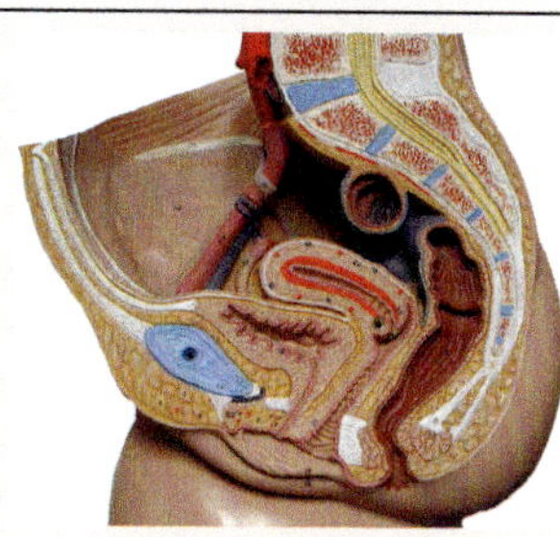

3.1. Concept of the Female Reproductive System

The intricate network of organs and tissues that make up the female reproductive system enables reproduction and supports the growth of the fetus during pregnancy. It consists of several essential parts, each with distinct roles and interactions that combine to form new life. The ovaries are two tiny, almond-shaped organs that are situated on either side of the pelvis and form the center of the female reproductive system. The main reproductive organs in females are the ovaries, which produce eggs (ova) through a process known as oogenesis. Ovulation is the process by which one egg is normally released from one of the ovaries once a month. The ovaries not only create eggs but also secrete hormones like progesterone and estrogen that control the menstrual cycle and preserve reproductive health.

The oviducts, or uterine tubes, are tubes that connect the ovaries to the body. Fertilization takes place in these thin tubes, which run from the ovaries to the uterus. Following ovulation, the released egg descends to the uterine tube, where it might come into contact with sperm that have penetrated the female reproductive system during sexual activity. If fertilization takes place, the resultant embryo moves down the uterine tube and into the uterus, where it starts to grow.

Nestled between the bladder and the rectum in the pelvic cavity, the uterus, also known as the womb, is a muscular and hollow organ. During pregnancy, it acts as the location of implantation and fetal development. Throughout the menstrual cycle, the endometrium, or inner lining of the uterus, experiences cyclical changes in response to hormonal fluctuations. The endometrium is shed during menstruation, signaling the start of a new cycle, if fertilization is unsuccessful. If fertilization takes place, the embryo implants into the thicker endometrial lining, where it grows into a fetus and gets nourishment and support. The lower part of the uterus that joins the vagina is called the cervix. It acts as an aperture through which menstrual blood leaves the uterus during menstruation and as a pathway for sperm to enter the uterus during sexual activity. Additionally, the cervix secretes a mucus that varies in consistency during the menstrual cycle, forming a barrier that, depending on the stage of the cycle, can either facilitate or inhibit sperm passage into the uterus.

Finally, the vagina is a muscular canal that connects the external genitalia to the cervix. It facilitates a variety of processes, such as childbirth, sex, and the removal of menstrual fluid from the body. Mucous membranes lining the vaginal walls create lubrication to lessen friction during sexual activity and keep the pH of the vagina slightly acidic to prevent infections. The female reproductive system, which is exquisitely crafted to facilitate the processes of reproduction and pregnancy, is a stunning illustration of biological complexity and adaptation. Reproductive health, fertility, and the treatment of gynecological disorders all depend on an understanding of the anatomy and function of each component. Prenatal care, contraception, and routine gynecological exams are crucial for preserving a woman's reproductive health over her lifetime.

The ovaries, also known as the female gonads or sexual glands, are the source of both the female sex hormones, progestogens, and estrogens, as well as ova (eggs). The uterus, which is located inside the lesser or true pelvis, receives eggs from the uterine tubes, or uterine, tubes. The cervical canal serves as the conduit between the uterus and the vagina. The vestibule, which contains the external genitalia collectively referred to as the vulva, is where the vagina opens.

3.1.1. External Genitalia

The structures surrounding the vaginal opening and the membrane that spans it, external to the hymen, are considered the female external genitalia. These include the labia majora, labia minora, the clitoris, the vestibule of the vagina, the vestibule bulb, the mons pubis (also known as the mons veneris), and the greater vestibular glands. The rounded protrusion in front of the pubic symphysis that is formed by fat tissue under the skin is called the mons pubis. When a child reaches puberty, they may have a few fine hairs; later in life, they become coarser and more numerous. Across the lower abdomen, the hairy region's upper limit is horizontal.

The labia majora are two distinct skin folds that run from the back of the perineum to the bottom of the mons pubis. They create the lateral limits of the vulval or pudendal cleft, which is where the urethra and vaginal openings are located. Every labium has an outer surface that is hairy and pigmented, and an inner surface that is smooth but has sebaceous glands. Sweat glands, fat, and loose connective tissue are all present in the labia majora. They have tissue like the dartos muscle and are corresponding to the male scrotum. The labium's tissue is where the round ligament ends. The two tiny, adipose-free skin folds known as the labia minora stretch backward on either side of the vaginal entrance. They are about 4 cm (1 and a half inches) long and rest inside the labia majora. The clitoris is the structure in the female that corresponds to the penis (apart from the urethra) in the male. On the front, an upper portion of each labium minus passes over the clitoris to form a fold called the prepuce of the clitoris, and a lower portion passes beneath the clitoris to form its frenulum. The fold that unfurls at childbirth connects the two labia minora at the back across the midline. The labia minora have sweat and sebaceous glands but no hair.

Two corpora cavernosa divided by a partition make up the clitoris, a tiny erectile structure. The glans clitoridis, a sensitive tip of spongy erectile tissue, is partially hidden beneath the forward ends of the labia minora. The urethra's external opening is situated right in front of the vaginal opening and about 2.5 cm (1 inch) behind the clitoris.

The cleft into which the urethra and vagina open is known as the vestibule of the vagina. The hymen vagina, a thin, morphologically variable fold of mucous membrane, is located at the vaginal opening. The little rounded elevations that remain after hymen rupture are referred to as carunculae hymenales. Two elongated masses of erectile tissue, one on each side of the vaginal opening, corresponding to the bulbs of the vestibule and the penis. The smaller mucous glands known as the greater vestibular glands are located at their posterior ends. A duct connects them to the groove that exists between each labium minus and the hymen. They line up with the male bulbourethral glands. The female blood and nerve supplies of these organs are comparable to those supporting corresponding male structures (Jaffe et al., 2017; Richards et al., 2018; Sikandar & Ali, 2020).

3.1.2. Internal Structures

3.1.2.1. The Vagina

The vagina, which derives from the word meaning "sheath," is the canal that runs from the vestibule between the labia minora to the cervix, or outer end, of the uterus inside the lesser pelvis. The hymen protects the orifice of the vagina. The vagina is in front of the rectum and anal canal and behind the bladder and urethra. Its walls are collapsed; the posterior wall is approximately 1.5 cm (0.6 inches) longer than the anterior wall, which measures about 7.5 cm (3 inches) in length. The vagina is pointed backward and upward in an oblique manner. The uterine and vaginal axes intersect at an angle greater than 90°. This angle changes significantly depending on the state of the rectum, the bladder, and pregnancy. The uterine cervix extends into the vagina for a brief distance, where it is typically pressed up against the posterior wall. As a result, the vagina has indentations in the front, back, and sides of the cervix. These are called the lateral fornices (at the sides), the anterior fornix (at the front of the cervix), and the posterior fornix (the largest, behind the cervix).

The recto-uterine pouch is formed when the peritoneum, or membrane, covering the upper portion of the posterior wall of the vagina, is folded back onto the rectum. There is a mass of tissue called the perineal body that separates the lower portion of the posterior vaginal wall from the anal canal.

The mucous membrane of the vagina is closely linked to an outer coat of smooth muscle. In the middle of the anterior and posterior walls of the mucous membrane, there is a longitudinal ridge. The ridges are referred to as the vaginal columns, and numerous rugae, or folds, branch out from them on either side. On the posterior wall, the furrows between the rugae are more noticeable and become particularly noticeable before childbirth. The membrane doesn't change much during the menstrual cycle—aside from the amount of glycogen, a complex carbohydrate that resembles starch—but in many mammals, there can be significant exfoliation or shedding of the surface cells. The uterine glands in the cervical canal have secreted the mucus that is present in the vaginal lining, which lacks glands. An outer longitudinal layer and a less developed inner circular layer make up the smooth muscle coat. The bulbospongiosus muscle, a striped muscle attached to the perineal body, encircles the lower part of the vagina.

The vagina receives its blood supply from multiple nearby vessels. These vessels include the internal iliac artery, which branches into the vaginal artery, as well as the uterine, middle rectal, and internal pudendal arteries. The uterovaginal plexus, inferior hypogastric plexus, and pudendal nerve supply the lower part of the vagina (Jaffe et al., 2017; Richards et al., 2018; Sikandar & Ali, 2020).

3.1.3. The Uterus

3.1.3.1. Uterine Structure

The uterus, or womb, is shaped like an inverted pear. It is a hollow, muscular organ with thick walls, and it has a glandular lining called the endometrium. In an adult, the uterus is 7.5 cm (3 inches) long, 5 cm (2 inches) in width, and 2.5 cm (1 inch) thick, but it enlarges to four to five times this size in pregnancy. The narrower, lower end is called the cervix, which projects into the vagina. The cervix is made of fibrous connective tissue and is of firmer consistency than the body of the uterus. The two uterine tubes enter the uterus at opposite sides, near its top. The part of the uterus above the entrances of the tubes is called the fundus; the part below is termed the body. The body narrows toward the cervix, and a slight external constriction marks the juncture between the body and the cervix.

The uterus is typically anteverted, or turned forward, to form roughly a right angle with the vagina rather than lying in line with it. The degree of distension in the rectum and bladder influences the position of the uterus. Pregnancy-related uterine enlargement pushes the organ up into the abdominal cavity and closer alignment with the vagina. The term "anteflexed" refers to the soft forward curve of the non-pregnant uterus. The diaphragm or muscular floor of the pelvis, certain fibrous ligaments, the other pelvic organs, and the peritoneal folds all support and hold the uterus in place. Two double-layered broad ligaments that each have a round ligament between their layers that corresponds to the male gubernaculum testis and a uterine tube along their upper free border is among the supporting ligaments. The uterus's position is also maintained by two ligaments on either side of the cervix, known as the cardinal (Mackenrodt) ligaments.

Relative to the size of the organ, the uterine cavity is remarkably small. The cavity is triangular and flattened, and the front and back walls touch, except for pregnancy. The triangle is inverted, with the apex located at the uterine isthmus—the opening leading into the cervix—and the base located at the top, between the apertures of the two uterine tubes. The cervix's canal is somewhat larger in the middle and flattened from front to back. It has two longitudinal ridges that cross it, and it has oblique folds that extend from each ridge in a pattern resembling a tree's branches. The external so of the uterus is the opening of the cervical canal, which is 2.5 cm (1 inch) long and opens into the vagina. The external so is tiny, frequently depressed, and nearly round. Following childbirth, the external so becomes more slit-like as it is surrounded by lips on both the front and back. A mucous membrane that lines the cervical canal is made up of many glands that release an alkaline, transparent mucus. This lining's upper portion experiences periodic changes that are like those seen in the body but less pronounced. In the mucous membrane of the cervical region, there are numerous tiny cysts known as Nabothian cysts. Cervical smears are taken from this area to look for early changes that could indicate cancer.

Three layers of tissue make up the uterus. The organ is partially covered on the outside by a serous coat of peritoneum, a membrane that secretes fluid like blood but without the clotting factor fibrinogen and cells. Only the cervix's body is covered in front; the portion above the vagina and extended onto the posterior vaginal wall is covered in back, where it is folded back to the rectum. The two broad ligaments of the uterus are formed by the peritoneal layers, which extend from the uterine margin to each side wall of the pelvis.

Most of the organ is made up of the muscular middle layer of tissue, or myometrium. It is made up of tightly packed, smooth, unstriped muscle fibers that are quite firm. There are also nerves, lymph vessels, and blood vessels. The muscle is composed of three layers of fibers that run in distinct directions. The outermost fibers have a longitudinal arrangement. The middle layer, which is the thickest, has strands that are dispersed randomly in all directions. The arrangement of the innermost fibers is circular and longitudinal.

The mucous membrane, also known as the endometrium, is the innermost layer of tissue in the uterus. It borders the uterus cavity to the uterus's isthmus, where it joins the cervical canal's lining. Embedded in the stroma, the cellular framework of the endometrium, are many uterine glands that open into the uterine cavity. There are also a lot of lymphatic spaces and blood vessels. The endometrium appears differently depending on the stage of reproductive development. After reaching puberty, it reaches full development and undergoes significant changes with every menstrual cycle. It experiences additional changes before, during, and following pregnancy, as well as during menopause and old age. Most of these alterations are caused by hormones and are managed by ovulation activity.

3.1.3.1. The Endometrium in the Menstrual Cycle

It is customary to think of the endometrium as being composed of three layers to comprehend the nature of the changes that occur in it during each menstrual cycle. Although they blend invisibly, they serve different functional purposes: the outer, or basal, layer stays in place against the innermost layer of the myometrium, while the inner two layers are shed during menstruation. The stratum compactum, stratum spongiosum, and stratum basale epidermidis are the names given to the three layers, in that order. The lining cells and uterine gland necks are in the stratum compactum, which is closest to the uterine cavity. Its stroma is rather dense. Beneath the lining cells lie superficial blood vessels. The broad middle layer is called the stratum spongiosum. The stromal cells are larger and more loosely arranged than in the stratum compactum; they contain the major parts of the uterine glands and the blood vessels that go with them. The bases of the uterine glands and blood vessels are in the stratum basale epidermidis, which is pressed up against the uterine muscle. Throughout the menstrual cycle, its stroma doesn't really change.

The menstrual cycle lasts roughly 28 days, with a normal range of 21 to 34 days, from the start of one menstrual flow to the start of the subsequent one. It reflects the ovarian cycle of changes, which is governed by the anterior lobe of the pituitary gland. The four phases of the menstrual cycle are post-menstrual, proliferative, secretory, and menstrual.

After ovulation, the secretory phase reaches its peak approximately one week later. Midcycle, or roughly 14 days before the start of the subsequent menstrual flow, is when ovulation happens. To accept a fertilized ovum, the endometrium has been primed and stimulated to a state of active secretion. The conditions are in place for the blastocyst, which is derived from a fertilized ovum, to adhere to the endometrium and then embed. The success of this procedure, known as implantation, depends on the endometrium being suitably prepared during both the proliferative and secretory phases. A hormone produced by specific blastocyst cells causes the corpus luteum to prolong and remain active after implantation. Menstruation is suppressed as a result, and the endometrium is maintained and further stimulated by progesterone, leading to increased endometrial thickness. The decidua refers to the endometrium in the early stages of pregnancy.

Menstruation is the end of the secretory phase in a cycle where the ovum has not been fertilized. Before implantation, certain conditions must be met by the endometrium. Menstruation starts once this phase is over. After repair, the endometrium is once again able to be stimulated to the crucial point at which implantation is possible.

3.1.3.2. Blood Supply and Innervation

The ovarian arteries, which connect with the ends of the uterine arteries and send branches to supply the uterus, and the two uterine arteries, which are branches of the internal iliac arteries, provide blood to the uterus. The sympathetic nerve fibers that cause uterine muscle contraction and vessel constriction, as well as the parasympathetic (sacral) nerve fibers that prevent muscle contraction and result in blood vessel dilatation, are the nerves that supply the uterus.

3.1.3.3. Uterine Tubes (Fallopian Tubes)

Ovum is transported from the ovaries to the uterine cavity by the uterine tubes, or uterine, tubes. On one end, each opens into the uterus, and on the other, into the abdominal cavity close to an ovary. The tubes are divided into three distinct sections: the isthmus, which opens into the uterus; the ampulla, which is the expanded and thin-walled intermediate portion; and the infundibulum, which is the funnel-shaped outer end. Fimbriae, or irregular projections, surround the infundibulum. Usually attached to the ovary, one fimbria is a little larger than the others.

The small aperture leading into the abdomen is located at the base of the infundibulum. The ampulla of the tube is where the ovum normally fertilizes. The fertilized egg is normally transferred to the uterus, but on rare occasions, it may stick to the tube and begin growing into an ectopic pregnancy, also known as a tubal pregnancy. The conceptus may extrude through the abdominal opening or may rupture the tube, resulting in hemorrhage, because the tube is unable to support this pregnancy.

The peritoneum surrounds the uterine tube except for the area next to the wide ligament on its border. The smooth muscle fibers of the uterus are continuous with the outer layer of smooth muscle and the inner circular layer. Numerous longitudinal folds in the inner lining are covered in ciliated columnar and secretory cells. Transport of sperm to the ampulla and a fertilized ovum toward the uterus is likely aided by muscular contraction, movement of the hair-like cilia, and passage of the watery secretions (Jaffe et al., 2017; Richards et al., 2018; Sikandar & Ali, 2020).

3.1.4. The Ovaries

3.1.4.1. Ovarian Structure

The two ovaries are the female gonads or primary sex organs; they are like the testes in males. Each is suspended from the back layer of the uterine broad ligament by a mesentery or fold of membrane. The almond-shaped ovary rests vertically against the ovarian fossa, a depression on the side wall of the lesser pelvis, in an unconceiving woman. This relationship changes both before and after conception. Each ovary is somewhat over 2.5 cm (1 inch) in length, 1.25 cm (0.5 inch) across, and slightly less in thickness, but the size varies much with age and with state of activity.

The ovarian artery and vein, lymphatic vessels, and nerve fibers are all located within the mesentery of the ovary, which aids in maintaining its position. The ovary's inner or medial surface is where the uterine tube curves downward after arching over it. The ovary's surface is smooth and covered in cubical cells, except for its hilum, which is where the nerve and blood vessels enter the ovary and where the mesentery is attached. The ovary's substance is separated into two parts below the surface: the medulla, which is the inner part, and the cortex, which is the outer part. The tunica albuginea, a thin zone of connective tissue, is formed by the outermost portion of the cortex, right beneath the outer covering. The follicles and corpora lutea, as well as stromal or framework cells encased in a fine network of fibers, make up the remaining portion of the cortex.

The ovarian follicles, also known as mature vesicular follicles (Graafian follicles), are rounded enclosures in the cortex that surround the developing ova near the ovary's surface. Primary or immature ovarian follicles are present in large numbers at birth and during childhood. Each is covered in a single layer of flattened cells and contains a primitive ovum or oocyte. A young female's two ovaries can contain up to 7,00,000 primary follicles. Before or after puberty, most of these degenerate.

3.1.4.2. Ovulation

There is a cyclic development of one or more follicles into a mature follicle every month from the onset of puberty until menopause (apart from during pregnancy). The primary follicle's covering layer thickens and separates into an outer vascularized theca interna and an inner membrana granulosa. The cells, primarily theca interna, generate estrogenic steroid hormones and have an impact on the uterine endometrium as well as other tissues. Follicle-stimulating hormone (FSH), produced by the anterior lobe of the pituitary gland, stimulates and maintains the follicle until it reaches maturity.

The luteinizing hormone (LH) works in tandem with FSH to trigger the maturing, fluid-filled follicle to release estrogens. LH also causes a ripe follicle (1.0–1.5 cm [0.4–0.6 inch] in diameter) to rupture, causing the liberation of the oocyte into the peritoneal cavity and thence into the uterine tube. This liberation of the oocyte is called ovulation; it occurs at about the midpoint of the reproductive cycle, on the 13th or 14th day of a 28-day cycle as measured from the first day of the menstrual flow.

The ruptured follicle collapses after ovulation due to the loss of its follicular fluid, and it quickly changes into the corpus luteum, also referred to as the "yellow body," a soft, well-vascularized glandular structure. The corpus luteum grows quickly, vascularizes in approximately four days, and is completely developed in nine days. Progesterone and a few other estrogens are produced by the gland. The luteinizing hormone both stimulates and sustains its activity. In the endometrium, progesterone stimulates glandular proliferation and secretion after estrogens prime the body.

The primary oocyte divides into a secondary oocyte and a small, primitive ovum known as the first polar body while the ovarian follicle matures. This happens around the time the follicle begins to form its cavity; additionally, the oocyte acquires the zona pellucida, a translucent acellular covering or envelope. The secondary oocyte, which has a diameter of 120–140 micrometers and is encircled by the zona pellucida and a few cell layers known as the corona radiata, is released during ovulation. At the moment of fertilization, the oocyte reaches its ultimate stage of development when the second polar body, a primitive ovum, forms.

The corpus luteum has a limited shelf life of roughly 14 days if fertilization is not achieved. Menstruation starts at the end of this phase, coinciding with the gland's degeneration. The corpus luteum shrinks, fibrous tissue develops, and it becomes a corpus albicans, a scar-like structure that lasts for several months. If fertilization and blastocyst implantation takes place, the blastocyst cells produce hormones, specifically human chorionic gonadotropin, to extend the corpus luteum's life. For the first two months of pregnancy at least, it remains active until the placental tissue assumes responsibility for producing hormones. By the time of parturition, the corpus luteum of pregnancy had also retrogressed and turned into a fibrous scar.

3.1.4.3. Blood Supply and Innervation

Similar to the testicular arteries, the ovarian arteries emerge from the front of the aorta and descend into the pelvic cavity at the lesser pelvic brim. Each artery enters the ovary through the suspensory ligament, travels through the broad ligament beneath the uterine tube, and exits the mesovarium to split into branches that are distributed throughout the ovary. One branch continues to anastomose with the uterine artery by continuing in the broad ligament. Each ovary gives rise to a network of ovarian veins, which eventually unite into a single vein with terminations resembling those of testicular veins. The ovarian nerve network on the ovarian artery is the source of the nerves.

3.1.5. Cervix

The cervix is a vital component of the female reproductive system, located at the base of the uterus and linking it to the vagina. This cylindrical organ has multiple functions in reproduction, menstrual cycles, and safeguarding the female reproductive system against harmful agents. Anatomically, the cervix can be divided into two sections: the endocervix, which extends into the uterus, and the ectocervix, which protrudes into the vagina. The boundary between these sections is known as the transformation zone, which is at high risk for developing conditions such as cervical cancer. Serving as a barrier between the uterus and the vagina is one of the cervix's main roles. It creates a physical barrier that lowers the chance of infections by keeping pathogens and other foreign objects out of the uterus. This includes bacteria. Furthermore, the cervix secretes a substance called cervical mucus or cervical fluid, which is essential for reproductive health and fertility. Hormonal fluctuations cause changes in the composition and consistency of cervical mucus during the menstrual cycle. During the menstrual cycle fertile window, estrogen causes cervical mucus to become thin, clear, and stretchy, resembling raw egg whites. This kind of mucus increases the likelihood of conception and promotes fertility by making it easier for sperm to pass through the cervix and into the uterus (Figure 3.1).

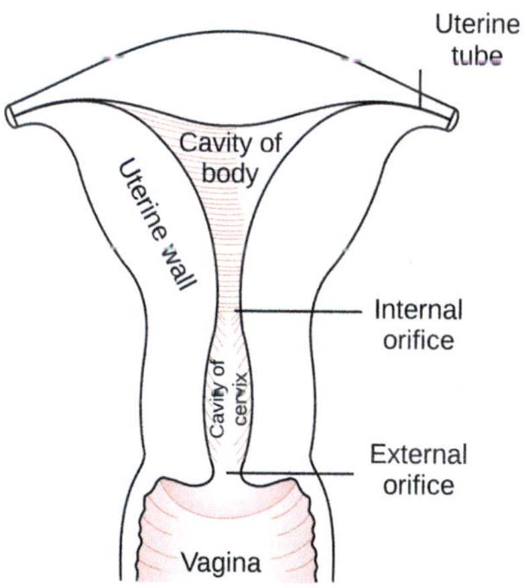

Figure 3.1. *The cervix is a donut-shaped organ that connects your uterus and vagina.*

Source: By Henry Vandyke Carter – Henry Gray (1918) Anatomy of the Human Body (See "Book" section below) Bartleby.com: Gray's Anatomy, Plate 1167. This is a retouched picture, which means that it has been digitally altered from its original version. Modifications: vectorization (CorelDraw). The original can be viewed here: Gray1167.png. Modifications made by Mysid., Public Domain, https://commons.wikimedia.org/w/index.php?curid=1420450.

Conversely, cervical mucus thickens and becomes less helpful for sperm transport during the infertile stages of the menstrual cycle, such as the pre-ovulation and post-ovulation periods. This shift in the consistency of mucus forms a barrier that prevents sperm from passing through, decreasing the chance of conception outside of the fertile window. Reproductive health and fertility depend on the cervix's capacity to produce and modify cervical mucus in response to hormonal cues.

The role of this part in childbirth is another important one. The cervix changes in several ways during pregnancy to get ready for labor and delivery. The cervix thins out (effaces) and dilates as the due date draws near, facilitating the fetus's passage through the birth canal during labor. Hormonal changes and uterine contractions aid in this process, which is called cervical ripening, and it culminates in the complete dilation of the cervix to allow for the birth of the child. The cervix is essential for gynecological health screenings, especially for the detection and prevention of cervical cancer, in addition to its reproductive roles. Frequent cervical cancer screening makes it possible to identify abnormal cervical cells or HPV infection early on, both of which are risk factors for cervical cancer. This is usually accomplished through Pap smears (Papanicolaou test) or HPV (human papillomavirus) testing. Cervical cancer prognosis and outcomes are greatly improved by early detection and intervention, underscoring the significance of cervical health education and screening programs.

An essential part of the female reproductive system, the cervix acts as a physical barrier, controls the production of cervical mucus, promotes fertility, aids in childbirth, and aids in gynecological health screenings. Maintaining fertility and preventing cervical diseases requires an understanding of the anatomy and functions of the cervix. Women's healthcare must include routine gynecological exams and cervical cancer screenings, which enable people to take proactive measures to protect their reproductive health.

3.1.6. Purpose of Your Cervix

Your cervix is a passage that allows fluids to flow inside and out of your uterus. It's also a powerful gatekeeper that can open and close in ways that make pregnancy and childbirth possible.

Your cervix plays important roles in the following:

1. **Menstruation:** The period of blood you shed each month as part of your menstrual cycle has to pass from your uterus and through your cervix before exiting your vagina.
2. **Pregnancy:** During penis-in-vagina sex, or intercourse, your partner may ejaculate (release) sperm into your vagina. The sperm must travel through your cervix to reach your uterus and uterine tubes to fertilize an egg.
3. **Fertility:** Your cervical mucus plays a role in how easily you can become pregnant. Around ovulation (when your body releases an egg), your cervix secretes mucus that's thinner and less acidic than usual, making it easy for sperm to pass through to your uterus. As a result, sperm can reach your egg and fertilize it more easily.
4. **Vaginal Delivery:** Your cervix controls when a baby exits your uterus during childbirth. During pregnancy, your cervix secretes a mucus plug that seals entry to your uterus. Once it's time for the baby to be born, the mucus plug dissolves, and your cervix becomes softer and thinner. Your cervix widens (dilates) so that the baby can exit your uterus. Your provider can estimate how long it will take for your baby to be born based on how much your cervix has dilated.
5. **Protecting Your Uterus:** Your cervix prevents objects inserted into your vagina, such as tampons or diaphragms, from slipping inside your uterus (Jaffe et al., 2017; Richards et al., 2018; Sikandar & Ali, 2020).

3.1.7. Structure of the Cervix

A component of the female reproductive system is the cervix. It is the narrower lower portion of the uterus that is continuous above the broader upper part, or body, of the uterus, measuring about 2–3 centimeters (0.8–1.2 in) in length. The vaginal portion of the cervix, also known as the ectocervix, is the lower end of the cervix that protrudes through the vaginal anterior wall, and the supravaginal portion of the cervix is the remaining portion of the cervix that is above the vagina. Its length is made up of a central canal called the cervical canal, which joins the vaginal lumen to the uterine cavity. The orifices are referred to as the uterine internal orifice (or external OS) and external orifice, respectively. The endocervix is the mucosa lining the cervical canal, and the exocervix is the mucosa covering the ectocervix. The cervix has a thick layer of smooth muscle and an inner mucosal layer. The supravaginal portion has a serosal covering made of connective tissue and peritoneum overlying it posteriorly (Figure 3.2).

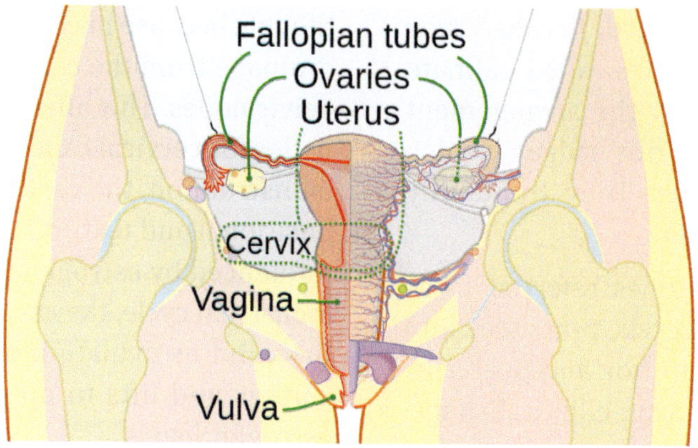

Figure 3.2. *Diagram of the uterus and part of the vagina. The cervix is the lower part of the uterus situated between the external OS (external orifice) and internal OS (internal orifice). The cervical canal connects the interior of the vagina and the cavity of the body of the uterus.*

Sources: https://upload.wikimedia.org/wikipedia/commons/thumb/9/95/Cervix_uteri%2C_breastfeeding_woman_after_2_births.jpg/1200px-Cervix_uteri%2C_breastfeeding_woman_after_2_births.jpg; By CDC, Mysid – Vectorized in Inkscape by User: Mysid from a CDC image (https://www.cdc.gov/cancer/nbccedp/cc_basic.htm), public domain. https://web.archive.org/web/20050206211444/http://www.cdc.gov/cancer/nbccedp/cc_basic.htm, Public Domain, https://commons.wikimedia.org/w/index.php?curid=2885139.

An adult's normal cervix is seen through the vagina with a bivalved vaginal speculum. Encircling the external OS, the functional squamocolumnar junction is discernible as the asymmetrical division between the paler and deeper pink mucosa tones (Figure 3.3).

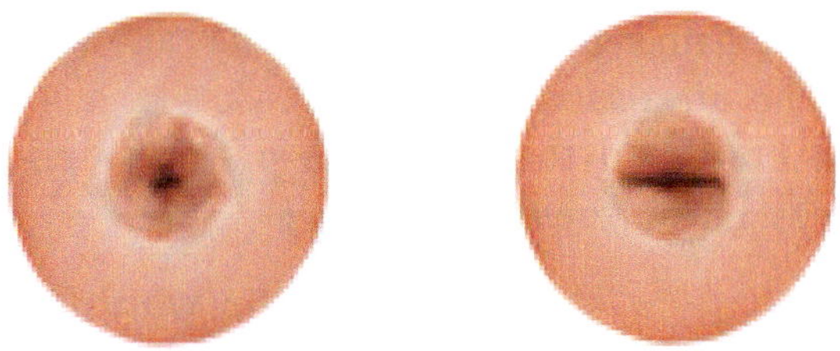

Figure 3.3. *Cervix before (left) and after vaginal birth (right).*

Source: https://upload.wikimedia.org/wikipedia/commons/c/cd/Cervix_birth.png.

The bladder is in front of the upper portion of the cervix. It is divided from it by the parametrium, a cellular connective tissue that also covers the cervix's sides. The recto-uterine pouch is formed by the peritoneum, which covers the supravaginal cervix from behind. It begins on the back of the vaginal wall, turns upward, and ends on the rectum. Compared to the remainder of the uterus, the cervix is more closely attached to the surrounding structures. The cervical canal's width and length can vary significantly between women or throughout a woman's life. In premenopausal adults, the canal's widest diameter is 8 mm, or 0.3 inches. It is narrower at each end and wider in the center. The canal's anterior and posterior walls feature a vertical fold, from which ridges extend laterally and diagonally upward. Because they resemble a palm leaf, these are called palmate folds. The canal is sealed by the arrangement of the anterior and posterior ridges, which interlock with one another. They frequently disappear after giving birth.

The ectocervix, sometimes referred to as the vaginal portion of the cervix, protrudes into the cervix between the anterior and posterior vaginal fornices. It has a convex, elliptical shape. There is a tiny, depressed external opening that connects the cervix and vagina on the rounded portion of the ectocervix. Age, hormonal state, and whether childbirth has occurred can all affect the size, shape, and internal opening of the ectocervix and external so. The external opening is small and circular in women who have not had a vaginal delivery, and it resembles a slit in women who have. The ectocervix measures 3 cm (1.2 in) in length and 2.5 cm (1 in) in width on average.

The uterine artery's descending branch supplies blood to the cervix, where it empties into the uterine vein. The S2–S3 pelvic splanchnic nerves emerge and send pain signals from the cervix to the brain. The uterosacral ligaments, which connect the uterus to the anterior sacrum, are the path taken by these nerves.

Lymphatic drainage from the cervix is facilitated by three channels. The external iliac lymph nodes and, eventually, the paraaortic lymph nodes are reached by the anterior and lateral cervix draining to nodes along the uterine arteries. This process is facilitated by the cardinal ligaments at the base of the broad ligament. The posterior segment of the cervix drains to the obturator and presacral lymph nodes, while the posterior and lateral cervix drains along the uterine arteries to the internal iliac lymph nodes and finally the paraaortic lymph nodes. There are differences, though, because in certain individuals, lymphatic drainage from the cervix goes to distinct sets of pelvic nodes. This affects the process of checking nodes for cervical cancer involvement. Following menstruation, the cervix experiences a range of positional and textural changes that are directly influenced by estrogen. Throughout most of the menstrual cycle, the cervix stays closed, low, and firm. But as ovulation draws nearer, the cervix softens and lifts to open due to the increased estrogen levels.

3.1.7.1. Where Is Your Cervix Located?

One crucial component of your reproductive anatomy is your cervix. Your cervix is situated three to six inches inside your vaginal canal inside your pelvic cavity. It extends downward onto the upper portion of your vagina from its starting point at the base of your uterus. Your ectocervix is the area where your cervix protrudes onto the topmost portion of your vagina. Your uterus, cervix, and vagina are situated in front of your rectum and anus (the organs that allow you to poop) and behind your bladder and urethra (the organs that allow you to pee).

3.1.7.2. What Does Your Cervix Look Like?

The Latin word for "neck" is where the word "cervix" originates. Your cervix, like your neck, is roughly shaped like a tube or cylinder that connects vital body parts. Your cervix connects your uterus to your vagina, whereas your neck connects your head to the rest of your body. The middle of your cervix is wider than the ends, which narrow to open into your uterus at the top and your vagina at the bottom.

Your cervix consists of the following parts:

- **Internal OS:** The opening that leads to your uterus. Your provider may refer to your internal OS during pregnancy.

- **Endocervical Canal:** A tunnel that extends from your Internal OS to your ectocervix.
- **Ectocervix:** The part of your cervix that bulges onto the top of your vagina.
- **External OS:** The opening that leads to your vagina.

The transformation zone (TZ) is the area where the ectocervix and endocervical canal overlap. The region of your cervix where cell changes most frequently occur is the TZ. It is the most typical location in the cervix where aberrant cells proliferate, suggesting diseases like cervical dysplasia or cervical cancer.

3.1.7.3. How Big Is Your Cervix?

You have an inch-long cervix. However, cervical sizes differ. After giving birth, your cervix usually enlarges. Those who are still fertile have larger cervixes than those who have gone through menopause. During childbirth, your cervix becomes noticeably shorter, making it easier for the baby to pass through your vagina and out of your uterus.

3.1.7.4. Can You Touch Your Cervix?

Yes following when your menstrual cycle occurs. Your longest finger should eventually come to a stop that prevents it from sliding in any farther if you insert it into your vaginal canal. Your cervix is this barrier. It could feel spongy and soft, or tight and firm. Whether or not you are ovulating affects the location and texture of your cervix. During ovulation, it is the hardest to reach and the softest. Make sure you wash your hands well with warm water and mild soap before attempting to touch your cervix. If not, you run the risk of infecting your cervix with bacteria.

3.1.7.5. What Is Your Cervix Made of?

Your cervix consists of strong fibromuscular tissue. Two main types of cells line your cervix:

- **Glandular Cells:** These cells line the endocervical canal, the innermost part of your cervix.
- **Squamous Cells:** These cells cover the ectocervix, the outermost part of your cervix, and your vagina.

These different cell types meet at the TZ, where cell changes frequently take place. This area is of particular interest to your provider during screenings for cervical cancer (Jaffe et al., 2017; Richards et al., 2018; Sikandar & Ali, 2020).

3.2. Oogenesis: Process of Egg Production

The outermost layers of the ovaries are where oogenesis takes place. Oogenesis, like the production of sperm, begins with a germ cell. This germ cell, known as an oogonium in oogenesis, develops during an individual's embryonic development. During mitosis, the oogonium generates one to 2 million oocytes at the time of birth.

Meiosis in primary oocytes starts prior to birth (Figure 3.4). But during the first prophase, the meiotic division is stopped in its tracks. All subsequent eggs are in prophase I at birth. This is not the case with the male reproductive system, where sperm are generated continuously during an individual's lifetime. An ovary develops a few follicles every month due to anterior pituitary hormones, which start to take effect in adolescence. As a result, the first meiotic division of a primary oocyte is completed. The cell divides unevenly, giving one cell—referred to as a secondary oocyte—most of its cytoplasm and organelles while giving the other cell only a single set of chromosomes and a small amount of cytoplasm. The second cell is known as a polar body, and it typically degrades. Once more, cell division is stopped, this time during metaphase II. This secondary oocyte is released during ovulation and passes through the oviduct on its way to the uterus. The cell proceeds through meiosis II if the secondary oocyte is fertilized, creating a second polar body and haploid egg that unites with the haploid sperm to form a fertilized egg (zygote) with all 46 chromosomes. Oogenesis occurs in the outermost layers of the ovaries. Oogenesis, like sperm production, starts with a germ cell called an oogonium (plural: oogonia). However, to multiply, this cell divides through mitosis, and the developing embryo eventually produces one or 2 million copies of itself.

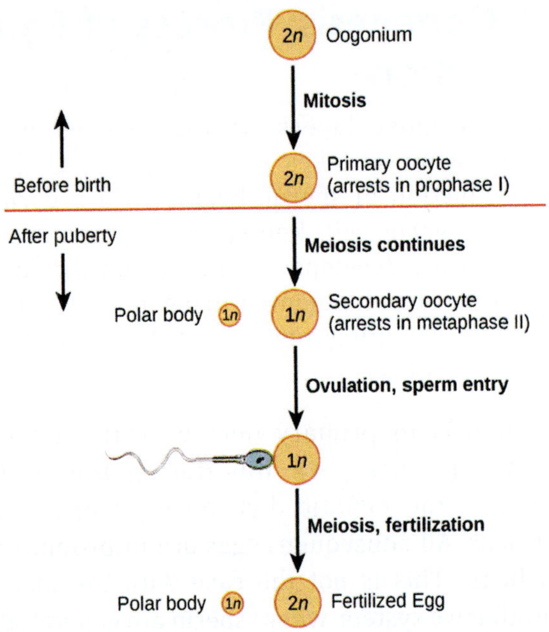

Figure 3.4. *The process of oogenesis occurs in the ovary's outermost layer.*

Source: https://s3-us-west-2.amazonaws.com/courses-images/wp-content/uploads/sites/1223/2017/02/09204044/Figure_43_03_06.jpg.

The process by which female germ cells, also called oogonia, mature into mature eggs, or ova, is called oogenesis. The primary reproductive organs in females, the ovaries, undergo a highly regulated and intricate process. Oogenesis usually results in the formation of one mature egg cell from each oogonium, as opposed to spermatogenesis, which yields four functional sperm cells from each spermatogonium.

The cell that starts meiosis is called the primary oocyte. This cell will initiate the first meiotic division, but it will cease to grow during the first prophase. When they are born, all future eggs are in the prophase stage. Adolescents experience the development of numerous ovarian follicles due to anterior pituitary hormones. The primary oocyte's first meiotic division is thus finished. When a cell divides unevenly, most of the cellular material and organelles go to one cell, known as a secondary oocyte, while only one set of chromosomes and a small amount of cytoplasm go to the other cell. The second cell usually dies and is called a polar body. Another meiotic arrest occurs during the metaphase II stage. During ovulation, this secondary oocyte will be released and travel toward the uterus via the oviduct. If the secondary oocyte fertilizes, the cell moves on to meiosis II, where it completes the process and produces a fertilized egg and second polar body with all 46 human chromosomes—half of which originate from the sperm.

Oogenesis starts in the fetus before birth, which is how it differs from spermatogenesis. The primordial gonad's cortex is colonized by primordial germ cells, which are derived from the embryo's yolk sac. Around 7 million copies of mitosis are replicated by mid-gestation (about 20 weeks). After this peak, there is a loss of cells, leaving about 2 million cells. Primary oocytes are formed during the prenatal stage of meiosis I. Therefore, the supply of ova is limited. In the gonads, primary oocytes are grouped together.

The flattened epithelial cells that envelop them are referred to as the primary follicle. More atresia (cell death) takes place during childhood, leaving about 40,000 eggs at puberty. Only one of the 15–20 primary oocytes that start to mature each month after puberty matures into an oocyte.

The primary oocytes undergo three stages:

- Pre-antral;
- Antral; and
- Preovulatory.

The mature ovum develops from the oogonia. This process is known as oogenesis. In the female ovary, millions of mother cells—also referred to as oogonia—are produced during fetal development. These mother cells undergo meiotic cell division, which results in the production of primary oocytes. At prophase I, the meiotic division ceases. Primary follicles have embedded primary oocytes on their outer layer. Secondary follicles are formed when primary follicles are surrounded by more granulosa cell layers. Secondary follicles go on to form the tertiary follicle. The tertiary follicles of a female reach puberty when the primary oocytes complete meiosis and divide unevenly to form haploid secondary oocytes and the polar body. Following specific structural and functional changes, the tertiary follicle gives rise to mature vesicular follicles. When a secondary oocyte completes a second meiotic division, an ovum is created. Ovum is released by the mature vesicular follicle during the menstrual cycle. The process by which an ovum is discharged from the mature vesicular follicle is called ovulation. Ovulation is controlled by the female reproductive hormone, which is produced by the pituitary gland.

1. **Pre-Antral Stage:** The primary oocyte will now grow significantly, even though it is still in meiosis I. As follicular cells proliferate and grow, a layered cuboidal epithelium is created. These cells are called glycoprotein-releasing granulosa cells. These materials form the zona pellucida, which envelops the primary oocyte. When surrounding connective tissue cells differentiate further, a specialized layer of surrounding cells called theca folliculi is formed. This layer is responsive to LH and can secrete androgens under its influence.
2. **Antral Stage:** As granulosa cells interact, they create fluid-filled cavities that merge to form a central space known as the antrum. This transformation signifies the transition from primary to secondary follicles. During each menstrual cycle, one secondary follicle becomes dominant, aided by hormones such as FSH, LH, and estrogen.
3. **Pre-Ovulatory Stage:** The LH surge causes this stage and meiosis I has now concluded. Within the follicle, two haploid cells with different sizes develop. One of the daughter cells becomes the first polar body and does not develop into an ovum because it has a lot less cytoplasm than the other. Another haploid cell, the secondary oocyte, is also generated. Following that, meiosis II is completed in both daughter cells. The original polar body will replicate to produce two polar bodies, but the secondary oocyte ceases to exist during meiosis II metaphase. This occurs three hours before the ovulation period (Jaffe et al., 2017; Richards et al., 2018; Sikandar & Ali, 2020).

3.2.1. Process of Oogenesis

The process of oogenesis can be divided into several distinct stages, each characterized by specific cellular changes and developmental events:

1. **Formation of Oogonia:** Oogonia are the primitive germ cells that give rise to eggs. They undergo mitotic divisions during fetal development to increase their numbers. These cells then differentiate into primary oocytes before birth.
2. **Meiotic Division I:** Meiosis in oogenesis begins during fetal development but arrests at prophase I of meiosis I until puberty. At puberty, under the influence of hormones such as follicle-stimulating hormone (FSH), some primary oocytes are activated to resume meiosis. During meiosis I, the primary oocyte divides asymmetrically, producing one large cell called a secondary oocyte and one smaller cell called a polar body. The polar body typically degenerates and does not participate in fertilization.
3. **Meiotic Division II:** Following meiosis, I, the secondary oocyte enters meiosis II but arrests at metaphase II. Completion of meiosis II occurs only if fertilization takes place. If fertilization occurs, the secondary oocyte completes meiosis II, producing a mature egg and another polar body. The mature egg contains a haploid set of chromosomes, ready to fuse with the sperm's haploid set during fertilization to form a diploid zygote.
4. **Maturation and Ovulation:** Throughout the menstrual cycle, several primary oocytes start to mature within fluid-filled sacs called follicles in the ovaries. Only one dominant follicle typically matures fully and releases a secondary oocyte during ovulation, which is the process of the egg being expelled from the ovary into the uterine tube. Ovulation is triggered by a surge in luteinizing hormone (LH) released by the pituitary gland.
5. **Fertilization:** If a sperm successfully fertilizes the secondary oocyte in the uterine tube, it completes meiosis II, resulting in the formation of a mature egg and a second polar body. The zygote then undergoes further divisions, ultimately leading to the formation of an embryo, which implants into the uterine wall for further development.

A strictly controlled process called oogenesis makes sure that mature eggs that can support fertilization and embryonic development are produced. The coordination of the different stages of oogenesis is greatly aided by hormonal regulation, particularly that of FSH and LH. Comprehending the oogenesis process is fundamental to understanding fertility, assisted reproductive technologies, and the physiology of female reproduction.

3.2.2. Oogenesis in Non-Human Mammals

In mammals, the first part of oogenesis starts in the germinal epithelium, which gives rise to the development of ovarian follicles, the functional unit of the ovary (Figure 3.5).

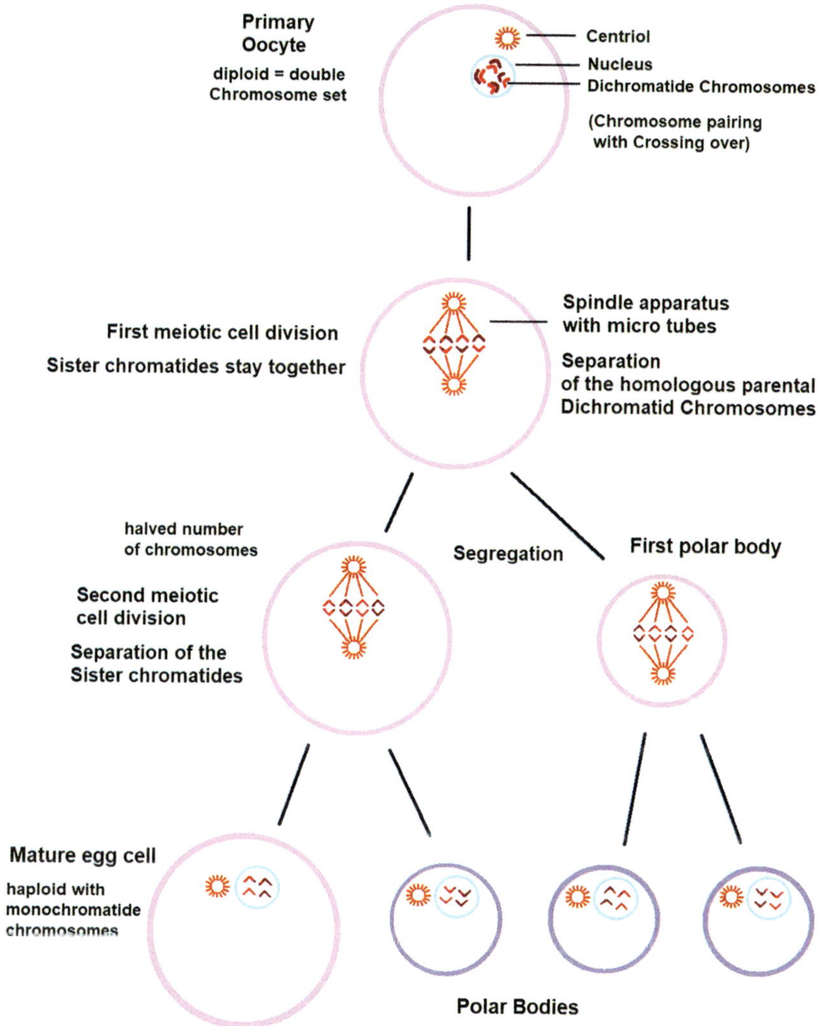

Figure 3.5. *Diagram showing the reduction in number of the chromosomes in the process of maturation of the ovum. (In mammals, the first polar body normally disintegrates before dividing, so only two polar bodies are produced.*

Source: https://upload.wikimedia.org/wikipedia/commons/3/31/Oogenesis_-_Meiosis.png.

Oogenesis consists of several sub-processes: oocytogenesis, ootidogenesis, and finally maturation to form an ovum (oogenesis proper). Folliculogenesis is a separate sub-process that accompanies and supports all three oogenetic sub-processes.

Oogonium – (Oocytogenesis) → Primary Oocyte – (Meiosis I) → First Polar body (Discarded afterward) + Secondary oocyte – (Meiosis II) → Second Polar Body (Discarded afterward) + Ovum.

Oocyte meiosis, important to all animal life cycles yet unlike all other instances of animal cell division, occurs completely without the aid of spindle-coordinating centrosomes.

3.2.2.1. The Creation of Oogonia

Traditionally, oogonia formation has been associated with the common process of gametogenesis, which in female humans starts with the processes of folliculogenesis, oocytogenesis, and ootidogenesis, rather than oogenesis proper. During the development of the embryo, oogonia go through meiosis and become oocytes. DNA replication and meiotic crossingover are the first steps in meiosis. The early prophase is when it ends.

3.2.2.2. Maintenance of Meiotic Arrest

Mammalian oocytes are kept in meiotic prophase arrest for extended periods—years in humans, and months in mice. First, insufficient cell cycle proteins to support meiotic progression cause the arrest. But as the oocyte develops, these proteins are produced, and cyclic AMP becomes necessary for meiotic arrest. Adenylyl cyclase located in the oocyte membrane is responsible for producing cyclic AMP. GPR3, a constitutively active G-protein-coupled receptor, and Gs, a G-protein found in the oocyte membrane, both maintain the activity of adenylyl cyclase.

A complex of cells called a follicle, which encircles the oocyte, is also necessary for the maintenance of meiotic arrest. Meiosis proceeds in the oocyte when it is removed from the follicle. The granulosa cells that make up the follicle are joined to one another by proteins called gap junctions, which permit small molecules to move between the cells. Cyclic GMP, a tiny molecule produced by the granulosa cells, diffuses into the oocyte via gap junctions. Cyclic GMP keeps meiotic arrest in place in the oocyte by preventing the phosphodiesterase PDE3 from breaking down cyclic AMP. The guanylyl cyclase NPR2 generates the cyclic GMP.

3.2.2.3. Reinitiation of Meiosis and Stimulation of Ovulation by Luteinizing Hormone

Follicles develop receptors for luteinizing hormone, a pituitary hormone that triggers the ovulation of a fertile egg and reinitiates meiosis in the oocyte. The follicle's granulosa cells' outer layers contain receptors that luteinizing hormone binds to, reducing the granulosa cells' cyclic GMP levels. Because gap junctions connect the granulosa cells and oocyte, the oocyte's cyclic GMP also decreases, which triggers the restart of meiosis. After that, meiosis moves on to the second metaphase, where it again pauses until fertilization. Additionally, luteinizing hormone increases the expression of genes that cause ovulation (Jaffe et al., 2017; Richards et al., 2018; Sikandar & Ali, 2020).

3.2.3. Human Oogenesis

The process of turning oogonia into primary oocytes, also known as oocytogenesis, is the first step in the development of primary oocytes, or oogenesis. Only one mature oocyte—accompanied by three additional cells known as polar bodies—will emerge from a single oogonium. Complete oocytogenesis occurs either before or soon after birth (Figure 3.6).

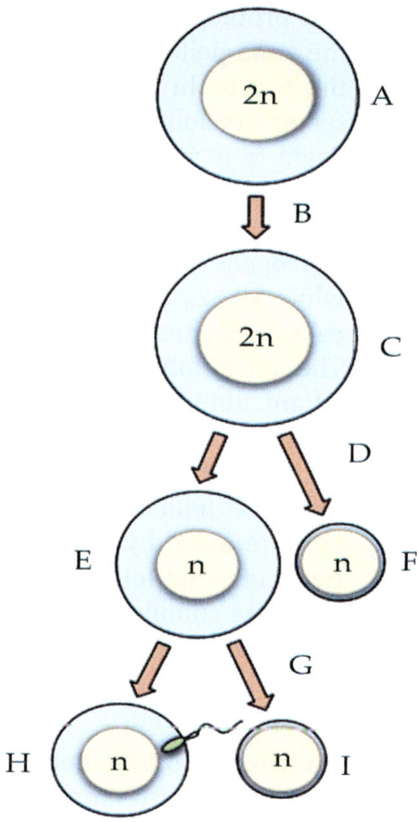

Figure 3.6. *Oogenesis in eukaryotic cells. (A) oogonium where the mitotic division occurs; (B) differentiation and meiosis I begins; (C) primary oocyte; (D) meiosis I is completed, and meiosis II begins; (E) secondary oocyte; (F) first polar body; (G) ovulation must occur and the presence of the sperm penetration (fertilization) induces meiosis II to completion; (H) ovum; and (I) second polar body.*

Source: https://upload.wikimedia.org/wikipedia/commons/thumb/1/1a/Oogenesis.svg/337px-Oogenesis.svg.png.

3.2.3.1. Number of Primary Oocytes

It's a common misconception that, unlike the male spermatogenesis process, which produces gametocytes continuously, oocytogenesis ends when no more primary oocytes are produced. Put another way, at about 20 weeks of gestation, when roughly 7 million primary oocytes have been created, primary oocytes reach their maximum development. By the time they are born, however, this number has already decreased to about 1–2 million per ovary. During adolescence, the quantity of oocytes diminishes even further, reaching roughly 60,000 to 80,000 per ovary. A woman's life will yield only approximately 500 mature oocytes; the remaining ones will experience atresia or degeneration.

The idea that there is a limited supply of oocytes around the time of birth has been refuted by two publications. It has been documented that in the postnatal mouse ovary, germline stem cells (derived from bone marrow and peripheral blood) can regenerate ovarian follicles. DNA clock measurements, on the other hand, do not show that oogenesis continues throughout the lifetimes of human females. Therefore, more research is needed to ascertain the actual dynamics of small follicle formation.

3.2.3.2. Ootidogenesis

When the original oocyte matures into an ootid, the process of ootidogenesis continues. Meiosis is the process that makes this happen. By definition, a primary oocyte is, in fact, a cell whose main purpose is to divide through the process of meiosis. Nevertheless, prophase I marks the end of this process, which started at prenatal age. All oocytes, still primary oocytes, have stopped developing at this point in the fetus's development, known as the dictyate. Only a small percentage of these cells continue to grow after menarche each menstrual cycle.

Ø **Meiosis I:** This of ootidogenesis starts in the embryonic stage and ends in the prophase I diplotene stage when the child reaches puberty. While DNA repair is not visible during the pre-dictyate (leptotene, zygotene, and pachytene) stages of meiosis, it is actively repaired by the mouse oocyte during the dictyate (prolonged diplotene) stage of meiosis. However, synapsis and tetrad formation occur in those primary oocytes that continue to develop during each menstrual cycle, allowing for chromosomal crossover. The primary oocyte has now transformed into the secondary oocyte because of meiosis I.

- Ø **Meiosis II:** The haploid secondary oocyte starts meiosis II right after meiosis I. However, until fertilization, if it happens at all, this process is also stopped at the metaphase II stage. The egg disintegrates and releases (menstruates) if it is not fertilized, and the secondary oocyte does not finish meiosis II and does not develop into an ovum. An ootid and another polar body are now formed after meiosis II is finished.

The polar body is small in size:

1. **Ovarian Cycle:** The ovarian cycle is divided into several phases:
    i. **Follicologenesis:** During ootidogenesis, the ovarian follicle progresses from a primordial stage to a preovulatory stage as the ootid develops. The primary follicle undergoes a series of transformations, taking four months to become preantral, two months to become antral, and finally maturing into a Graaf follicle. The primary follicle's oocyte-lining cells change from a flat to a cubic shape, leading to increased metabolic activity. This results in the release of glycoproteins and proteoglycans that form the zona pellucida surrounding the oocyte. In the preantral secondary follicle, theca cells begin to form internally and externally. Aromatase produced by follicular cells converts androgens to estrogens, while LH stimulates theca cells to produce androgens. The antral follicle contains an antrum with follicular fluid containing estrogen, allowing for the transition to the Graaf follicle. The oocyte is surrounded by the zona pellucida, and follicular cells form the cumulus oophorus. At this stage, the oocyte produces cortical granules containing acid glycoproteins.

    ii. **Dominant Follicle Selection:** The follicle with more FSH receptors will be more favored, simultaneously inducing the death of the other follicles (3–10 antral follicles that enter this phase each month). Low concentrations of estrogen will inhibit further production of FSH by the pituitary gland with negative feedback, so the follicles left behind will accumulate in the follicular antrum instead of androgens.

    iii. **Mature Vesicular Follicle (Graafian Follicle):** Estrogen at other concentrations induces LH release, with the peak of LH called LH surge, which induces stages that will lead to follicle burst. LH receptors also appear on follicular cells, which stimulate the oocyte to become a secondary oocyte, blocked in metaphase, waiting for fertilization. LH also stimulates oophore cumulus cells to release progesterone.

iv. **Ovulation:** Bursting of the follicle, oocyte leakage with pellucid zone, and radiated corona cells. The lining membrane is thinned on the ovary where the follicle bursts and the cells attached to it emerge from the stigma. The ovary is collected from the uterine tube, where fertilization can take place in the ampullate zone.

v. **Formation of the Corpus Luteum:** The corpus luteum develops from the follicle's remaining structures. First, there is a clot, which is later replaced by loose connective tissue; follicular cells, as well as cells of the outer (Tecali lutein cells) and internal (granulosa cells) theca, form solid cords. LH continually stimulates progesterone, which the luteal body raises in concentration. The corpus luteum degenerates (body albicans) if the egg is not fertilized; if implanted, it remains until three months of pregnancy, at which point the placenta takes over by producing progesterone and estrogen. Human chorionic gonadotropin takes the place of LH, which is required to maintain the viability of the corpus luteum.

2. **Uterine Cycle:** This cycle occurs parallel to the ovarian cycle and is induced by estrogen and progesterone. The endometrium, formed by a monostratified cylindrical epithelium, with uterine glands (simple tubular), connective with a functional superficial layer (divided into a spongy layer, a compact layer, and a deeper basal layer, which is always maintained, presents four phases:

   i. **Proliferative Phase:** From the 5th to the 14th day of the ovarian cycle, it is conditioned by estrogens. The functional layer of the uterus is restored, with mitotic division of the basal layer.

   ii. **Secretive Phase:** From the 14th to the 27th day of the ovarian cycle, influenced by the progesterone produced by the corpus luteum. Cells become hypertrophic, and tubular glands begin to produce glycogen.

   iii. **Ischemic Phase:** Beginning of the menstrual phase from 27 to 28 days.

   iv. **Regressive or Desquamative Phase:** From 1 to 5 days, the spiral-shaped arteries undergo ischemia, and the functional layer detaches.

If, instead, there is fertilization, the uterine mucosa is modified to accommodate the fertilized egg and the secretive phase is maintained (Jaffe et al., 2017; Richards et al., 2018; Sikandar & Ali, 2020).

3.2.3.3. Maturation into Ovum

After Meiosis II, both polar bodies separate, leaving only the ootid, which subsequently matures into a mature ovum. The process of polar body formation serves to eliminate the excess haploid sets of chromosomes that arise from meiosis.

3.2.3.4. In Vitro Maturation

The process of allowing ovarian follicles to mature *in vitro* is known as "*in vitro* maturation" (IVM). It might be carried out ahead of an IVF. Under these circumstances, ovarian hyperstimulation is not necessary. Instead, before IVF, oocytes can mature outside of the body. Therefore, the body doesn't need to receive an injection of gonadotropins, or not at all, at a lower dose. *In vitro* maturation of immature eggs has been achieved with a 10% survival rate; however, the technique is not yet clinically available. This method may make it possible to create oocytes that can go straight through *in vitro* fertilization from cryopreserved ovarian tissue.

3.2.4. Ovarian Aging

It is a complex process that involves multiple cell types, precise follicular cell-oocyte reciprocal interactions, a variety of nutrients and combinations of cytokines, and specific growth factors and hormones depending on the developmental stage. By definition, it means to recapitulate mammalian oogenesis and produce fertilizable oocytes *in vitro*. These conditions, when combined with *in vitro* procedures that seem to reproduce effectively, enable the production of a sizable number of fertilizable oocytes that can develop into viable mouse offspring entirely in a dish. This method is especially useful for cancer patients whose ovarian tissue is currently cryopreserved to maintain fertility. Creating culture systems that aid in oocyte development from the primordial follicle stage is a viable method of restoring fertility as an alternative to autologous transplantation. To better support the three main phases of ovarian tissue culture – (i) primordial follicle activation; (ii) isolation and culture of growing preantral follicles; and (iii) removal from the follicle environment and maturation of oocyte cumulus complexes—many studies have been carried out over time. Although mice have successfully undergone complete oocyte development *in vitro* through the production of live offspring, despite decades of effort, higher mammals have not yet achieved the goal of obtaining oocytes of sufficient quality to support embryo development.

During meiosis, the ATM and BRCA1 proteins are used to repair DNA double-strand breaks. It seems that these proteins are essential for preventing ovarian aging. However, in human and other species' oocytes, homologous recombinational repair of DNA double-strand breaks mediated by BRCA1, and ATM becomes less effective with age. Compared to women without BRCA1 mutations, women with these mutations have lower ovarian reserves and menopause earlier. Ovarian aging is linked to ovarian reserve depletion and menopause in women without specific BRCA1 mutations as well, albeit at a slower rate than in those with such mutations. Despite the decline in ovarian reserve, older premenopausal women seem to have enough meiotic recombinational repair capacity to prevent deterioration of their germline, as they typically produce normal offspring. During the decades-long period in humans between early oocytogenesis and the meiotic stage (dictyate stage), when homologous chromosomes are effectively paired, DNA damage can occur in the germline. It has been proposed that processes reliant on chromosome pairing, like homologous recombination, may be largely responsible for undoing such DNA damage (Fabbri et al., 2018).

A Closer Look

The Labia Minora

The inner labia, or labia minora, are small skin folds that are located inside the vulva, next to the urethral and vaginal openings. Their sensitivity is partly due to the abundance of blood vessels and nerve endings in them. The labia minora, in contrast to the labia majora, lack hair follicles but are packed with sebaceous glands that secrete oil to keep the delicate tissue hydrated. The appearance of the labia minora varies greatly between people; variances in symmetry, size, shape, and color are all perfectly normal. Hormonal changes, aging, and childbirth are some of the factors that can cause these variations to alter.

The labia minora are essential for preventing physical irritation and infections at the urethral and vaginal openings. They swell as a result of increased blood flow during sexual arousal, which improves sensation and increases sexual pleasure. They also help to control the urine's flow. Both inner labia's typical presentations—extending outside of or staying tucked inside the outer labia—are possible. Promoting body positivity and sexual health requires an appreciation of the inherent diversity of the labia minora (Jaffe et al., 2017; Richards et al., 2018; Sikandar & Ali, 2020).

Summary

- The female reproductive system is a complex network of organs and structures that work together to facilitate the process of reproduction and support the development of a fetus during pregnancy.
- The vagina (the word means "sheath") is the canal that extends from the cervix (outer end) of the uterus within the lesser pelvis down to the vestibule between the labia minora. The orifice of the vagina is guarded by the hymen. The vagina lies behind the bladder and urethra and in front of the rectum and anal canal.
- To understand the nature of the changes in the endometrium during each menstrual cycle it is usual to consider the endometrium to be composed of three layers. They blend imperceptibly but are functionally distinct: the inner two layers are shed at menstruation, and the outer or basal layer remains in position against the innermost layer of the myometrium.
- The cervix is a crucial structure within the female reproductive system, situated at the lower end of the uterus and connecting it to the vagina. This cylindrical-shaped organ plays multifaceted roles in reproduction, menstruation, and protecting the female reproductive tract from pathogens.
- Oogenesis occurs in the outermost layers of the ovaries. As with sperm production, oogenesis starts with a germ cell. In oogenesis, this germ cell is called an oogonium and forms during the embryological development of the individual. The oogonium undergoes mitosis to produce about one to two million oocytes by the time of birth.
- Oogenesis starts with the process of developing primary oocytes, which occurs via the transformation of oogonia into primary oocytes, a process called oocytogenesis.

References

1. Fabbri, R., Zamboni, C., Vicenti, R., MacCiocca, M., Paradisi, R., & Seracchioli, R. (2018). Update on oogenesis in vitro. *Minerva Ginecologica, 70*(5), 588–608.
2. Jaffe, L. A., & Egbert, J. R. (2017). Regulation of mammalian oocyte meiosis by intercellular communication within the ovarian follicle. *Annual Review of Physiology, 79*(1), 237–260. https://doi.org/10.1146/annurev-physiol-021115-105305.
3. Johnson, J., Bagley, J., Skaznik-Wikiel, M., et al. (2005). Oocyte generation in adult mammalian ovaries by putative germ cells in bone marrow and peripheral blood. *Cell, 122*(2), 303–315. https://doi.org/10.1016/j.cell.2005.06.031.
4. Lobo, R. A. (2003). Early ovarian aging: A hypothesis. What is early ovarian aging? *Human Reproduction, 18*(9), 1762–1764.
5. Manandhar, G., Schatten, H., & Sutovsky, P. (2005). Centrosome reduction during gametogenesis and its significance. *Biology of Reproduction, 72*(1), 2–13.
6. Mehlmann, L. M., Saeki, Y., Tanaka, S., Brennan, T. J., Evsikov, A. V., Pendola, F. L., & Jaffe, L. A. (2004). The Gs-linked receptor GPR3 maintains meiotic arrest in mammalian oocytes. *Science, 306*(5703), 1947–1950. https://doi.org/10.1126/science.1105018.

7. Norris, R. P., Ratzan, W. J., Freudzon, M., Mehlmann, L. M., Krall, J., Movsesian, M. A., & Jaffe, L. A. (2009). Cyclic GMP from the surrounding somatic cells regulates cyclic AMP and meiosis in the mouse oocyte. *Development, 136*(11), 1869–1878. https://doi.org/10.1242/dev.031898.

8. Richards, J. S., & Ascoli, M. (2018). Endocrine, paracrine, and autocrine signaling pathways that regulate ovulation. *Trends in Endocrinology & Metabolism, 29*(5), 313–325. https://doi.org/10.1016/j.tem.2018.02.002.

9. Shuhaibar, L. C., Egbert, J. R., Norris, R. P., Lampe, P. D., Nikolaev, V. O., Thunemann, M., & Jaffe, L. A. (2015). Intercellular signaling via cyclic GMP diffusion through gap junctions restarts meiosis in mouse ovarian follicles. *Proceedings of the National Academy of Sciences, 112*(17), 5527–5532. https://doi.org/10.1073/pnas.1506463112.

10. Sikandar, A., & Ali, M. (2020). Micro-architecture of the female reproductive system. IntechOpen. https://doi.org/10.5772/intechopen.88023.

11. Wang, J.-J., Ge, W., Liu, J.-C., Klinger, F. G., Dyce, P. W., De Felici, M., & Shen, W. (2017). Complete in vitro oogenesis: Retrospects and prospects. *Cell Death & Differentiation, 24*(11), 1845–1852. https://doi.org/10.1038/cdd.2017.129.

12. Zhang, M., Su, Y.-Q., Sugiura, K., Xia, G., & Eppig, J. J. (2010). Granulosa cell ligand NPPC and its receptor NPR2 maintain meiotic arrest in mouse oocytes. *Science, 330*(6002), 366–369. https://doi.org/10.1126/science.1193572.

Chapter 4

GAMETOGENESIS

Contents

Unit Introduction

The formation of sperm and eggs, known as gametogenesis, occurs through the process of meiosis. This process involves two nuclear divisions that separate paired chromosomes in the nucleus, as well as separate chromatids that were formed earlier in the cell's life cycle. Meiosis and its accompanying cell divisions result in the creation of haploid cells containing half of the normal pairs of chromosomes found in diploid cells. Sperm production is referred to as spermatogenesis, while egg production is known as oogenesis.

A complex and tightly controlled biological process called gametogenesis transforms germ cells into mature gametes and is necessary for sexual reproduction. In humans, the gonads—the ovaries in females and the testes in males—are where gametogenesis takes place. The process starts with the mitotic division of primordial germ cells, which gives rise to the development of oogonia in females and spermatogonia in males. Spermatogenesis in males is a sequence of mitotic, meiotic, and morphological changes that result in the development of mature sperm cells. Primary spermatocytes are created by mitotic divisions of spermatogonia, and secondary spermatocytes are created by meiosis I. After that, haploid spermatids are formed by meiosis II. Further morphological changes in these spermatids result in the formation of mature spermatozoa, including the formation of a head with the nucleus and acrosome, a midpiece with mitochondria for energy production, and a tail for motility.

The process of oogenesis in females is more intricate and is marked by a shorter time frame and fewer germ cells. Oogonia divide mitotically to produce primary oocytes, which are then stopped in prophase I of meiosis and remain that way until puberty. A cohort of primary oocytes is stimulated to resume development during each menstrual cycle, but only one of these usually completes meiosis I, giving rise to the formation of a polar body and a secondary oocyte. Only when fertilization takes place and a mature ovum and another polar body are formed, is meiosis II finished. Oocytes are created before birth and exist in a limited supply that gets smaller over time, in contrast to sperm, which are produced continuously throughout the reproductive life.

Hormonal signals, growth factors, and cell-cell interactions are some of the factors that control the development and maturation of germ cells during gametogenesis. By promoting gonadal development, follicular growth, and steroidogenesis, hormones like follicle-stimulating hormone (FSH), luteinizing hormone (LH), estrogen, and testosterone are essential in coordinating the intricate processes of gametogenesis. The highly regulated and orchestrated process of gametogenesis is necessary for both male and female sexual reproduction. Although the fundamentals of gametogenesis are the same for both sexes, spermatogenesis and oogenesis differ significantly in terms of timing, mechanisms, and results. Determining the mechanisms underlying fertility and reproductive disorders and creating treatments to maximize reproductive health require an understanding of the complexities of gametogenesis (Fertility Basics, 2015; Conception and Pregnancy: Ovulation, Fertilization, and More, 2016).

Orientation and Directional Terms:

Terms	Definition	Illustration
Chromosomes	Chromosomes are threadlike structures made of protein and a single molecule of DNA that serve to carry the genomic information from cell to cell.	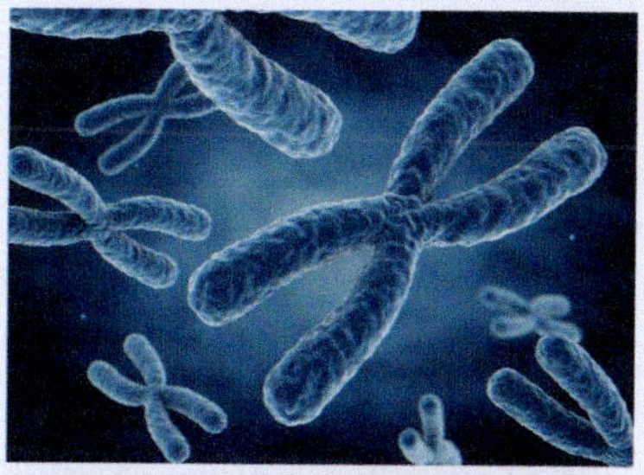
Spermatogenesis	Spermatogenesis is the process of sperm cell development. Rounded immature sperm cells undergo successive mitotic and meiotic divisions (spermatocytogenesis) and a metamorphic change (spermiogenesis) to produce spermatozoa. Mitosis and meiosis.	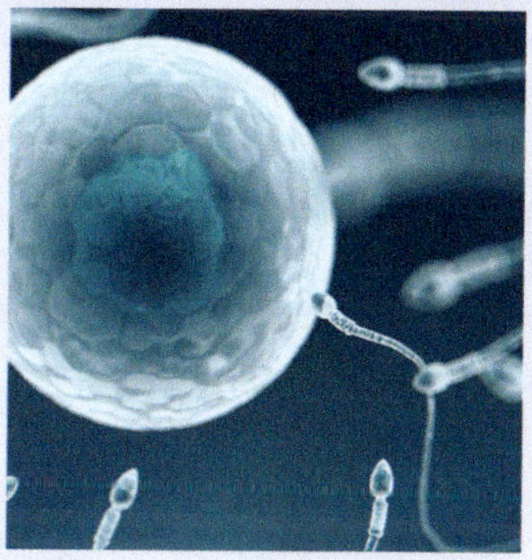
Oogenesis	Oogenesis, also known as ovogenesis or oögenesis, is the process of developing a female gamete, or ovum, from a primordial germ cell (PGC).	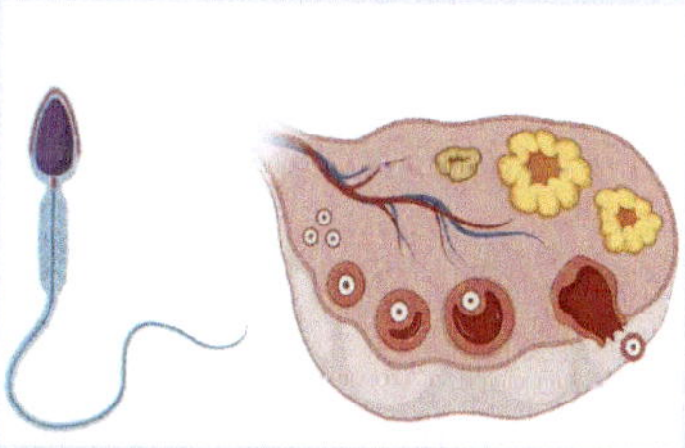
Mitochondria	Mitochondria are membrane-bound cell organelles (mitochondrion, singular) that generate most of the chemical energy needed to power the cell's biochemical reactions.	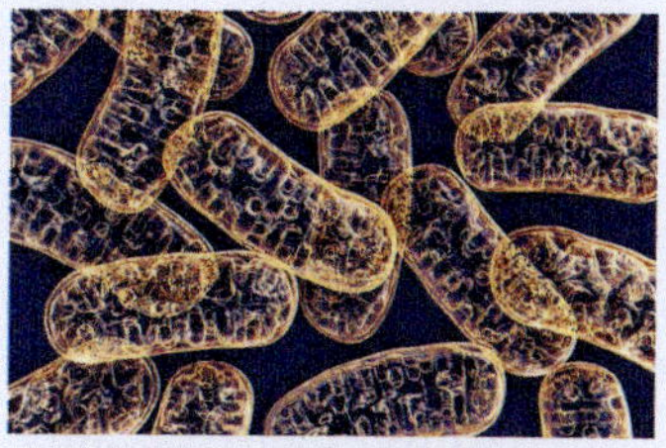
Follicle-stimulating hormone	Follicle-stimulating hormone (FSH) is a hormone that plays a significant role in sexual development and reproduction by affecting the function of the ovaries and testes.	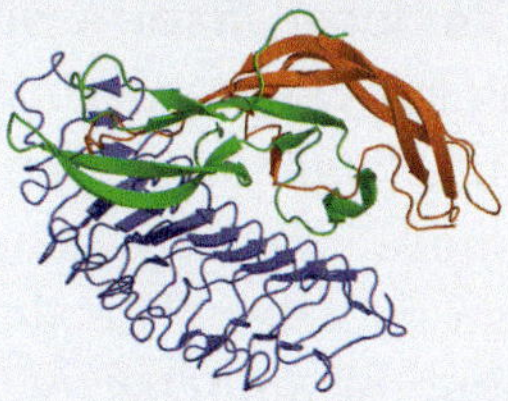

4.1. Comparison of Spermatogenesis and Oogenesis

The two unique processes of gametogenesis that take place in the female and male reproductive systems, respectively, are oogenesis and spermatogenesis. Even though both processes result in the development of haploid gametes, which are required for sexual reproduction, there are some clear distinctions between them in terms of timing, location, regulation, and final products. Timing and duration are two of the main ways that spermatogenesis and oogenesis differ from one another. Spermatogenesis, which produces millions of spermatozoa every day in males, starts during puberty and lasts the duration of the male reproductive lifespan. On the other hand, oogenesis begins in the womb with the development of primary oocytes, which are halted during meiosis's first prophase until puberty. A group of primary oocytes resume development during each menstrual cycle, but usually only one of them completes meiosis I, giving rise to a secondary oocyte and a polar body. Only fertilization, which results in the creation of a mature ovum and another polar body, completes meiosis II. In contrast to sperm, which are constantly produced, oocytes are found in a limited supply that gradually decreases, causing menopause in females.

Additionally, spermatogenesis and oogenesis differ in location. Within the seminiferous tubules of the testes, spermatogonia go through mitotic divisions, meiosis, and morphological changes to form mature spermatozoa. This process is known as spermatogenesis. On the other hand, oogenesis takes place inside the ovaries, more precisely inside organs known as ovarian follicles. The developing oocytes are housed in follicles, which also supply the microenvironment and hormone signals required for their maturation.

Though both processes are governed by hormones, there are differences in the regulation of oogenesis and spermatogenesis. The secretion of luteinizing hormone (LH), follicle-stimulating hormone (FSH), and gonadotropin-releasing hormone (GnRH) is how the hypothalamic-pituitary-gonadal (HPG) axis controls spermatogenesis in males. The anterior pituitary gland releases LH and FSH in response to stimulation from GnRH. These hormones then act on the testes to promote spermatogenesis and increase testosterone production. In turn, testosterone produces a negative feedback loop that controls the release of FSH, LH, and GnRH. The regulation of oogenesis in females is more intricate and includes cyclical fluctuations in the levels of GnRH, LH, FSH, estrogen, progesterone, and inhibin in the menstrual cycle. These hormones control ovulation, the development of follicles, and the lining of the uterus becoming ready for possible implantation.

Additionally, there are differences between the results of oogenesis and spermatogenesis regarding gamete function and production. Numerous, tiny, and extremely motile spermatozoa that are best suited for fertilization are produced during spermatogenesis. Sperm have three main body parts: a tail for movement, a midpiece with mitochondria for energy production, and a head with the nucleus and acrosome. Oogenesis, on the other hand, results in comparatively few, large, and immotile ova. The cytoplasm of oocytes is rich and full of nutrients and organelles that are essential for the early development of the developing embryo after fertilization. Although the primary objective of both spermatogenesis and oogenesis is the production of haploid gametes for sexual reproduction, there are clear distinctions in their timing, locations, regulations, and final products. Comprehending these distinctions is imperative in clarifying the mechanisms behind fertility and reproductive disorders, as well as in formulating interventions aimed at enhancing reproductive health (Fertility Basics, 2015; Conception and Pregnancy: Ovulation, Fertilization, and More, 2016).

4.1.1. Processes of Spermatogenesis and Oogenesis

Because gametogenesis produces genetically diverse progeny, which ensures the survival of the species, it is a necessary process for sexual reproduction. Male and female gametes develop through a process called gametogenesis, and when these gametes combine to form a zygote, the process of creating a new individual begins.

Gametogenesis, the process by which gametes are created, is a crucial component of sexual reproduction in all living things, including plants and animals. This involves the development of specialized reproductive cells called gametes, which are carried by ova (male and female gametes), respectively. Half of the genetic material required for progeny is carried by each gamete. After a series of intricate cellular processes known as gametogenesis, viable, functional gametes that are prepared for fertilization mature. In spermatogenesis and oogenesis, gametogenesis is the process by which a diploid gamete cell divides to produce haploid sperm and egg cells, respectively.

4.1.2. Spermatogenesis

Male immature germ cells are produced in the testes. During puberty, male spermatogonia, or immature germ cells, develop into sperm through a process called spermatogenesis. Spermatogonia are diploid cells that proliferate and multiply during mitosis. Primary spermatocytes undergo meiosis to produce haploid cells known as secondary spermatocytes. These secondary spermatocytes undergo a second meiotic division to produce immature sperm or spermatids. These spermatids go through spermiogenesis to become sperm. A variety of hormones are involved in spermatogenesis promotion, including androgens, LH, FSH, and GnRH.

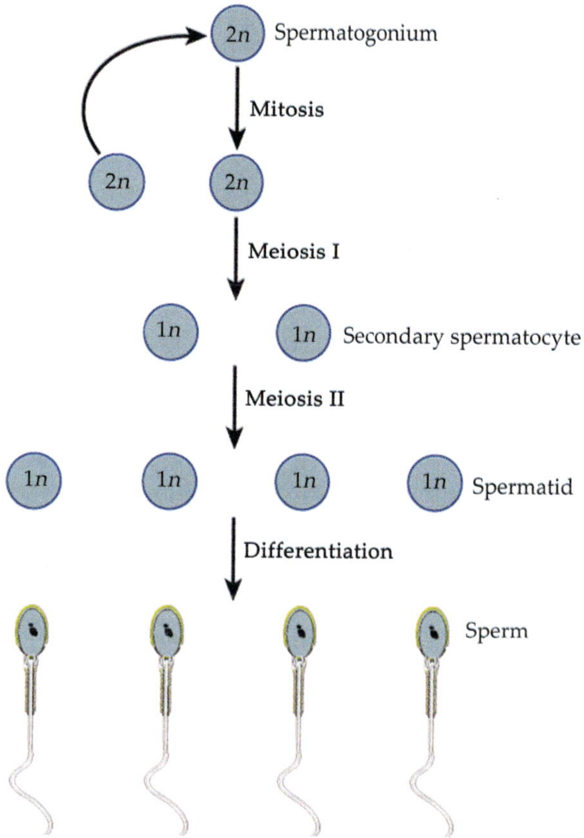

Figure 4.1. *Spermatogenesis: During spermatogenesis, four sperm are formed from each primary spermatocyte, which divides into two haploid secondary spermatocytes; these cells will go through a second meiotic division to produce four spermatids.*

Source: https://s3-us-west-2.amazonaws.com/courses-images/wp-content/uploads/sites/1223/2017/02/09204014/Figure_43_03_05.jpg.

Spermatozoa are found in the lumen of the tube, and stem cells are found at the tube's periphery, where spermatogenesis occurs in the wall of the seminiferous tubules. Directly beneath the tubule's capsule are the diploid, undifferentiated cells. These stem cells, called spermatogonia (plural: spermatagonium), divide into two progenies during the process of mitosis. One of the progenies matures into a sperm cell, while the other generates the next round of sperm (Figure 4.1).

Meiosis is initiated by an organism referred to as a primary spermatocyte. An additional spermatocyte is a haploid cell that develops after the first meiotic division. This haploid cell requires one more meiotic cell division. A spermatid is an endosome that is created during meiosis. When a cell enters the tubule lumen and grows a flagellum or tail, it is referred to as a sperm cell. Four sperm are produced by each primary spermatocyte that goes through meiosis. Stem cells are present from birth until the onset of adolescence and are deposited during gestation, despite being dormant. These cells are activated by gonadotropic hormones that the anterior pituitary produces during adolescence, which leads to the production of viable sperm.

4.1.2.1. In the Beginning

When males hit puberty, which occurs between the ages of 10 and 16 on average, they begin to produce sperm. Approximately 200 million sperm are produced daily by biological males. By doing this, the chance that sperm will get to the egg after ejaculation is increased. The seminiferous tubules in the male testes are where sperm production takes place. To keep the tubules apart from systemic circulation, a blood-testis barrier forms in the testicles.

4.1.2.2. Protecting the Sperm

Sertoli cells make up the blood testis barrier. This is essential to prevent blood chemicals from influencing the development of the sperm. Among these products are waste materials and hormones. It is also important because, due to their genetic differences and expression of distinct surface antigens, the sperm are not recognized as foreign by the male's immune system.

4.1.2.3. Forming Functional Sperm

Through mitosis, the initial population of diploid cells, referred to as spermatogonia, divides to yield two identical cells. One of these A1 spermatogonia cells will be used to repopulate the spermatogonia population. Males maintain their fertility into adulthood as a result of this replenishment of spermatogonia.

Mature sperm will eventually form from the other cell, the type B spermatogonium. Primary spermatocytes are identical diploid cells formed by the multiple mitotic replications of type B spermatogonia, which are connected by cytoplasmic bridges.

Primary spermatocytes then undergo meiosis:

- **Meiosis I:** This produces two haploid cells, known as secondary spermatocytes.
- **Meiosis II:** This produces four haploid cells, known as spermatids.

4.1.2.4. Maturation

When the cytoplasmic bridges break down, the process known as spermiation occurs, releasing the spermatids into the seminiferous tubule lumen. The process of remodeling and differentiating into mature spermatozoa is known as spermiogenesis, and it occurs as the spermatids travel along the seminiferous tubules toward the epididymis. From the seminiferous tubule to the rete testis, cells will migrate.

Eliminating surplus fluid aids in concentrating the sperm. Following that, cells move to the epididymis, which houses and develops sperm during its final stages. Multiple spermatogenic processes must occur simultaneously within a single seminiferous tubule for sperm production to be continuous rather than intermittent, as spermatogenesis takes approximately 70 days. Every 16 days, or every 16 spermatogenic cycle, new groups of spermatogonia form. Each of these populations of spermatogenic cells will be at a different stage of spermatogenesis.

4.1.2.5. Following Ejaculation

Remember that as soon as sperm exit the male body and enter the female reproductive system, they are rendered incapable of reproducing. For the sperm cell to adhere to the zona pellucida of the egg cell, its head must be free of cholesterol and glycoproteins (Fertility Basics, 2015; Conception and Pregnancy: Ovulation, Fertilization, and More, 2016).

4.2. Structure and Function of Male and Female Gametes

Male and female gametes, also known as sperm and egg cells, respectively, are specialized reproductive cells with distinct structures and functions tailored to their roles in sexual reproduction.

4.2.1. Structure of Male Gametes (Sperm)

1. **Head:** The head of a sperm cell contains the genetic material (chromosomes) in the form of tightly packed DNA. At the tip of the head is the acrosome, a structure filled with enzymes that aid in penetrating the egg's protective layers during fertilization.
2. **Midpiece:** Following the head is the midpiece, which contains mitochondria responsible for providing energy (in the form of ATP) for the sperm's movement.
3. **Tail (Flagellum):** The tail, or flagellum, is a long, whip-like structure that propels the sperm forward, enabling it to swim through the female reproductive tract towards the egg.

4.2.1.1. Function of Male Gametes (Sperm)

The primary function of sperm cells during fertilization is to transfer genetic material from the male to the female gamete (egg). Sperm can enter the female reproductive system and reach the egg due to their unique motility. When sperm approach an egg, they undergo an acrosome reaction that releases enzymes that aid in the breaching of the egg's protective layers. After successful fertilization, the sperm and egg combine genetic material to form a zygote, marking the beginning of the embryonic development process.

4.2.2. Structure of Female Gametes (Eggs)

1. **Plasma Membrane:** The egg cell is surrounded by a plasma membrane, which serves as a barrier and regulates the passage of molecules in and out of the cell.
2. **Cytoplasm:** Within the egg cell, the cytoplasm contains organelles such as mitochondria for energy production and ribosomes for protein synthesis.
3. **Nucleus:** Like all cells, the egg cell contains a nucleus that houses the genetic material (DNA) necessary for fertilization and embryonic development.

4.2.2.1. Function of Female Gametes (Eggs)

The primary function of egg cells during fertilization is to transfer the genetic material of the mother to the developing zygote. Eggs are significantly larger than sperm and contain a large amount of cytoplasm and other organelles that are vital for the early stages of embryonic development. The nuclei of the sperm and the egg unite during fertilization to create a diploid zygote, which then divides into several cells to form an embryo.

Male and female gametes each have distinct structures and purposes that are adapted to their particular roles in sexual reproduction. Sperm cells are specialized for motility and delivering the male genetic material, whereas egg cells are provided with nutrients and organelles to aid in fertilization and the initial stages of embryonic development. These gametes unite during fertilization to initiate the process of generating new life.

4.2.3. Mechanisms of Fertilization and Formation of the Zygote

The complicated process of fertilization, which unites sperm and egg, is necessary for the zygote to form—the first stage of embryonic development.

This intricate process involves several key steps and molecular mechanisms:

1. **Sperm Activation and Capacitation:** Upon ejaculation, spermatozoa are released into the female reproductive tract. They undergo a process called capacitation, involving biochemical and physiological changes that render them capable of fertilizing an egg. Capacitation involves the removal of proteins from the sperm's surface, changes in membrane fluidity, and increased motility, enabling the sperm to swim efficiently through the female reproductive tract.
2. **Sperm Migration:** Sperm must navigate through the female reproductive tract to reach the site of fertilization, typically the ampulla of the uterine tube where the egg is released during ovulation. Chemotactic signals released by the egg and the female reproductive tract guide sperm migration towards the egg. Sperm also undergo hyperactivation, a vigorous motility pattern, to penetrate the egg's protective layers.
3. **Egg Activation:** At the same time, the released egg undergoes a series of changes known as egg activation. This process includes the resumption of meiosis, the release of cortical granules from the egg's cytoplasm to prevent polyspermy (fertilization by more than one sperm), and the formation of the egg's pronucleus.
4. **Sperm-Egg Recognition and Binding:** The final step involves the recognition and binding of the sperm to the egg's zona pellucida, an extracellular matrix surrounding the egg. Specific molecules on the surface of the sperm, such as sperm receptors, interact with glycoproteins on the zona pellucida, facilitating sperm egg binding. This interaction triggers the acrosome reaction, during which enzymes released from the sperm's acrosome help penetrate the zona pellucida.

5. **Fusion of Sperm and Egg:** Once a sperm successfully penetrates the zona pellucida, it binds to receptors on the egg's plasma membrane, triggering membrane fusion between the sperm and egg. This fusion allows the sperm's genetic material, contained within the sperm head, to enter the egg's cytoplasm.
6. **Formation of the Zygote:** The fusion of sperm and egg nuclei results in the formation of a zygote, which contains a complete set of chromosomes from both parents. This single-cell embryo undergoes rapid cell division through mitosis, forming a blastocyst as it travels down the uterine tube toward the uterus for implantation.

The process of embryonic development begins with the successful union of genetic material from both parents during fertilization and zygote formation, which is made possible by the precise coordination of molecular and cellular events. Any of these mechanisms that are disrupted can affect early embryonic development and fertilization, which can result in abnormal development or infertility (Fertility Basics, 2015; Conception and Pregnancy: Ovulation, Fertilization, and More, 2016).

4.3. Hormonal Regulation of Gamete Production

Hormonal signals play a crucial role in controlling the development and maturation of germ cells into viable sperm and eggs, a process known as gametogenesis. This process starts in the embryonic stage of human development and lasts the entirety of the reproductive life. To coordinate the intricate chain of events that result in the production of mature gametes, hormone regulation is essential.

Gonadotropin-releasing hormone (GnRH), luteinizing hormone (LH), follicle-stimulating hormone (FSH), testosterone, and inhibin are the main hormones in males that are involved in gametogenesis. The hypothalamus secretes GnRH, which causes the anterior pituitary gland to release FSH and LH. To maintain and develop male reproductive tissues and to produce sperm cells through spermatogenesis, LH acts on the interstitial cells in the testes to stimulate the production of testosterone. FSH, on the other hand, supports sperm maturation and speeds up the spermatogenesis process by acting on the sustentacular cells inside the seminiferous tubules. Additionally, testosterone controls the secretion of GnRH, LH, and FSH by acting as a negative feedback loop on the hypothalamus and pituitary. Furthermore, the pituitary receives negative feedback from the Sertoli cell-produced inhibin, which specifically inhibits FSH secretion and influences spermatogenesis.

In females, a complex cyclic interplay of hormones, mainly GnRH, LH, FSH, estrogen, progesterone, and inhibin, regulates gametogenesis. The anterior pituitary is stimulated to secrete LH and FSH by the hypothalamus' release of GnRH. Rising FSH levels during the menstrual cycle promote the development and growth of ovarian follicles, each of which contains an oocyte. The follicles produce more estrogen as they get older, which encourages the uterine lining to thicken in anticipation of possible implantation. Additionally, estrogen stimulates the hypothalamus and pituitary with positive feedback, which increases LH secretion and initiates ovulation. In addition, the LH surge causes the ruptured follicle to change into the corpus luteum, which secretes progesterone to keep the uterine lining intact and ready for implantation. The corpus luteum regresses in the absence of fertilization, which lowers progesterone and estrogen levels and causes menstruation and the start of a new cycle. The granulosa cells of the growing follicles secrete an inhibitor that acts as a negative feedback loop to the pituitary, specifically preventing the release of FSH and controlling the development of follicles.

Hormonal regulation maintains the appropriate timing and coordination of processes necessary to produce viable gametes throughout both male and female gametogenesis. Hormonal imbalances can result in several reproductive disorders, including hypogonadism, polycystic ovary syndrome (PCOS), and infertility. Comprehending the complex hormonal processes that regulate gametogenesis is essential for identifying and managing these disorders, and eventually enhancing fertility and reproductive health.

4.3.1. Hormonal Control of Reproduction

Hormones from the anterior pituitary and hypothalamus interact with hormones from reproductive tissues and organs to regulate the cycles of reproduction in both male and female humans. The hypothalamus controls and initiates the anterior pituitary gland hormone release in both sexes. The anterior pituitary receives a gonadotropin-releasing hormone (GnRH) from the hypothalamus when the reproductive hormone is needed. Follicle-stimulating hormone (FSH) and luteinizing hormone (LH) are released into the bloodstream as a result of this from the anterior pituitary. These hormones are produced in both sexes and are crucial in regulating reproduction, despite being named after their roles in female reproduction. In the reproductive systems of both men and women, other hormones serve particular purposes.

4.3.2. Male Hormones

The hypothalamus releases FSH and LH into the male system for the first time at the onset of puberty. FSH enters the testes and initiates the promotion of spermatogenesis by stimulating the sustentacular cells found in the walls of the seminiferous tubules (Figure 4.2). Additionally, LH enters the testes and triggers the production and release of testosterone into the bloodstream and testes by the Leydig interstitial cells, which are found between the walls of the seminiferous tubules.

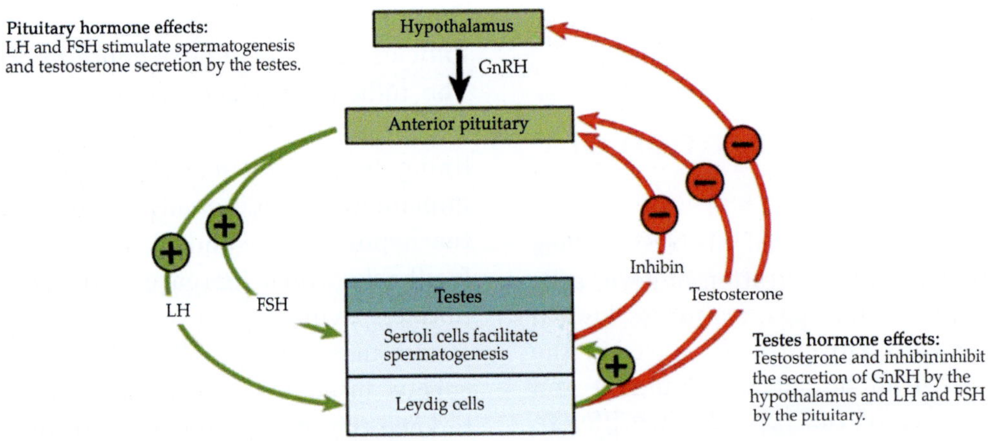

Figure 4.2. *Hormones control sperm production in a negative feedback system.*

Source: https://opentextbc.ca/biology/wp-content/uploads/sites/96/2015/10/Figure_43_04_01-1024x436-1-768x327.jpg.

Testosterone promotes the production of sperm and is also accountable for the development of secondary sexual traits in males during puberty. These traits include a deeper voice, the growth of facial, underarm, and pubic hair, an increase in muscle mass, and the onset of sexual desire.

Rising testosterone levels in men cause the anterior pituitary and hypothalamus to block the release of GnRH, FSH, and LH, creating a negative feedback loop. Furthermore, the hormone inhibin is produced by the sustentacular cells and is released into the bloodstream when the sperm count is excessively high. This stops FSH and GnRH from being released, which slows down spermatogenesis. The sperm count increases when the sustentacular cells stop releasing inhibin when it falls below 20 million/mL.

4.3.3. Female Hormones

In females, the regulation of reproduction is more intricate. The menstrual cycle and the ovarian cycle make up the female reproductive cycle. The menstrual cycle controls the development and upkeep of the uterine lining, whereas the ovarian cycle controls the release of eggs and the preparation of endocrine tissues (Figure 4.3). These cycles, which have an average duration of 28 days, are synchronized over a 22–32-day cycle. Similar to a male, the anterior pituitary releases FSH and LH in response to GnRH from the hypothalamus. Furthermore, the growing follicles release progesterone and estrogen. Similar to testosterone in men, estrogen is in charge of a woman's secondary sexual traits. These include the development of the breasts, hip flaring, and a shortened time for bone growth.

4.3.3.1. The Ovarian Cycle and the Menstrual Cycle

The hormones of the hypothalamus, pituitary, and ovaries regulate the ovarian and menstrual cycles, as shown in Figure 4.3. The fluctuation of these hormones drives the progression of these cycles, which occur simultaneously. The follicular phase, the first half of the ovarian cycle, is initiated by increasing levels of FSH that stimulate follicle growth on the surface of the ovary. This growth prepares the egg for ovulation. As the follicles develop, they release estrogen. The start of this phase coincides with menstruation, the shedding of the functional layer of the uterus's endometrium. After around five days, estrogen levels increase, marking the beginning of the proliferative phase of the menstrual cycle. During this time, the endometrium regenerates, replenishing the blood vessels and glands that were lost at the end of the previous cycle.

Around day 14, or just before the middle of the cycle, high levels of estrogen cause FSH, and especially LH, to rise quickly before falling. The most mature follicle bursts and releases its egg in response to the LH spike. It's ovulation right now. The eggs from the follicles that did not burst degenerate. When the extra follicles degenerate, the amount of estrogen drops. The luteal phase of the ovarian cycle and the secretory phase of the menstrual cycle, which last from roughly day 15 to day 28, begin after ovulation. The ruptured follicle undergoes modifications during the luteal and secretory phases. Physical alterations occur in the follicle's cells, resulting in the formation of the corpus luteum. Progesterone and estrogen are produced by the corpus luteum. Progesterone suppresses the release of additional FSH and LH while promoting the regeneration of the uterine lining. When a fertilized egg becomes available during this cycle, the uterus is getting ready to receive it. Progesterone is increased while FSH and LH inhibition stops more eggs and follicles from developing. Over the course of the following few days, the corpus luteum produces an increased amount of estrogen that stabilizes.

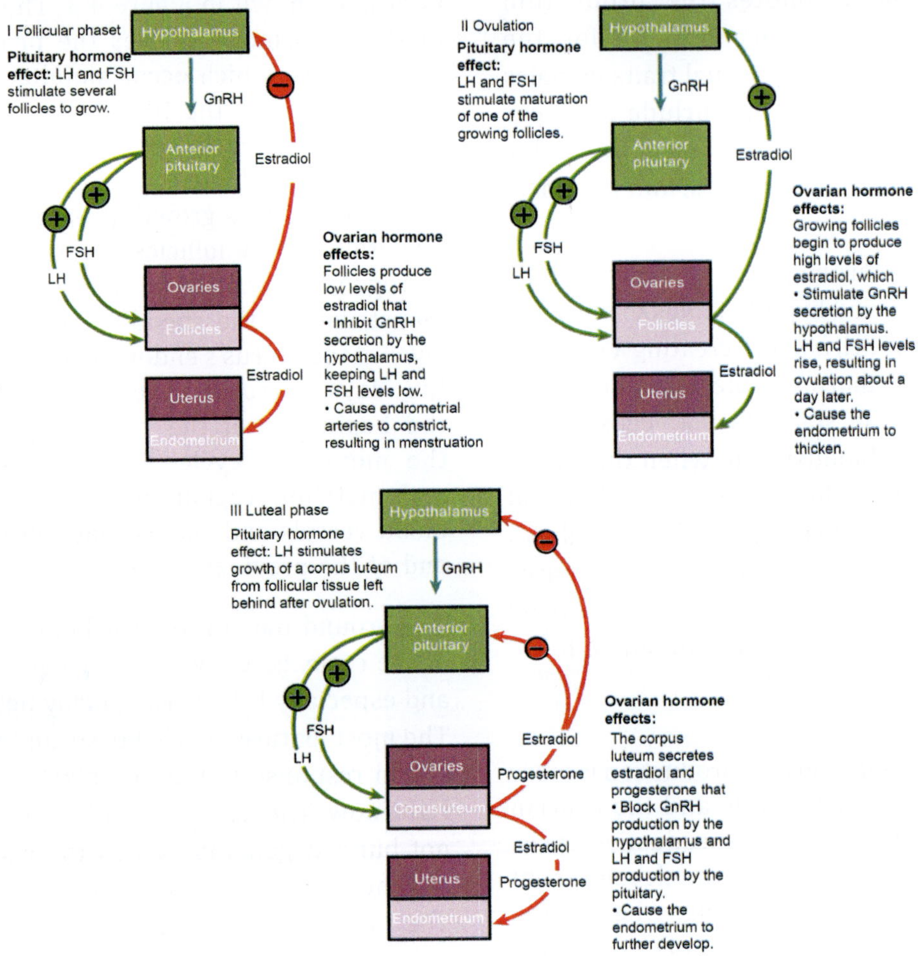

Figure 4.3. *The ovarian and menstrual cycles of female reproduction are regulated by hormones produced by the hypothalamus, pituitary, and ovaries.*

Source: https://opentextbc.ca/biology/wp-content/uploads/sites/96/2021/03/Figure_43_04_02f-768x779.png.

The corpus luteum degenerates and estrogen and progesterone levels drop in the uterus in the absence of a fertilized egg being implanted. As progesterone levels decline, the endometrium starts to deteriorate, which starts the subsequent menstrual cycle. Progesterone declines also enable the anterior pituitary to receive GnRH from the hypothalamus, which releases FSH and LH and recommences the cycles.

4.3.3.2. Reproductive Endocrinologist

A doctor who treats a range of hormone disorders associated with reproduction and infertility in men and women is known as a reproductive endocrinologist. Menstrual issues, infertility, miscarriage, sexual dysfunction, and menopause are among the disorders. Physicians may treat patients with assisted reproductive technologies (ART), fertility medications, or surgery. *In vitro* fertilization is one technique used in assisted reproductive technology (ART) to modify the egg or sperm to facilitate reproduction.

Reproductive endocrinologists complete three years of fellowship training in reproductive endocrinology after completing a four-year obstetrics and gynecology residency. The doctor needs to pass written and oral exams in both areas to become board-certified in this field (Fertility Basics, 2015; Conception and Pregnancy: Ovulation, Fertilization, and More, 2016).

4.3.4. Gestation

The fertilization of an egg initiates pregnancy, which lasts until the baby is born. The gestation period, or duration of pregnancy, is 266 days in humans and comparable in other great apes. The egg and sperm nuclei fuse 24 hours after fertilization when the egg nucleus has completed meiosis.

The cell is referred to as a zygote after fusion. The developing embryo passes through the oviduct and into the uterus once the zygote starts the process of cleavage. Within seven days, the developing embryo must implant into the uterine wall; otherwise, it will degrade and perish. By breaking down the endometrial cells, the blastocyst, or developing embryo, grows into the endometrium. The blastocyst is then sealed into the tissue by the endometrium healing. Human beta chorionic gonadotropin (β-HCG) is released by the chorion, another layer of the blastocyst, and it travels to the corpus luteum to maintain its activity. This guarantees sufficient progesterone levels to preserve the uterine endometrium and support the growing embryo. The level of β-HCG in urine or serum is determined by pregnancy tests. The test is positive if the hormone is present.

Three equal periods, or trimesters, make up the gestation period. The endometrial lining uses diffusion to manage nutrition and waste during the first two to four weeks of the first trimester. The placenta develops and the outer layer of the embryo starts to fuse with the endometrium as the trimester goes on. The placenta assumes responsibility for the embryos and fetus's nutritional and waste needs; nutrients are transferred to and eliminated from the placenta by the mother's blood. The mother's liver breaks down and excretes substances from the fetus, including bilirubin. A portion of the mother's immunoglobulins will cross the placenta and offer passive protection from a few possible infections.

During the first trimester, internal organs and body structures start to develop. The liver, heart, eyes, and limb buds have all essentially developed by week five. The body is essentially formed by eight weeks, at which point the term "fetus" applies (Figure 4.4).

The person is roughly two inches (five centimeters) long, and many of their organs, including their liver and lungs, are still developing. Since all the body's organs and structures are still developing during the first trimester, exposure to toxins is particularly risky during this time. The viability of the fetus may be severely impacted by anything that tampers with chemical signaling during that stage of development. During the second trimester, the fetus grows to about 30 cm (about 12 inches). It becomes active and the mother usually feels the first movements. All organs and structures continue to develop. The placenta has taken over the functions of nutrition and waste elimination and the production of estrogen and progesterone from the corpus luteum, which has degenerated. The placenta will continue functioning up through the delivery of the baby. During the third trimester, the fetus grows to 3 to 4 kg (6.5–8.5 lbs.) and is about 50 cm (19–20 inches) long. This is the period of the most rapid growth during the pregnancy as all organ systems continue to grow and develop.

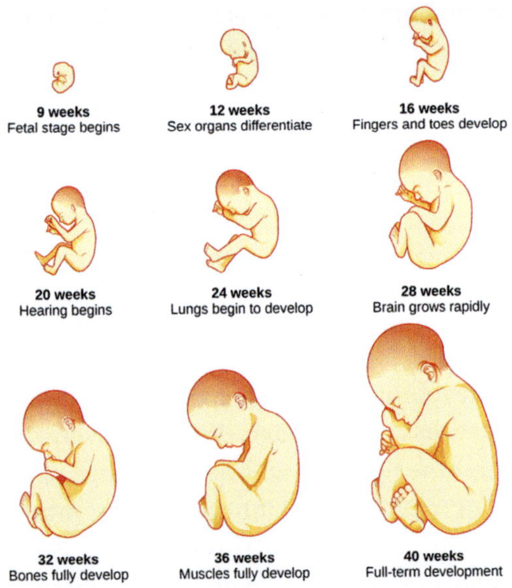

Figure 4.4. *During the fetal stage, the baby's brain develops and the body adds size and weight until the fetus reaches full-term development.*

Source: https://courses.lumenlearning.com/suny-hvcc-lifespandevelopment4/chapter/prenatal-development/.

The contraction of muscles to remove the placenta and fetus from the uterus is known as labor. Estrogen stimulates the development of uterine wall receptors that bind the hormone oxytocin towards the end of the third trimester. At this point, the baby turns around, facing downward and forward, and engages the cervix (uterine opening) with its back or crown. As a result, the cervix contracts, and the hypothalamus receives nerve impulses that trigger the posterior pituitary gland to release oxytocin. The uterine wall's smooth muscle contracts in response to oxytocin. Prostaglandins are released into the uterus by the placenta at the same time, intensifying contractions. To ensure an adequate supply of oxytocin, a positive feedback relay takes place between the posterior pituitary, hypothalamus, and uterus. The force and intensity of the contractions increase with the recruitment of additional smooth muscle cells.

Labor occurs in three stages. The cervix dilates and thins during the first stage. For the baby and placenta to be expelled during birth, this is required. Eventually, the cervix enlarges to a length of roughly 10 cm. The baby is discharged from the uterus in stage two. To facilitate delivery, the mother compresses her abdominal muscles, pushes, and her uterus contracts. After the baby is born and the placenta has fully detached from the uterine wall, the placenta passes through the final stage. Pitocin, a synthetic form of oxytocin, can be used to induce and sustain labor if it stops before stage two is reached (Fertility Basics, 2015; Conception and Pregnancy: Ovulation, Fertilization, and More, 2016).

A Closer Look

Oogenesis

Oogenesis is the process by which oocytes, or female gametes, are produced in the ovaries of female animals. This intricate process begins before birth, during fetal development. Primordial germ cells differentiate into oogonia, which undergo mitosis to form primary oocytes. These primary oocytes enter the first meiotic division but are arrested in the prophase I stage until puberty. Each primary oocyte is encased in a follicle, forming a primordial follicle.

With the onset of puberty and the influence of hormonal cycles, a primary oocyte resumes meiosis I each menstrual cycle, but typically, only one completes this stage, resulting in a secondary oocyte and a smaller polar body due to asymmetric cytokinesis. The secondary oocyte begins meiosis II but halts at metaphase II and is released during ovulation. If fertilization occurs, the secondary oocyte completes meiosis II, forming a mature ovum and another polar body. If no fertilization takes place, the secondary oocyte degenerates.

Oogenesis differs from spermatogenesis, the male counterpart, in several key aspects. While spermatogenesis results in four viable sperm cells from each spermatogonium, oogenesis produces only one viable ovum from each oogonium, with the other products being non-functional polar bodies. This disparity is due to the need to provide the ovum with ample cytoplasm and organelles to support early embryonic development.

The hormonal regulation of oogenesis is complex, involving the hypothalamus, pituitary gland, and ovaries. Follicle-stimulating hormone (FSH) stimulates follicle growth while luteinizing hormone (LH) triggers ovulation and the formation of the corpus luteum. Estrogen and progesterone, produced by the ovaries, further regulate the menstrual cycle and prepare the endometrium for the potential implantation of a fertilized egg. Oogenesis is a meticulously controlled process essential for female fertility and the perpetuation of species, highlighting the elegance and complexity of reproductive biology (Fertility Basics, 2015; Conception and Pregnancy: Ovulation, Fertilization, and More, 2016).

Summary

- Gametogenesis, the production of sperm and eggs, involves the process of meiosis. During meiosis, two nuclear divisions separate the paired chromosomes in the nucleus and then separate the chromatids that were made during an earlier stage of the cell's life cycle.
- Meiosis and its associated cell divisions produces haploid cells with half of each pair of chromosomes normally found in diploid cells
- Gametogenesis is the process by which male and female gametes develop, and fertilization is the joining of these gametes to form a zygote, which starts the process of creating a new individual.
- The female gametophyte, sometimes referred to as the embryo sac, is the site of fertilization and the development of female gametes, and it is essential to the reproductive process of flowering plants.
- The process of gamete production, known as gametogenesis, is intricately regulated by hormonal signals that orchestrate the development and maturation of germ cells into functional sperm and eggs. In humans, this process begins during embryonic development and continues throughout reproductive life.
- Pregnancy begins with the fertilization of an egg and continues through to the birth of the individual. The length of time of gestation, or the gestation period, in humans is 266 days and is similar in other great apes.

References

1. Alikani, M., Calderon, G., Tomkin, G., Garrisi, J., Kokot, M., & Cohen, J. (2000). Cleavage anomalies in early human embryos and survival after prolonged culture in-vitro. *Human Reproduction, 15*(12), 2634–2643.
2. Amano, T., Kato, Y., & Tsunoda, Y. (2001). Full-term development of enucleated mouse oocytes fused with embryonic stem cells from different cell lines. *Reproduction, 121*(5), 729–733.
3. Barritt, J. A., Brenner, C. A., Willadsen, S., & Cohen, J. (2000, July). Spontaneous and artificial changes in human ooplasmic mitochondria. *Human Reproduction, 15*(Suppl 2), 207–217.
4. Bavister, B. D., & Squirrell, J. M. (2000). Mitochondrial distribution and function in oocytes and early embryos. *Human Reproduction, 15*(Suppl 2), 189–198.

Chapter

REPRODUCTIVE HORMONES

5

Contents

Unit Introduction

Reproductive hormones are essential for controlling the intricate processes involved in human reproduction, including the growth and operation of reproductive organs, the creation of gametes, and the female menstrual cycle. The complex interactions between these hormones, which are produced by specialized glands including the pituitary, ovaries, testes, and hypothalamus, guarantee the healthy operation of the reproductive system. The brain region known as the hypothalamus, which releases gonadotropin-releasing hormone (GnRH), is at the center of the reproductive hormone system. Follicle-stimulating hormone (FSH) and luteinizing hormone (LH), two important hormones, are secreted by the adjacent pituitary gland in response to GnRH stimulation. FSH is the hormone that causes ovarian follicles, which house developing egg cells, to begin growing and maturing in females. Ovulation, or the release of a mature egg from the ovary, is caused by LH. LH stimulates the production of testosterone in males, whereas FSH stimulates the production of sperm cells in the testes. The female ovaries are important reproductive organs that produce ova and sex hormones like progesterone and estrogen. The production of estrogen, which is mostly produced by the ovarian follicles, is essential for the maintenance of the uterine lining during pregnancy, the development of secondary sexual characteristics in females, and menstrual cycle regulation. Progesterone helps sustain pregnancy by preparing the uterus for the implantation of a fertilized egg and is mainly produced by the corpus luteum following ovulation.

The testes are the main reproductive organs in males, where they produce testosterone and sperm cells. FSH and testosterone both promote spermatogenesis, the process of producing new eggs. The androgen hormone testosterone is essential for the development of secondary sexual traits in males, including muscular mass, deep voice, and facial hair. It also contributes to mood and libido regulation.

In females of reproductive age, the menstrual cycle is a recurring process that is controlled by a complex interaction of hormones. The luteal phase, ovulation, and follicular phase are the three phases of the cycle, which start with menstruation, or the shedding of the uterine lining. Ovulation, the development of ovarian follicles, and alterations in the uterine lining to get ready for a possible pregnancy are all impacted by fluctuations in estrogen and progesterone levels throughout the menstrual cycle.

Reproductive disorders and other health problems can result from imbalances in the reproductive hormones. Hormonal imbalances can lead to conditions like endometriosis, male hypogonadism, and polycystic ovarian syndrome (PCOS). Furthermore, changes in reproductive hormones during menopause and andropause (the male counterpart of menopause) can substantially alter an individual's physiology and mental state. Both male and female reproductive systems depend on the reproductive hormones to function properly. Their complex regulation facilitates the menstrual cycle, gamete development, and maintenance of secondary sexual traits, all of which are necessary for human reproduction.

Orientation and Directional Terms:

Terms	Definition	Illustration
Hypothalamus	Hypothalamus is a gland in your brain that acts like your body's thermostat. It takes in signals from organs in your hormone (endocrine) system and other areas of your brain and sends hormones to your pituitary gland.	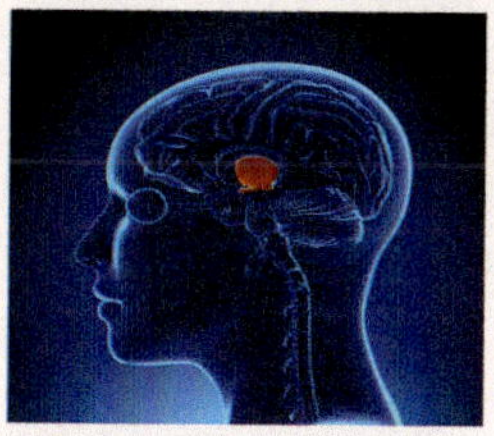
Luteinizing hormone	Luteinizing hormone (LH) is a chemical in your body that triggers important processes in your reproductive system. LH spurs ovulation and helps with the hormone production needed to support pregnancy.	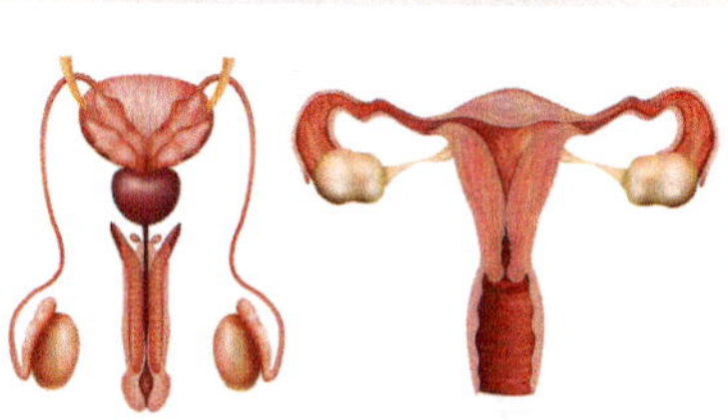
Pregnancy	Pregnancy is the term used to describe the period in which a fetus develops inside a woman's womb or uterus. Pregnancy usually lasts about 40 weeks, or just over 9 months, as measured from the last menstrual period to delivery. Health care providers refer to three segments of pregnancy, called trimesters.	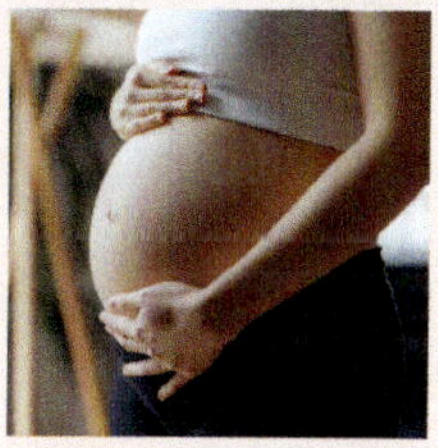
Polycystic ovarian syndrome	PCOS is a common hormone problem in women of childbearing age. Women with PCOS may not ovulate, and have abnormal hormone levels.	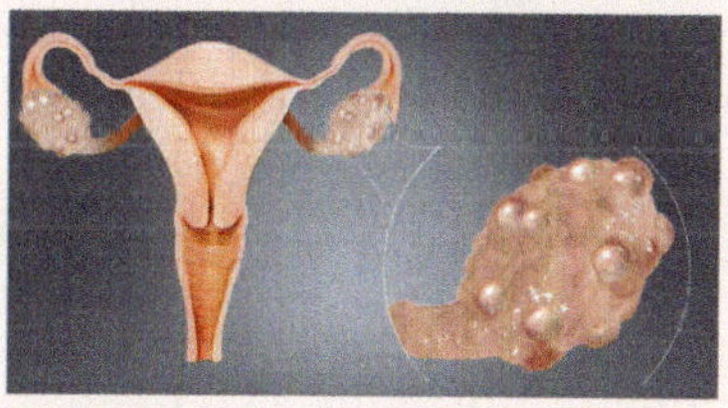
Menopause	Menopause is the time that marks the end of your menstrual cycles. It's diagnosed after you've gone 12 months without a menstrual period.	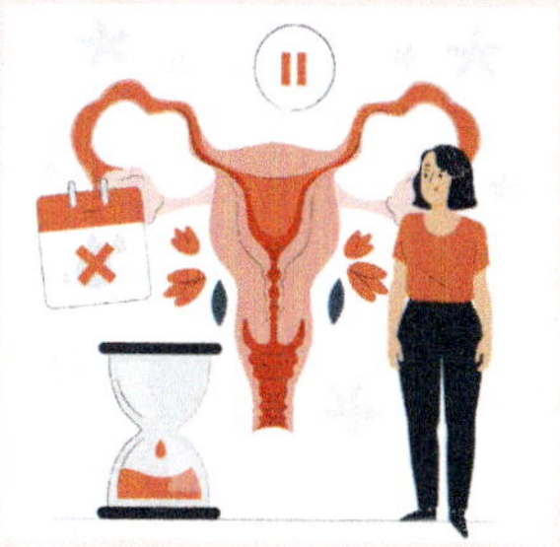

5.1. Endocrine Glands Involved in Reproductive Function

The body's numerous endocrine glands produce a complex interplay of hormones that control the intricate processes involved in human reproduction. Together, these glands—which include the testes, ovaries, pituitary, and hypothalamus—coordinate the development and operation of female reproductive organs, gamete production, and the menstrual cycle.

The primary controller of the reproductive hormone system is the hypothalamus, a part of the brain located directly above the pituitary gland. It generates gonadotropin-releasing hormone (GnRH), a crucial hormone that triggers the release of follicle-stimulating hormone (FSH) and luteinizing hormone (LH) from the adjacent pituitary gland. These hormones are essential for controlling the female and male reproductive systems.

The main reproductive organs in females are the ovaries, which also produce female sex hormones like progesterone and estrogen. The hormone known as follicle-stimulating hormone (FSH) promotes the development and maturation of ovarian follicles, which are the precursor cells of eggs. In the meantime, luteinizing hormone (LH) causes the ovary to release a mature egg during ovulation. The corpus luteum, a transitory endocrine structure that secretes progesterone to prime the uterine lining for the possible implantation of a fertilized egg, develops from the remnants of the ovarian follicle after ovulation.

The testes are the main reproductive organs in males, where they produce testosterone, the hormone associated with masculinity, and sperm cells. In the seminiferous tubules of the testes, spermatogenesis—the process of producing sperm cells—is triggered by follicle-stimulating hormone or FSH. Concurrently, the production of testosterone is stimulated by luteinizing hormone (LH) in the interstitial cells of the testes. Male secondary sexual traits like the development of muscles, the deepening of the voice, and the growth of facial and body hair are all significantly influenced by testosterone. In males, it also controls sperm production, libido, and general reproductive health.

The pituitary gland, also known as the master gland, secretes FSH and LH in response to signals from the hypothalamus and is thus a key player in controlling reproductive function. The anterior and posterior pituitary lobes make up the pituitary gland, which is located directly below the hypothalamus. While the posterior pituitary stores and releases hormones like oxytocin, which is involved in lactation and labor, the anterior pituitary generates and releases FSH and LH.

Furthermore, tiny amounts of the sex hormones androgens and estrogens are produced by the adrenal glands, which are situated atop the kidneys. The adrenal glands contribute to total androgen production in both males and females, even though the testes are the main source of androgens (including testosterone) in males. Comparably, in females, the ovaries are the main source of estrogen; however, small amounts of estrogen are also produced by the adrenal glands, especially during menopause when ovarian estrogen production decreases.

The numerous endocrine glands work together to secrete different hormones that control reproductive function. Follicle-stimulating hormone (FSH) and luteinizing hormone (LH) is released by the pituitary gland in response to gonadotropin-releasing hormone (GnRH), which is produced by the hypothalamus to start the reproductive hormone cascade. In turn, these hormones control the development of gametes, the release of sex hormones, and the reproductive systems in both males and females. The significance of hormonal balance in preserving reproductive health and fertility is highlighted by the fact that malfunctions or imbalances in these endocrine glands can result in reproductive disorders and health complications (Davey & Grossmann, 2016; Whirledge & Cidlowski, 2019).

5.1.1. Hypothalamus

The hypothalamus, a small yet vital area located deep in the brain, acts as a central control center for managing numerous physiological processes necessary for keeping the body in balance and governing intricate behaviors. Positioned below the thalamus and above the pituitary gland, the hypothalamus is commonly referred to as the body's chief regulator because of its crucial function in merging neural and hormonal cues to harmonize different bodily functions such as regulating temperature, hunger, thirst, sleep patterns, and reproductive activities.

Being an intermediary between the endocrine and neurological systems is one of the hypothalamus' main roles. The secretion of different neurohormones acts upon the pituitary gland to regulate the release of pituitary hormones, which in turn regulate the activity of other endocrine glands throughout the body, enabling it to accomplish this. For example, the pituitary gland releases follicle-stimulating hormone (FSH) and luteinizing hormone (LH), two important regulators of reproductive function, in response to the production of gonadotropin-releasing hormone (GnRH) from the hypothalamus.

Furthermore, the hypothalamus is essential for maintaining the body's internal balance by monitoring and responding to fluctuations in blood pressure, body temperature, and nutrient levels. This is achieved through specific nuclei within its structure that receive input from different body parts and process it to trigger appropriate physiological reactions. For instance, the preoptic area of the hypothalamus houses neurons that can detect changes in body temperature, allowing the hypothalamus to implement thermoregulatory responses like sweating or shivering to keep the body temperature at an optimal level.

The hypothalamus is not only responsible for maintaining physiological balance, but also plays a crucial role in regulating behaviors like hunger, thirst, and sleep-wake cycles. Specialized nuclei within the hypothalamus, such as the arcuate nucleus and ventromedial nucleus, monitor nutrient and energy levels to adjust feeding behavior accordingly. Neurons within the arcuate nucleus respond to hunger signals like ghrelin, leptin, and insulin to regulate appetite and food intake based on energy balance.

Furthermore, the hypothalamus controls thirst and fluid balance by secreting vasopressin, or ADH, to conserve water and maintain proper hydration levels. Dysfunction in this regulation can lead to conditions like diabetes insipidus, which causes excessive thirst and urination due to impaired ADH secretion or response.

In addition, the hypothalamus plays a key role in controlling sleep-wake cycles and circadian rhythms by communicating with the suprachiasmatic nucleus (SCN), which acts as the body's internal clock. The SCN receives signals from light-sensitive cells in the eyes and helps coordinate biological rhythms with external factors. Problems with hypothalamic control of circadian rhythms can result in sleep disorders like insomnia or circadian rhythm sleep-wake disorders.

The hypothalamus is primarily responsible for controlling a broad range of physiological functions and actions that are necessary to preserve homeostasis and guarantee the survival of the organism. The hypothalamus integrates sensory information, initiates appropriate responses, and coordinates the activities of various bodily systems through its complex connections with the nervous system and endocrine system. The hypothalamus is a crucial regulator of behavior and physiological processes, and any dysfunction in this area can have a significant impact on one's health and overall well-being (Davey & Grossmann, 2016; Whirledge & Cidlowski, 2019).

5.1.2. Pituitary Gland

The pituitary gland, also known as the master gland, is a pea-sized organ that is housed inside the sella turcica, a bony structure at the base of the skull, at the base of the brain. Despite its diminutive size, the pituitary gland secretes hormones that affect specific organs all over the body, helping to regulate a host of biological processes. The anterior pituitary (adenohypophysis) and posterior pituitary (neurohypophysis), which make up this gland, are each in charge of different functions.

The anterior pituitary gland produces and releases hormones that oversee growth, metabolism, reproduction, and stress response. One essential hormone it produces is growth hormone (GH), which promotes growth, cell multiplication, and restoration in humans and animals. Imbalances in GH secretion can cause conditions like gigantism or dwarfism. Another crucial hormone from the anterior pituitary is adrenocorticotropic hormone (ACTH), which prompts the adrenal glands to create cortisol, a stress hormone that assists in the body's reaction to stress and metabolic regulation.

Thyroid-stimulating hormone (TSH), which is also produced by the anterior pituitary, controls the thyroid gland's secretion of thyroid hormones necessary for growth, metabolism, and energy production. Another hormone that the anterior pituitary releases is called prolactin, which affects reproductive processes and increases milk production in nursing moms. Gonadotropins are vital for sexual development and reproduction because they control the activities of the gonads, which are the female ovaries and the male testes. These hormones include luteinizing hormone (LH) and follicle-stimulating hormone (FSH).

Conversely, the hypothalamus produces two hormones that are stored and released by the posterior pituitary gland: vasopressin (also known as antidiuretic hormone, or ADH) and oxytocin. Numerous physiological processes, such as uterine contractions during childbirth, milk ejection during breastfeeding, and social bonding, are facilitated by oxytocin. Vasopressin helps to maintain blood pressure and prevent dehydration by regulating the body's water balance through the kidneys' regulation of water reabsorption. The hypothalamus, a part of the brain situated directly above the pituitary, closely controls the hormones secreted by the pituitary gland. The hypophyseal portal system, a system of blood vessels, allows the hypothalamus to release and inhibit hormones that are sent to the pituitary gland. These hormones from the hypothalamus either stimulate or inhibit the release of particular hormones, which regulates the anterior pituitary's hormone secretion.

Hormone imbalances resulting from disorders of the pituitary gland can cause many health issues. For instance, malignant or benign pituitary tumors can produce too much or too little of a certain hormone, which can result in symptoms like irregular growth, infertility, weight gain or loss, and mood swings. Radiation therapy, surgery, and medication are frequently used in conjunction to treat pituitary disorders to relieve symptoms and restore hormonal balance.

The pituitary gland secretes hormones that affect growth, metabolism, reproduction, stress response, and water balance, thereby acting as an essential regulator of many physiological processes. Its complex relationship with the hypothalamus guarantees appropriate hormone regulation, and any problems with this system can have serious negative effects on health. Thus, correctly diagnosing and treating endocrine disorders requires an understanding of the pituitary gland's function.

5.1.3. Gonads

The reproductive organs known as gonads are in charge of synthesizing sex hormones and producing gametes, which are eggs in females and sperm in males. The gonads are the testes in males and the ovaries in females.

5.1.3.1. Testes

The testes, located in the scrotum outside the abdominal cavity, are the male reproductive glands. They contain seminiferous tubules where spermatogenesis, the production of sperm, takes place. Spermatogenesis is a complex process involving germ cells developing into mature spermatozoa with the support of sustentacular cells within the tubules.

Apart from sperm production, the testes also secrete testosterone, the primary male sex hormone. Testosterone is an androgen that is vital for the development of male reproductive tissues like the testes and prostate, as well as secondary sexual characteristics such as facial hair growth, deepening of the voice, and muscle mass development. It also influences libido and contributes to overall male physiology and behavior.

5.1.3.2. Ovaries

The female gonads, or ovaries, are found in the pelvic cavity on either side of the uterus. Thousands of follicles, each containing an immature egg cell (oocyte) encircled by supporting cells, are found within them. Follicles mature during the menstrual cycle, and during ovulation, one dominant follicle releases a mature egg. Follicle-stimulating hormone (FSH) and luteinizing hormone (LH), which are secreted by the pituitary gland, control this process.

Aside from producing eggs, the ovaries also produce estrogen and progesterone, which are the main female sex hormones. Estrogen, primarily produced by the ovarian follicles, is important for the growth of female reproductive organs, regulating the menstrual cycle, and keeping bone density. Progesterone, produced by the corpus luteum post-ovulation, readies the uterine lining for a fertilized egg and supports pregnancy if fertilization happens.

The ovaries and testes work together to regulate the reproductive system and maintain general health. Reproductive disorders, hormonal imbalances, and infertility can result from any abnormalities or dysfunctions in gonadal function. It is essential to comprehend the physiology and regulation of the gonads to diagnose and treat disorders that impact both male and female fertility and reproductive health (Davey & Grossmann, 2016; Whirledge & Cidlowski, 2019).

5.2. Role of Hormones Such as Testosterone

Testosterone, commonly known as the "male hormone," has a diverse impact on the human body that goes beyond just masculinity. It is produced mainly in the testes in males and in smaller quantities in the ovaries and adrenal glands in females, belonging to a group of hormones called androgens. While it is most linked to male reproductive health and traits, testosterone also plays an important role in metabolism, bone density, muscle mass, mood regulation, and cognitive function in both men and women. For the development of primary and secondary sexual characteristics in males during puberty and beyond, testosterone is essential. It causes the male reproductive organs to enlarge, the voice to become deeper, and facial and body hair to grow. Additionally essential to the development of strength and muscle mass, testosterone shapes the typical male physique. Testosterone levels rise during puberty, causing physical changes that signal the passage from childhood to adulthood.

Beyond its function in the development of the body, testosterone affects many physiological functions all through life. It is essential for controlling sexual desire or libido in both men and women. Testosterone levels are frequently associated with sexual drive and arousal, but the precise mechanisms underlying this association are intricate and multidimensional. Additionally, testosterone aids in the body's metabolic functions. It affects how fat is distributed, encouraging the growth of lean muscle mass, and preventing the deposition of fat. Thus, low testosterone levels in men have been linked to metabolic diseases like insulin resistance and type 2 diabetes, as well as increased body fat and decreased muscle mass.

Furthermore, testosterone promotes bone mineralization and growth, which contributes to bone health. Reduced bone density is linked to low testosterone levels, which can raise the risk of osteoporosis and fractures, especially in older men. Thus, it's critical to maintain optimal testosterone levels to protect bone health and lower the risk of fractures and complications from osteoporosis.

Beyond its physiological effects, testosterone affects behavior, mood, and thought processes. Research has indicated that testosterone levels may affect mood regulation; low levels have been linked to fatigue, irritability, and depressive symptoms in both men and women. Additionally, testosterone might be involved in cognitive function, specifically regarding verbal fluency, memory, and spatial ability. Research on the precise connection between testosterone and cognitive function is still ongoing, though.

Additionally, testosterone has been linked to the control of emotions and social conduct. Although the degree to which testosterone influences aggression, dominance, and risk-taking behavior varies from person to person and is influenced by a variety of factors, including genetics, upbringing, and environmental circumstances, research indicates that testosterone may have an impact on these traits.

Even though testosterone is essential for many physiological functions, abnormalities in its levels can have negative health effects. Hypogonadism, or low testosterone levels, can cause symptoms like erectile dysfunction, weariness, and loss of muscle mass. On the other hand, high testosterone levels, especially in women, can cause hirsutism, or excessive hair growth, acne, and irregular menstruation.

In addition to affecting bone health, metabolism, mood regulation, behavior, and sexual characteristics, testosterone has a wide range of effects on the human body. For general health and well-being, maintaining optimal testosterone levels is crucial, and imbalances in testosterone can have serious physiological and psychological repercussions (Davey & Grossmann, 2016; Whirledge & Cidlowski, 2019).

5.2.1. Estrogen and Progesterone

Two vital hormones, estrogen and progesterone, are mostly produced by the ovaries in females, though the adrenal glands and the placenta can also synthesize smaller amounts of these hormones during pregnancy. These hormones are essential for controlling several physiological processes that occur during the female reproductive cycle. These processes affect not only reproductive function but also many other bodily systems.

Estrogen comes in various forms, the most potent of which is estradiol. It is commonly referred to as the primary female sex hormone. It is in charge of secondary sexual traits like breast development and body fat distribution, as well as the growth and maintenance of female reproductive structures like the uterus, uterine tubes, and vagina. In addition, estrogen supports cardiovascular health, brain function, and bone density.

Phases of the menstrual cycle, which are controlled by the interaction of progesterone and estrogen, are distinguished by distinct physiological events and varying hormone levels. Rising estrogen levels during the follicular phase, which lasts for the first half of the cycle, encourage the endometrium, or lining of the uterus, to develop in anticipation of the possible implantation of a fertilized egg. In addition, estrogen causes the pituitary gland to release luteinizing hormone (LH), which in turn causes ovulation—the release of a mature egg from the ovary.

The ruptured follicle becomes the corpus luteum, a transitory endocrine structure that secretes progesterone and estrogen, during the luteal phase that follows ovulation. This phase is dominated by progesterone, which is vital in promoting the thickening and vascularization of the endometrium in preparation for possible implantation. Menstruation and the shedding of the uterine lining result from a decline in estrogen and progesterone levels following fertilization and implantation.

Apart from their functions in the menstrual cycle, progesterone and estrogen have an impact on conception and delivery. The placenta assumes responsibility for producing these hormones during pregnancy, maintaining their levels to aid in gestation. The growth of fetal organs and the development of the reproductive system are two aspects of fetal development that estrogen helps control. Progesterone inhibits the mother's immune system to prevent the fetus from being rejected and preserves the uterine lining, which helps to avoid contractions that could cause premature labor.

Estrogen and progesterone have systemic effects on the body's tissues and organs in addition to their reproductive effects. For instance, estrogen lowers the risk of osteoporosis in women by promoting calcium absorption and preventing bone resorption, which helps maintain bone density. Additionally, it affects lipid metabolism, encouraging positive modifications to cholesterol levels. Furthermore, estrogen possesses neuroprotective properties that may lower the likelihood of cognitive deterioration and neurodegenerative illnesses like Alzheimer's.

Progesterone plays a role in promoting relaxation and sleep in addition to its reproductive activities. It also has calming and sedative effects on the central nervous system. Additionally, it regulates the immune system, guaranteeing the mother's tolerance to the growing fetus throughout her pregnancy. Progesterone has also been linked to breast health; in fact, some research indicates that it may even prevent the onset of breast cancer.

Essential hormones like progesterone and estrogen control many facets of female reproduction, such as the menstrual cycle, getting pregnant, and giving birth. These hormones affect a variety of tissues and organs systemically, influencing immune regulation, lipid metabolism, bone health, and cognitive function in addition to reproduction. Comprehending the functions of estrogen and progesterone is essential for managing hormone-related disorders, reproductive health, and general women's health throughout their lives.

5.2.2. Follicle-Stimulating Hormone (FSH)

One important hormone that the anterior pituitary gland, a pea-sized organ at the base of the brain, produces and releases is called follicle-stimulating hormone (FSH). It is essential for controlling the reproductive system in both males and females, mostly through promoting the development of gametes (eggs in females and sperm in males) and the synthesis of sex hormones. In females, the ovarian cycle, which controls the maturation of eggs and the production of ovarian hormones, is largely dependent on FSH.

FSH levels rise in the early follicular phase of the menstrual cycle, promoting the development and growth of ovarian follicles, each of which contains an immature egg (oocyte). FSH stimulates the granulosa cells' ability to proliferate within the follicles and produce more estrogen. A negative feedback loop results in the follicles secreting more and more estrogen as they get older, which in turn prevents them from secreting more FSH.

FSH in females plays a key role in the development and maturation of ovarian follicles, a process known as folliculogenesis. FSH helps multiple follicles grow, but usually, only one becomes dominant and reaches ovulation. This process is triggered by a surge in LH, stimulated by increasing estrogen levels. Ovulation is the release of a mature egg from the ovary. After ovulation, FSH levels decrease and the remaining follicles regress, preparing for the next menstrual cycle.

FSH acts on the sustentacular cells in the testes' seminiferous tubules, where it promotes spermatogenesis—the process of producing new sperm cells—in males. Initiating signaling cascades that promote the growth and differentiation of germ cells into mature spermatozoa, FSH binds to receptors on sustentacular cells. In conjunction with testosterone, another necessary component for spermatogenesis, FSH guarantees the uninterrupted generation of sperm, thereby preserving male fertility.

The pituitary gland, gonads, and hypothalamus all have feedback mechanisms in place to control the intricate process of regulating FSH secretion. The hypothalamus secretes gonadotropin-releasing hormone (GnRH), which causes the anterior pituitary gland to release more FSH and LH. The hypothalamus and pituitary receive feedback from the levels of sex hormones, specifically testosterone in men and estrogen in women, which regulate the secretion of GnRH, FSH, and LH in a precisely calibrated regulatory system.

Both male and female infertility and a variety of reproductive disorders can result from disturbances in FSH activity or levels. Low levels of FSH may be linked to hypothalamic or pituitary dysfunction, whereas high levels may suggest ovarian failure or decreased ovarian reserve in women. Abnormal FSH levels in men have been linked to male infertility and spermatogenic disorders. Follicle-stimulating hormone (FSH) stimulates the development of gametes and coordinates the production of sex hormones, which in turn controls reproductive function in both males and females. Normal reproductive health and fertility depend on its exact control and balanced activity.

5.2.3. Luteinizing Hormone (LH)

The anterior pituitary gland is a pea-sized structure at the base of the brain that secretes the hormone luteinizing hormone (LH). LH is essential for controlling the reproductive system in both males and females, working in tandem with follicle-stimulating hormone (FSH) to mainly stimulate the production of sex hormones and initiate ovulation in females. LH affects the ovaries in females during the menstrual cycle, which has multiple phases, such as the luteal, ovulation, and follicular phases.

Positive feedback inhibits the release of both LH and FSH during the follicular phase, which is the first half of the menstrual cycle. This is due to growing ovarian follicles' production of estrogen. But when the follicles get older, estrogen levels rise, which sets off a positive feedback loop that causes an abrupt spike in LH secretion—a phenomenon called the LH surge.

Ovulation, or the release of a mature egg from the ovary, is caused by the LH surge and usually occurs in the middle of the menstrual cycle. An essential step in the reproductive process, ovulation enables sperm to fertilize eggs, which leads to the development of embryos. The ruptured follicle becomes the corpus luteum, a transitory endocrine structure that secretes progesterone, another crucial hormone that aids in the uterus's preparation for the possible implantation of a fertilized egg, after ovulation.

Male sex hormone testosterone is produced and secreted in response to interstitial cells in the testes being activated by LH. Testosterone is essential for male reproductive function, which includes the growth and maintenance of secondary sexual traits like the development of muscle mass, facial and body hair, and deepening of the voice. Additionally, it promotes spermatogenesis, which is the process by which sperm are produced in the testes' seminiferous tubules. Robust feedback mechanisms involving the hypothalamus, pituitary gland, and gonads regulate the secretion of LH. The hypothalamus secretes gonadotropin-releasing hormone (GnRH), which causes the anterior pituitary gland to release more LH and FSH. The release of GnRH and LH is regulated by feedback from sex hormones like testosterone and estrogen, which helps to preserve the delicate balance in the reproductive system.

Hormonal imbalances and a variety of reproductive disorders can result from abnormalities in LH activity or levels. Elevated levodopamine levels could be a sign of diseases like primary testicular failure (hypogonadism) in men or polycystic ovarian syndrome (PCOS) in women. On the other hand, low levels of LH may be linked to pituitary or hypothalamic dysfunction, which can result in reduced testosterone production in men and infertility or irregular menstruation in women. LH stimulates the production of testosterone in men and ovulation in women, and it is an essential regulator of reproductive function in both sexes. Normal reproductive health and fertility depend on exact control and balanced activity (Davey & Grossmann, 2016; Whirledge & Cidlowski, 2019).

5.3. Role of Sex Hormones in the Human Body

The hormone known as gonadal steroid (GSH) is involved in both the non-reproductive and reproductive systems. Gonadads are initially visible in the fifth week of pregnancy and develop on the medial surface of mesonephric ridges due to this early effect on the fetus. Thus, the kind of hormones and gonads that are present determine sexual development and discrimination. GSH has a significant impact on sexual behavior and function. Androgen and estrogen receptors can be found in several central nervous system structures, including the hypothalamus, midbrain, amygdala, cortex, and anterior pituitary gland. For a cellular response to occur, the GSH needs to bind to particular receptors. Receptor-antagonist binding typically results in the deactivation of these receptors.

5.3.1. Physiological Effects of Sex Hormones

Sex hormones are a class of steroidal hormones that function as chemical messengers in the body. Their chemical structures are derived from cholesterol. Steroid hormones act through receptors on extracellular proteins that are members of the nuclear substances family. These receptors alter the transduction of signals in a context-specific way by both genomic and non-genomic means.

Sex hormones, such as progesterone, estrogen, and testosterone, have a multitude of physiological effects on different parts of the body, including the reproductive system and other systems and processes.

These hormones are essential for growth, metabolism, cardiovascular health, bone health, brain function, and mood regulation:

1. Reproductive System:
   - Estrogen and progesterone regulate the menstrual cycle, ovulation, and the maintenance of pregnancy in females.
   - Testosterone is essential for spermatogenesis in males and the development and maintenance of male reproductive tissues.
2. Secondary Sexual Characteristics:
   - Estrogen promotes the development of female secondary sexual characteristics such as breast development, widening of the hips, and the growth of pubic and axillary hair.
   - Testosterone is responsible for the development of male secondary sexual characteristics such as facial and body hair growth, deepening of the voice, and increased muscle mass.
3. Bone Health:
   - Estrogen plays a crucial role in maintaining bone density by inhibiting bone resorption and promoting calcium absorption. Estrogen deficiency, as seen in menopause, can lead to osteoporosis.
   - Testosterone also contributes to bone health in both men and women by stimulating bone formation and mineralization.
4. Metabolism:
   - Estrogen influences lipid metabolism, promoting favorable changes in cholesterol levels by increasing high-density lipoprotein (HDL) cholesterol and decreasing low-density lipoprotein (LDL) cholesterol.
   - Testosterone helps regulate metabolism by promoting muscle growth and fat metabolism, contributing to overall body composition and energy expenditure.
5. Cardiovascular Function:
   - Estrogen has cardioprotective effects, helping to maintain healthy blood vessels, reduce inflammation, and improve endothelial function. It may lower the risk of cardiovascular disease in premenopausal women.
   - Testosterone may also have cardioprotective effects by improving cardiac function and reducing the risk of atherosclerosis and coronary artery disease.
6. Cognition and Mood Regulation:
   - Estrogen influences cognitive

function and mood regulation, with some evidence suggesting it may enhance memory, attention, and mood stability.

- Testosterone is associated with cognitive function, mood regulation, and spatial abilities, although the mechanisms are not fully understood.

7. Immune Function:
   - Sex hormones play a role in modulating immune function, with estrogen generally enhancing immune responses and testosterone exerting immunosuppressive effects.
8. Skin Health:
   - Estrogen contributes to skin health by maintaining skin thickness, collagen production, and elasticity. It also influences hair growth and hydration.
   - Testosterone regulates sebum production and hair growth, affecting skin texture and acne development.

Overall, sex hormones have a variety of effects on bodily physiological functions, underscoring their significance beyond the reproductive system. These hormones can cause a variety of health problems if they are out of balance or deficient, which highlights the importance of managing and regulating them properly.

5.3.2. Estrogen Receptor

5.3.2.1. Genomic Activity

Estrogen binds to SHBG in the blood and in the interstitial fluid, where it penetrates the cell membrane enters the cell nucleus, and binds to receptors. These 2 genes are encoded for 2 estrogen isoforms α and β.

The hormone-receptors structure forms dimers (usually ERα-ERα, ERβ-ERβ, or Erα-ERβ) that bind to a specific nucleotide sequence, namely, Estrogen-response elements (EREs) in regions that control different gene regulation of transcription (*see* Figure 5.1).

Estrogen functions via several nuclear receptors. The vagina, the breast, and the endometrium are all impacted by estrogen. Furthermore, it interacts with interleukin, parathyroid hormone, vitamin D, and calcitonin. The growth and division of skin cells, connective tissue, and mucosal membranes are stimulated by estrogen.

5.3.2.2. Non-Genomic Activities

Non-genomic mechanisms mediate the fast actions of estrogen, including the elimination of Ca^{2+} granular cells and uterine blood flow. The non-genomic activity takes place without binding to estrogen receptors in cells. One significant non-genomic effect of estrogen is its beneficial effects on blood vessels.

It affects the cerebral, coronary, and carotid arteries in addition to the blood vessels in the reproductive system. Nitrous oxide synthesis mediates endothelial protection and vasodilation. In addition, estrogen promotes the synthesis of prostacyclin, which has vasodilator and anti-platelet properties. Additionally, acetylcholine dilates blood vessels exclusively when estrogen is present (Davey & Grossmann, 2016; Whirledge & Cidlowski, 2019).

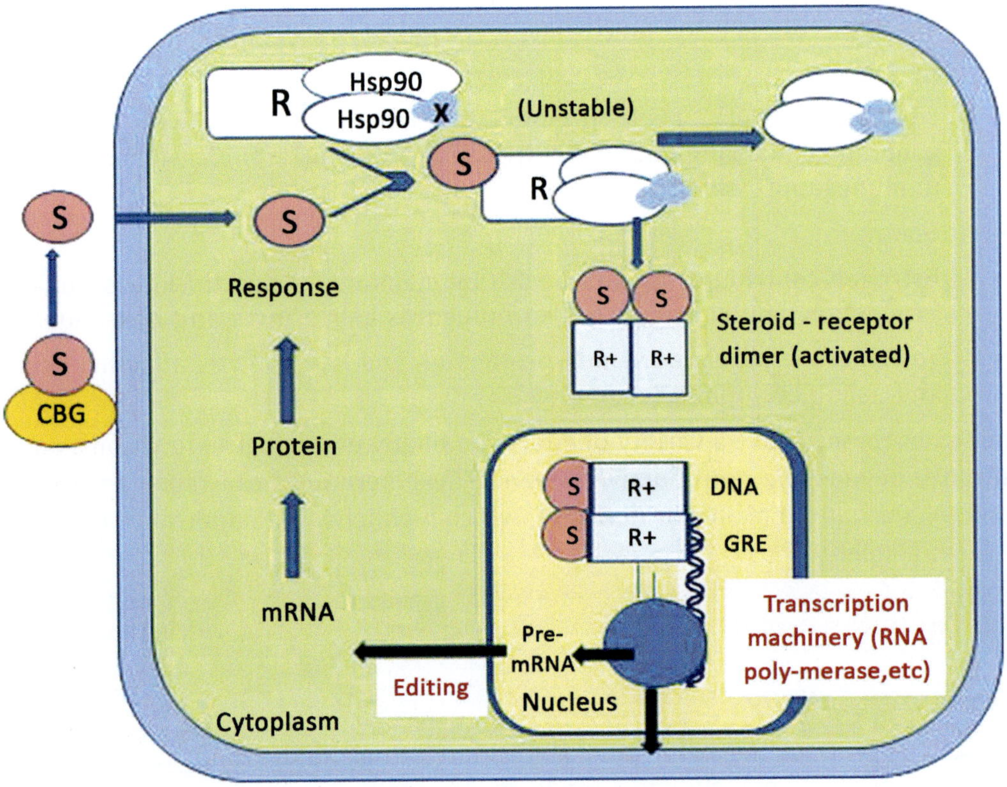

Figure 5.1. *Genomic action of steroid hormones (estrogen) in the cell.*

Source: Malik, A. N., (2021). Role of Sex Hormones in the Human Body. IntechOpen. doi: 10.5772/intechopen.95778.

5.3.3. Progesterone Receptors

Similar to estrogen, progesterone acts through nuclear receptors, specifically the PR-A and PR-B isoforms of progesterone receptors. The B-upstream segment, which is an additional 164 amino acids at the N-terminal region of PR-B that is absent from PR-A, is the difference between these two isoforms. Furthermore, loss of PRB-specific gene regulation activity results from any mutations in the amino acids in the B-upstream segment. PR-A and PR-B are typically found in equal amounts in human tissues, but disruptions in this ratio regulation can result in tissue abnormalities, such as those seen in breast cancers. Like estrogen progesterone receptors have genomic and non-genomic activities as shown in Figure 5.2.

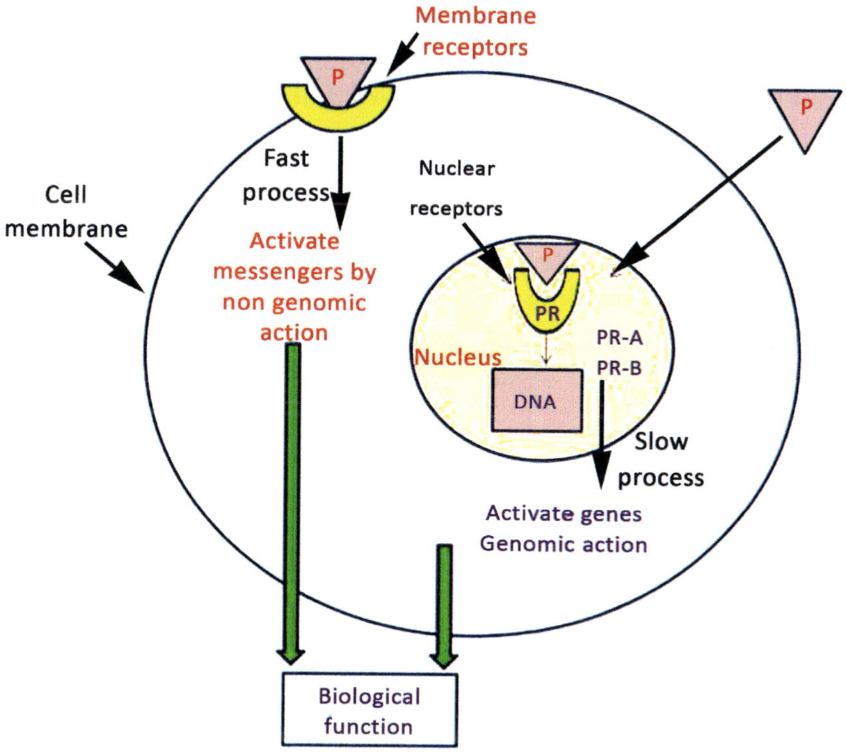

Figure 5.2. *Mode of progesterone action by genomic and non-genomic actions.*

Source: Malik, A. N., (2021). Role of sex hormones in the human body. IntechOpen. doi: 10.5772/intechopen.95778.

5.3.4. Androgen Receptors

Androgen belongs to the steroid hormone nuclear receptor family. The location of androgen receptors is on the X chromosome. These receptors are composed of 3 functional domains: the ligand binding domain, the DNA binding domain, and the N-terminal transcriptional regulation domain (Figure 5.3).

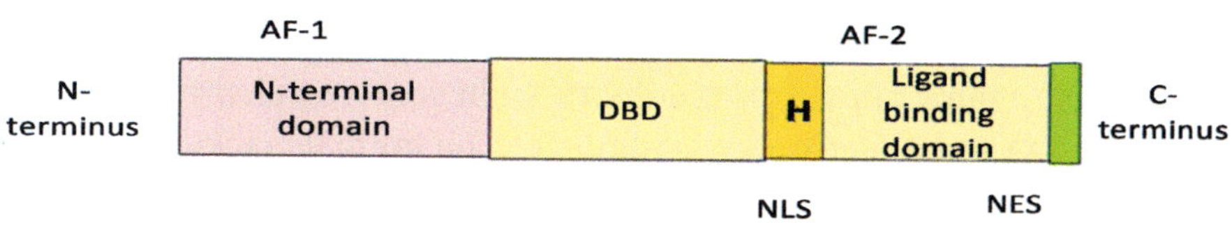

Figure 5.3. *Functional domains of the androgen receptor (AR): N-terminal domain, DNA binding domain (DBD), ligand binding domain. [AF-1: Transcriptional activating function 1; AF-2: transcriptional activating function 2; H: hinge region; NLS: nuclear localization signal; and NES: nuclear export signal].*

Source: Malik, A. N., (2021). Role of sex hormones in the human body. IntechOpen. doi: 10.5772/intechopen.95778.

Among the different types of steroid hormone receptors in the nucleus, the DBD is the most highly protected region, whereas the N-terminal domain of the androgen receptor is the most variable. Furthermore, this will cause a specific activation of the androgen receptors because of the highly protected DNA binding domain among steroid hormone receptors (nuclear receptors), which also contain selective androgen response elements.

When compared to testosterone, dihydrotestosterone binds to androgen receptors with a twofold greater affinity and a roughly fivefold lower dissociation rate. Similar to estrogen and progesterone, androgen receptors function through two different mechanisms: genomic (DNA-dependent) and non-genomic (DNA-independent) binding (Figure 5.4).

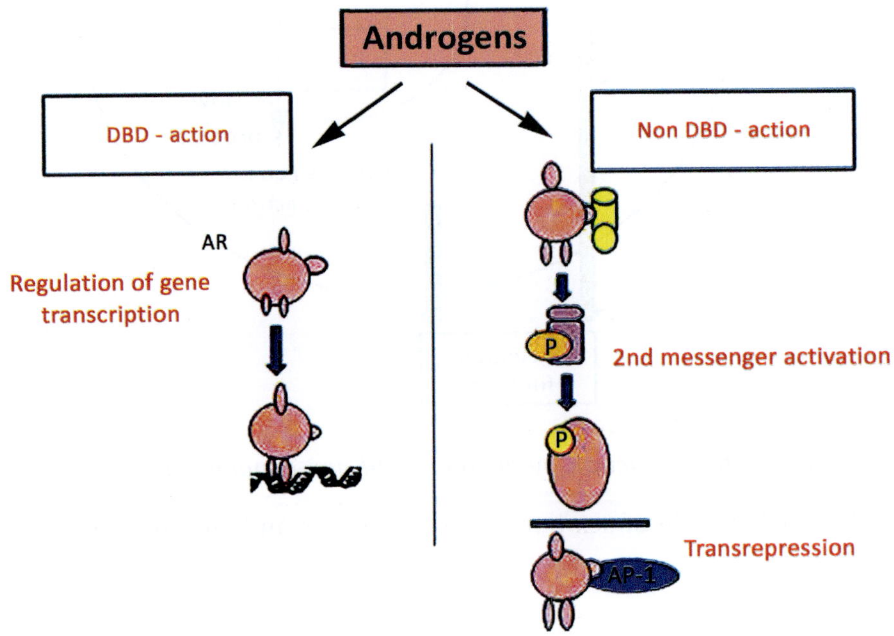

Figure 5.4. *Mechanisms of ligand-dependent androgen receptor (AR) action.*

Source: Malik, A. N., (2021). Role of sex hormones in the human body. IntechOpen. doi: 10.5772/intechopen.95778.

The biological effects of androgens on the muscle, bone, adipose tissue, prostate, nervous system, cardiovascular system, immune system, and hematopoietic system are critical. The biological effects of the AR mutation cause men's androgen receptors to become insensitive, which feminizes the male's external genitalia (XY female). Research conducted on animals lacking AR has demonstrated that a higher frequency of women experiencing premature ovarian senility due to follicular atresia is linked to androgenic signaling. Further examination of AR-free mice revealed abnormalities in the luteinization process of the ovarian follicle.

This is largely because androgens are transported to the prostate and play a role in metabolism, cell cycle formation, and growth factor signaling regulation. Furthermore, separate from the parasitic AR signal in the stroma, the epithelial AR signal in the prostate is associated with an "infection." AR is a crucial treatment for prostate cancer because it promotes VEGF-related angiogenesis and prostate growth. It has been demonstrated that AR signaling causes cancers in the breast, bladder, pancreas, ovary, and endometrium, among other organs.

5.3.5. The Biological Effects of Sex Steroids

Although estradiol and progesterone levels vary during menstruation, estrogen and progesterone levels are always higher in women than in men (Table 5.1).

Table 5.1. *Normal Ranges of Sex Steroids in Males and Females*

Gonadal Steroids	Normal Range, Conventional Units
Estradiol	• Women, basal 20–60 pg./mL. • Women, ovulatory surge >200 pg./mL. • Men <50 pg./mL.
Progesterone	• Women, luteal phase 2–20 ng/mL. • Women, follicular phase <2 ng/mL. • Men <2 ng/mL.
Dihydrotestosterone	• Women 0.05–0.3 ng/mL. • Men 0.25–0.75 ng/mL.
Testosterone	• Women <1 ng/mL. • Men 3–10 ng/mL.

Source: Malik, A. N., (2021). Role of sex hormones in the human body. IntechOpen. doi: 10.5772/intechopen.95778.

Depending on how they relate to the venereal system, estradiol and progesterone can have a variety of effects. The ovaries, uterine tubes, uterus, external genitalia, hypothalamus, and pituitary gland are all greatly impacted by steroid hormones. Non-reproductive tissues are significantly impacted by the hormones androgen, progesterone, and estrogen.

5.3.6. Cardiovascular System

Men and postmenopausal women have higher CVD risks, whereas premenopausal women have a significantly lower risk. The production of estrogen stimulates angiogenesis and supports the vasodilation effect by relaxing the smooth muscle and increasing nitric oxide production, which helps maintain low platelet activity.

Changes in susceptibility to hereditary cardiovascular diseases, which can be caused by several factors, are indicated by variations in the epidemiology, incidence, and sequelae of cardiovascular diseases in both sexes. In other instances, gender variations play a significant role in gene expression (particularly in X-chromosome genes), heart disease incidence, and the fact that, as previously mentioned, cardiovascular disease affects more men than women of the same age.

Thus, it has been proposed that the primary influence on the pathophysiology of cardiovascular disease comes from variations in sex steroid hormones. The primary sex hormones in men and women are androgens and estrogens, which are found in different amounts and have distinct biological effects on the body. Estrogens have a protective effect, in contrast to androgens, which are harmful because they increase the risk of atherosclerosis and heart disease.

As a matter of fact, during menopause (which typically lasts between 51 and 52 years), a drop in plasma estrogen and an increase in androgen are linked to a higher risk of cardiovascular disease in both men and women. This suggests that women who are going through menopause or who are developing hyperandrogenism have an increased risk of developing cardiovascular disease.

5.3.6.1. Characteristics of the Action of Sex Hormones on the Cardiovascular System, Development of Atherosclerosis and Coagulation

Due to their metabolic and vasoactive properties, sex hormones directly or indirectly affect cardiac function through genomic and non-genomic mechanisms. This effect mainly depends on the receptors, such as estrogen/testosterone are found in different cardiac cells in humans and animals. The contractions of the vascular walls were the same in male rats (in normal and castrated), but it was more evident in females with removed ovaries, indicating specific differences in vascular tone with estrogen in both sexes.

5.3.6.1.1. Oestrogenic Effects

Vascular function is impacted by estrogen via both genomic and non-genomic mechanisms. In actuality, vascular dilatation brought on by estrogen administration *in vivo* happens 5 to 20 minutes after ingestion and is unrelated to changes in gene expression. The answers appeared to be connected to sex. In this sense, intracoronary administration of estradiol has been shown to increase coronary blood flow in female patients with coronary diseases, but not in male patients.

The acute vasodilation effect of estrogen is endorsed by endothelial-dependent and independent mechanisms. The properties related to estrogen retention and transport of secondary ions (antagonist action of this hormone on Ca^{2+}), while the endothelial-dependent mechanism is highly dependent on the types of endothelial cells associated with the active estrogen receptor (EPs) by the activity of endothelial nitric oxide.

In addition, the effects of 17β-estradiol on endothelial, NO synthesis, and releases have been suggested to happen through ER alpha activation, while ER-β shows a stronger role in the non-genomic effects of estrogen including changes in blood vessels. The expression of extracellular genes and proteins is initiated by two different nuclear ERs (α and β). Both ERα and ER β have significant physiological effects on blood vessels. Animal studies have shown that ERα protects against vascular damage and atherosclerosis. ER – also controlled genes participate in the regulation of blood volume and blood pressure.

Furthermore, although this activity is low in postmenopausal women, ER intensity decreases dramatically in women with cardiovascular and cerebrovascular disease. These changes in vascular response to sex may be related to specific receptor density in vascular tissue, as the expression of sex hormone receptors may vary with sex and type of gonad.

These findings might point to a decline in estrogen's protective properties in women who have been long deprived of it. In actuality, the length of time from the onset of menopause determines the impact of estrogen on endothelial function, not the menopausal age. Estrogen generally dilates the systemic arteries, enhances peripheral and coronary endothelial function, inhibits endothelial secretion in women with coronary heart disease, and prevents coronary artery spasms. In males, blood vessels are impacted by estrogen as well. Atherosclerosis and vascular endothelial dysfunction have been linked to defective mutations in estrogen synthesis or receptor expression, according to prior research.

The production of androgen determines the levels of estrogen in men. In men, androstenedione and testosterone aromatization produced about 80% of the plasma 17-estradiol that is now known to be estrogen. Furthermore, male blood vessels directly produce estradiol, which activates endothelial smooth muscle cells' ERs. It has been observed that in men with atherosclerosis who have aromatase deficiency and endothelial dysfunction, low doses of estrogen enhance endothelial function.

Moreover, aromatase inhibitor-treated normal men experience endothelial dysfunction. The number of vasomotor tones can be influenced by sex hormones, which can change how the body reacts to vascular factors like aldosterone, angiotensin II (AII), and norepinephrine. Women are less likely than men to experience blood vessel constriction as a result of norepinephrine. Because of its vasodilation effect, endogenous estrogen aids in the regulation of blood pressure in premenopausal women.

After roughly 10 years, women start to experience high blood pressure, which is more common in older women than in men of the same age. Research on humans and animals has demonstrated that gender has an impact on atherosclerosis. Regardless of gender or weight, male or female obesity and hypertension are common causes of early and severe symptoms in animal models of atherosclerosis.

The metabolic, hemodynamic, and humeral effects that are influenced by estrogen and androgen also influence the CV profile. Furthermore, through a variety of blood stimuli, these hormones can directly influence the development of atheromas. In women, artery hardening is linked to estrogen loss (during menopause or following surgery). The severity of atherosclerosis lowers when estrogen/hormone therapy is initiated right after menopause.

When HRT begins in women who are 50–59 years old, there is a decreased risk of cardiovascular events and a lower death rate within the first 10 years following menopause. Because of this, the beneficial and detrimental effects of exogenous estrogen on blood vessels can occasionally be balanced. Hormone replacement therapy keeps the arteries from hardening. Only when hormones are started before the onset of atherosclerosis, and only then can atherosclerosis progress over time following menopause. According to current theory, there exists a "window of opportunity" during the perimenopausal or early postmenopausal years where hormonal replacement therapy may lower the risk of cardiovascular disease and its fatality by preventing atheroma formation. The significant effects of estrogen can only be achieved with oral medicines that are caused by first liver passages of hormones, which stimulate enzyme activity in the organs. In some patients, antithrombin III decreases, and factor VII and X show dose-dependent increases.

5.3.6.1.2. Mediated Effects of Testosterone

Numerous studies have failed to clarify the role of endothelium-derived NO in testosterone-induced vasodilation. Some studies have used endothelium-denuded tissue and inhibitors of NO synthesis, and these studies have suggested a partial role for NO; however, other studies have not found a connection between NO and testosterone-induced vasodilation. Testosterone-induced relaxation appears to involve the opening of K+ channels and the blockage of L-type calcium channels. It is an endothelium-independent relaxation that is not gender-specific or mediated by hormonal receptors.

The bloodstream expression of androgen receptors varies with the amount of estrogen present, indicating the density of distinct types of receptors in men and suggesting a sex-related response to androgen. While the full impact of testosterone on males remains unclear, the relationship between estrogen levels and the effects of androgens on females is less evident. The same plasma concentration is seen in transgender women who change their sexual orientation to become male and receive long-lasting testosterone. The shape and pattern of the brachial arteries are similar to those of females of the same age, but the diameter is larger due to impaired nitrate-induced vasodilation. Blood testosterone concentrations in postmenopausal women receiving estrogen therapy are roughly five times higher than normal levels, and vasodilation is enhanced. In women, testosterone has an effect similar to that of estrogen. The androgenic effects of women with atherosclerosis are largely determined by the ratio of estradiol to testosterone, rather than the levels of estrogen. In men having coronary angiography, there is a negative correlation between free testosterone levels and coronary heart disease. Furthermore, men with thicker intima-media have been found to have lower levels of androgen.

Women with serious medical conditions, like PCOS, provide observations that are used to evaluate potential androgenic effects in women. Due to high testosterone levels, women with PCOS have atherosclerosis and heart disease. They also have an increased risk of myocardial infarction (MI). This risk factor was compared to (132) females of the same age who did not have PCOS. The risk factor sample was established from independent risk factors for MI in a prospective population study conducted in Göteborg, Sweden, involving 1,462 female participants. The factors included increased waist/hip circumference ratio (central obesity), age, diagnosed hypertension, diabetes mellitus, and serum triglyceride levels. Compared to normal females of the same age, females with polycystic ovary syndrome had a frequently elevated risk (relative risk of 7.4) of developing MI (Davey & Grossmann, 2016; Whirledge & Cidlowski, 2019).

5.3.7. Lipid Metabolism and Sex Hormones

Sex hormones can influence lipid profiles, lipoprotein, HDL, LDL, and triglycerides—the latter two of which are crucial for the development of CVD—either directly or indirectly. The main cause of this is reduced estrogen production. In the liver, estrogen promotes the production of HDL, apolipoprotein A-I, and decreased triglyceride levels. Additionally, it enhances the reversion of cholesterol transport. Consequently, these hormones raise HDL levels while lowering triglyceride, LDL, and total cholesterol levels as well. Because of its unique androgenic properties and its function as an aromatization substrate for estradiol (E2), testosterone can have an impact on fat metabolism.

Heart disease is more common in both sexes, and elevated plasma testosterone levels are thought to affect the lipoprotein profile. According to data on men, plasma testosterone levels are inversely correlated with total cholesterol, LDL, triglycerides, fibrinogen, and PAI-1, and positively correlated with HDL-c serum levels. Clinical research has revealed that testosterone treatment has no effect on HDL cholesterol in older men, but several studies indicate that the overall effect on fat metabolism is a component of the unexplained effects on excess weight and insulin resistance.

These advantageous effects have the required result. Estradiol/testosterone ratio and estrogen levels determine how testosterone therapy affects the lipid profile of women, primarily by lowering HDL cholesterol. On the other hand, low HDL-c is androgenic. Because HDL-c can show a reduction in subfraction of HDL3, it is not directly linked to a significant reduction in cholesterol transport, and thus should not be regarded as a direct pro-atherogenic risk factor.

5.3.8. Obesity

Sex hormones are linked to variations in body fat distribution between genders. Even though androgens have been connected to the development of belly fat. The distribution of fat in Android is linked to androgen deficiency. The quantity and distribution of fat in women are correlated with ovarian function. Women gain weight during their periods; the fat is distributed in the gynoid region, with peripheral obesity, and the middle region (abdomen) during menopause.

High waist/hip ratios and abdominal circumference are indicators of the distribution of fat in androids in both sexes. These markers are linked to insulin resistance, serum triglycerides, low-density lipoprotein cholesterol, hypertension, and an increase in sympathetic drive, among other negative metabolic changes. Because androids do not produce sex hormones, they also have an impact on hormonal metabolism.

Supplements for male testosterone are made to decrease abdominal fat, promote lipolysis, and prevent the buildup of fat. Because testosterone also improves metabolic markers like lipid and glucose metabolism, hormone replacement treatment makes women gain weight and stops menopausal pattern body fat from spreading. Most people are unaware of the precise mechanism underlying this effect.

5.3.9. The Effect of Sex Hormones on Bone Regeneration and Resorption

Osteoporosis is brought on by a deficiency of the hormone estrogen (E2) in postmenopausal women and is partly responsible for osteoporosis in older men. Osteoclast cells (OC) proliferate more when there is an E2 deficiency, and their activity also increases concurrently with a decrease in apoptosis. Functional estrogen receptors have been present since the development of osteoblasts (*see* Figure 5.5).

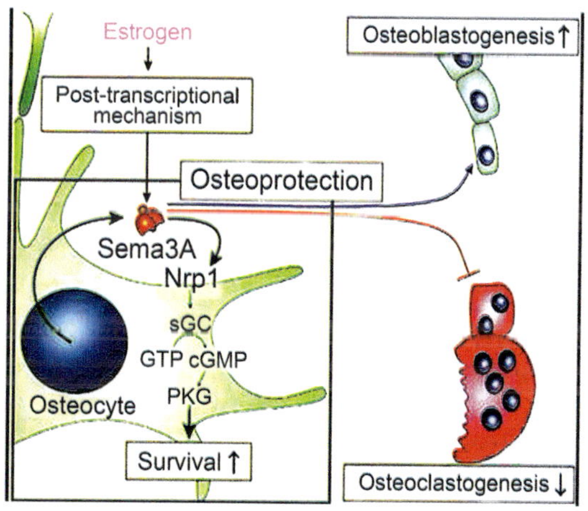

Figure 5.5. *The biological effects of estrogen on the bone.*

Source: Malik, A. N., (2021). Role of sex hormones in the human body. IntechOpen. doi: 10.5772/intechopen.95778.

The molecular underpinnings of estrogen activity have been rapidly but incompletely understood since 1988. The unique functions of cytokines, such as IL-1, IL-6, TNF-A, granulocytes, macrophage stimulating factor (M-CSF), and prostaglandin E2 (PGE2), which raise OC volume and activity in bone marrow, are the main reasons metabolism is important. Instead of producing more TNF, TNF-a-producing T cells in T cell-deficient OVX mice can produce more T cells overall. In this instance, bone marrow monocytes do not regulate tumor necrosis factor-α. It enhances M-CSF by increasing the production of RANKL-dependent OC. TNF-a directly affects precursors of OC. The bone-protective effects are altered by estradiol B (E2), which lowers the estrogen signal, particularly in bone cells in males and females. To transform bone cells into bone marrow, ER A is required. But it's challenging to form osteocytes that need estrogen.

5.3.10. Sex Hormones and Their Role in the Skin

Progesterone and estrogen preserve the dermal and epidermal layers' normal thickness while also promoting soft, healthy skin. Estrogen stimulates, proliferates, and inhibits keratinocyte apoptosis. Progesterone inhibits matrix metalloproteases in response to estrogen's increase in collagen synthesis in the skin, which works in tandem with estrogen to reduce the breakdown of collagen. In the dermis, estrogen promotes the synthesis and build-up of glycosaminoglycan.

Additionally, estrogen encourages wound healing. Numerous investigations have demonstrated the protective role of estrogen and its positive effects on skin physiology. It has been demonstrated that they quicken skin lesions' healing process. Pregnancy helps most women heal from inflammatory skin diseases like psoriasis, and estrogen may also have some protective effects against photoaging of the skin.

5.3.11. Effect of Sex Hormones on the Uro-Genital Tract

In the fourth week of intrauterine life, females' urogenital tracts first developed from their primitive urogenital sinuses. Both systems contain estrogen receptors, with varying blood levels of each receptor. There are a variety of symptoms associated with menstruation, most of which arise during pregnancy or after menopause when vaginal and lower urinary tract symptoms, as well as genital atrophy, are common. However, these alterations could be impacted by aging, which makes it challenging to establish causality.

5.3.11.1. Pathophysiology

Estrogen receptors are consistently found in the squamous epithelium of the vagina, urethra, and bladder trigone in areas with metaplasia. However, they are not present in the epithelium of the transitional dome of the bladder, indicating the origins of this tissue. The pelvic floor is also influenced by estrogens. In the lower urinary tract of women, estrogen increases cell cycle activity, increasing the number of superficial and intermediate cells. These changes are similar to vaginal changes seen in postmenopausal women.

Changes in the cytology of the urinary tract and vaginal tract during menstruation are nearly identical. Sediment changes following estrogen therapy are also observed. The urethral pressure profilometry (UPP) can identify regular variations in the symptoms related to urination during the menstrual cycle.

With mid-menstruation and an earlier luteal phase, the functional, anatomical, and physiological length of the urethra increases, indicating changes in the concentration of estrogen in the serum. Pregnancy also brings about changes, which validates a corresponding rise in urine output and gravid uterine pressure. A recent publication from the University of London School of Medicine raised the prospect of progesterone-mediated hormone influence on the bladder. The expression of progesterone receptors in the lower urinary tract may be linked to a woman's estrogenic status. Female bladders and urinary tracts contain androgen receptors; however, it is currently unknown what these receptors do.

5.3.11.1.1. Estrogen and Urinary Incontinence

Women, during menopause usually complain of frequent symptoms in the urinary system. The most common are frequent micturition, bed wetting, stress and urge incontinence, they may also experience urinary tract infections and vaginal symptoms, such as itching or dryness. The specific diagnosis of the underlying pathology is based on a comprehensive clinical study and the study of urodynamics. There are many causes for urinary incontinence; these include bladder dysfunction, instability with constipation, excessive urination, fistula (between the vagina and the bladder, or between vagina and ureter or with urethra), or diverticulum or immobility. The causes of transient enuresis in the elderly include urinary tract infections, estrogen deficiency, restricted mobility, medications, and depression. The two most common symptoms are stress and\ or urge incontinence.

Because of its significant role in the storage mechanism, the tissues of the pelvis and urinary tract are sensitive to estrogen. The pressure in the urethra must be higher than the pressure in the bladder for a woman to be on the continent. Because estrogen affects the epithelium, blood vessels, muscles, and connective tissues, it helps maintain positive pressure in the urethra, which is made up of four functional layers.

There have been reports of extracellular alterations in the urinary epithelial layer in response to estrogen. There is some evidence that estrogen influences the system's blood vessels and can treat female urogenital incontinence through increased sensitivity of the bladder, increased pressure in the urethra, stimulation of collagen production surrounding the urinary tract, and hypersensitivity to the alpha-adrenergic receptors of the ureteral smooth muscles.

5.3.11.1.2. Estrogen to Prevent and Treatment of Enuresis

The use of estrogen in treating enuresis is debatable, although less research has been done in this area. Some have produced consistent results, but this might be because of variations in estrogens, dosages, and duration of instructions. It is more challenging to treat this illness. To make the situation clearer, there are now two meta-analysis techniques. It was the Hormones and Urogenital Therapy (HUT) Committee's first report.

It has been discussed that postmenopausal women with enuresis can be treated with estrogen. It was not the case that only six of the 166 English-language articles published between 1969 and 1992 were taken into consideration. The findings demonstrated that for every patient with urine incontinence, actual stress is a significant psychological development. Urine volume did not change, according to the target parameters analysis. Only one test has a significant impact on the outcome, despite an increase in the maximum pressure required to close the urethra. Potentially controlled cases and 14 indirect studies of estrogen therapy were taken into consideration in the second meta-analysis. Additionally, they discovered that while estrogen therapy does not reduce stress, it can help with acute and persistent symptoms. For women in need of surgery or with low levels of stress, this approach may be helpful. Although estrogen has long been used to treat menopause and prevent frequent urination, numerous controlled studies have demonstrated its advantages. Urinary retention was lessened in 7 out of 11 women who took a combination of 2 mg of estradiol and 1 mg of estriol (Imagine Daily) as opposed to 1 in 10 who received a placebo.

5.3.11.1.3. Estrogen for Urinary Tract Infections

Women who have given birth are more likely to get a urinary tract infection (UTI) due to changes in urine production, particularly during sexual activity. The vaginal pH rises and its lactobacilli count falls as a result of colonization, which releases pathogenic Gram-negative bacteria into the urine. Estrogen can be used as a treatment or preventative measure in response to these changes, which can happen in adult women who regularly take steroids (Davey & Grossmann, 2016; Whirledge & Cidlowski, 2019).

5.3.12. Effects of Testosterone on Erythropoietin (EPO) and on Muscle

Elevated testosterone levels are crucial for hemoglobin and hematocrit, as well as for promoting EPO and lowering cellular fatigue. Testosterone stimulates EPO, improves red blood cell iron absorption, and fixes hemoglobin bound to EPO. After birth, a significant amount of DNA builds up in adult muscles, which are composed of satellite cells—which are crucial for regulating protein in muscle fibers and controlling muscle growth—and dependent cells. As a blood transporter that binds directly to muscles, testosterone raises protein levels.

5.3.13. Sex Hormones and Brain

Throughout life, estrogen participates in a variety of processes. For instance, differences in sexual behavior resulting from synaptic and neurological development. Estrogen controls both long-term and fast neuroplastic processes in the central nervous system, including synaptic-cyclical alterations, while progesterone is crucial for the synthesis of neurosteroids.

Numerous neurological processes and behaviors, including mood, pain sensitivity, blood pressure regulation, cognitive function, motor coordination, and motor coordination, are influenced by estrogen. There are subtle differences between these traits based on gender that raise questions about hormones and genetic factors, such as the mitochondrial genome.

Aging of the brain is frequently linked to numerous nervous system disorders brought on by problems at work. According to recent research, estrogen replacement therapy may lower a woman's chance of developing degenerative illnesses like Alzheimer's and cognitive decline. The largest class of medications used to stop Alzheimer's disease (AD) is estrogen.

It has been demonstrated that these steroids, which are potent neurotransmitters both *in vivo* and *in vitro*, have comparable protective effects against attention deficit disorder. The use of estrogen to reduce stress at the onset of menopause and treat Alzheimer's disease is supported by epidemiological evidence. This includes suppressing the amyloid expression of the pro-amyloid protein (A).

Epidemiological studies have shown that women develop Parkinson's disease (PD) 1.5 to 2 times lower than men, indicating a protective effect of estrogen. Experimental data show that estradiol has a protective effect on neurons and dopaminergic proteins. Studies have shown that higher levels of estrogen are associated with fewer symptoms of Parkinson's disease and an increased risk of Parkinson's disease in postmenopausal women. These data indicate that estrogen may have a protective effect on dopaminergic neurons.

5.3.13.1. Neuroprotective Effect of Estrogen

Naturally, estrogen serves additional purposes as well, such as energizing nerve cells and shielding them from external stimuli brought on by illnesses like Alzheimer's, stroke, and seizures. Although the precise function of the cellular nuclear ERs found to have an inhibitory effect on neurons is unknown, one important factor is that E2 promotes the expression and release of neuropeptide Y (NPY), which has antiexcitatory properties. The ability of E2 to translocate ER-β to mitochondria and sequester mitochondrial Ca^{2+} ions, including Bcl-2 translocation, is the second reason it is neuroprotective.

Research has demonstrated that the brain can produce cholesterol and possibly estrogen and that estrogen may be able to prevent stroke as well as fight Alzheimer's and Parkinson's disease. Pyramidal neurons are a significant subset of CA1 AR nuclei, and, like E2, androgens have a protective effect on nerve cells. In men, cholinergic activity rather than NMDA may be a major factor in the development of spinal synapses caused by nuclear ARAS.

5.3.13.2. The Behavioral Effects of Sex Hormones

Gender disparities are caused by sexual steroids, which have an impact on children's brains, particularly the hypothalamus. The sexual propensities of the three families of steroid hormones in the nervous system—estrogen, androgen, and progesterone—are linked to the behavioral differences between men and women. The elements that function as transcription factors following the disintegration of layers, nuclear translation, and the hormonal effects of DNA are linked to the classic family of receptors. Gender differences in the brain are usually anatomical, neurochemical, or molecular.

Neurotransmitters, enzymes, or regional hormones are the neurochemical targets of the sex-related neurochemical shift. Every gender difference in the hypothalamus is accompanied by molecular changes in sex, gene expression, and epigenetic modifications in phase signaling, all of which are controlled by the regulatory actions of estradiol. It has long been recognized that estrogen has a psychoactive effect. As a result, it's thought that improper estradiol metabolism could contribute to the emergence of mental illness. Variations in the area, size, number, or intensity of the brain's cells (such as variations in the size of the cells, the complexity or morphology of the brain, the length of the dendritic cells, and the number of contacts) (Davey & Grossmann, 2016; Whirledge & Cidlowski, 2019).

5.3.14. The Effect of Sex Hormones on the Immune System

About 15 years ago, the role that estrogen plays in the negotiations between the immune system and the internal system was described. Effects of estrogen: lymphoid tissue expresses CD8+ lymphocytes, macrophages, and ERF3 B lymphocyte rings, which can be membranes connected to receptors. Lymphocytes also contain anti-estrogen binding sites (AEBS) and estrogen binding sites.

Regarding cytokines: TNF levels in endotoxin coatings increase significantly with estrogen, while levels of IL-6 (due to ethylene 17 in the blood) decrease. Active ER stimulates nuclear transcription factors and maintains NF-IL6, NF-ICB, and C/EBPf3. Physiological levels of estradiol in cultured human cells significantly increase the activity of the IL-1 receptor antagonist (mRNA) but it is suppressed by higher estradiol concentrations. Estradiol 17F3 produces IL-5 mRNA *in vitro*. Estradiol and glucocorticoids activate secretory substances that prevent leukemia, sagging, and overuse in humans. Additionally, uterine epithelial cells in the uterus maintain uterine E2 cells and promote antigen secretion. Adults treated *in vitro* with 17G3-estradiol have increased natural killer cell activity. In classic ER, estradiol increases the sensitivity of human natural prostate killer cells. The cytotoxic potential of CD4+ cells is dependent on estrogen.

At physiological concentrations of estradiol (10-IOM), human polymorphonuclear leukocytes exhibit significantly less chemotactic activity. To put it briefly, antiestrogens impact the nervous and endocrine systems, target cells, or tissues in the transplant system by acting on particular estrogen receptors and lymphocytes.

Immune system alterations lead to changes in the nervous system and vice versa as they both produce a regulatory response. For instance, the thymus, an organ that produces the steroid hormone, enabled the use of this phrase. Furthermore, steroid precursors can be transformed into active hormones by the immune system.

Most of the immune system regulation is attributed to steroid hormones, which can regulate nuclear transcription factor-mediated signaling. It is unclear, nevertheless, if estrogen is required for the immune system to operate normally or if it has a variable impact on the primary estrogen levels that regulate vaccinations. The possible distinctions between the various steroid and estrogen receptors in the immune system are unknown. In men and women, estrogen regulates immune function in different ways.

Building the body's defenses against viral infections depends on estrogen. It has been demonstrated that immune modifications against the influenza virus and pneumonia are regulated and mediated by the stabilization of the cytokine storm. Women have lower levels of SARS-CoV-2 than men do because of the effects of estrogen. Some people think that SARS-CoV-2 shortens the infection by causing stress in the endoplasmic reticulum (ER).

Building the body's defenses against viral infections depends on estrogen. It has been demonstrated that immune modifications against the influenza virus and pneumonia are regulated and mediated by the stabilization of the cytokine storm. Women have lower levels of SARS-CoV-2 than men do because of the effects of estrogen. Some people think that SARS-CoV-2 shortens the infection by causing stress in the endoplasmic reticulum (ER) (Davey & Grossmann, 2016; Whirledge & Cidlowski, 2019).

A Closer Look

Parkinson's Disease

Parkinson's disease is a progressive neurodegenerative disorder that affects movement control. It was first described by James Parkinson in 1817 and has since become one of the most prevalent neurological disorders globally, affecting millions of people, predominantly those over the age of 60. However, early-onset cases can occur, albeit less frequently. The disease primarily manifests through a range of motor symptoms, including tremors, bradykinesia (slowed movement), rigidity, and postural instability. These symptoms result from the loss of dopamine-producing neurons in a region of the brain called the substantia nigra, which is responsible for regulating movement. As dopamine levels decrease, the communication between the brain and the body becomes disrupted, leading to characteristic motor impairments.

Aside from motor symptoms, Parkinson's disease can also present non-motor symptoms, such as cognitive impairment, depression, anxiety, sleep disturbances, and autonomic dysfunction. These non-motor symptoms can significantly impact a patient's quality of life and are often challenging to manage. The exact cause of Parkinson's disease remains elusive, although both genetic and environmental factors are believed to play a role. Mutations in certain genes, such as SNCA, LRRK2, and PARKIN, have been linked to familial cases of the disease, while exposure to toxins like pesticides and herbicides may increase the risk of developing Parkinson's in some individuals.

Currently, there is no cure for Parkinson's disease, but various treatment options aim to alleviate symptoms and improve quality of life. Medications such as levodopa, dopamine agonists, and MAO-B inhibitors can help manage motor symptoms by replenishing dopamine levels or mimicking its effects. Additionally, physical therapy, occupational therapy, and speech therapy can assist patients in maintaining mobility, independence, and communication skills as the disease progresses. Research into Parkinson's disease continues to advance, with ongoing studies exploring potential disease-modifying treatments and a better understanding of the underlying mechanisms. Early diagnosis and intervention remain crucial in managing the condition effectively and improving outcomes for individuals living with Parkinson's disease (Davey & Grossmann, 2016; Whirledge & Cidlowski, 2019).

Summary

- Reproductive hormones play a vital role in regulating the complex processes of human reproduction, orchestrating the development and functioning of reproductive organs, gamete production, and the menstrual cycle in females.
- The hypothalamus, a small but crucial region nestled deep within the brain, serves as a central hub for regulating a myriad of physiological processes essential for maintaining homeostasis and orchestrating complex behaviors.
- Testosterone, often dubbed the "male hormone," plays a multifaceted role in the human body, influencing various physiological processes beyond just masculinity. Produced primarily in the testes in males and in smaller amounts in the ovaries and adrenal glands in females, testosterone belongs to a class of hormones called androgens.
- Follicle-stimulating hormone (FSH) is a key hormone produced and released by the anterior pituitary gland, a pea-sized organ located at the base of the brain.
- It plays a crucial role in the regulation of reproductive function in both males and females, primarily by stimulating the development of gametes (sperm in males and eggs in females) and the production of sex hormones.
- Gonadal Steroid hormones (GSH) play an important role in reproductive and non-reproductive systems. As this effect occurs early in the fetus' life, gonads are initially present at the fifth weeks and developed on the medial surface of mesonephric ridges.
- Estrogen is involved in many processes throughout life. Minds of men and women. For example, neurological developmental and synaptic changes resulting in sexual behavioral differentiation. Progesterone is important for synthesis of neurosteroid, and estrogen regulates rapid and prolonged neuroplastic processes in the central nervous system, including synaptic-cyclical changes.

References

1. Anderson, G. L., Limacher, M., Assaf, A. R., et al. (2004). Effects of conjugated equine estrogen in postmenopausal women with hysterectomy: The Women's Health Initiative randomized controlled trial. *JAMA, 291*(14), 1701–1712.
2. Arnal, J. F., Scarabin, P. Y., Tremollieres, F., Laurell, H., & Gourdy, P. (2007). Estrogens in vascular biology and disease: Where do we stand today? *Current Opinion in Lipidology, 18*(5), 554–560.
3. Ashcroft, G. S., & Ashworth, J. J. (2003). Potential role of estrogens in wound healing. *American Journal of Clinical Dermatology, 4*(11), 737–743.
4. Carr, M. C. (2003). The emergence of the metabolic syndrome with menopause. *Journal of Clinical Endocrinology and Metabolism, 88*(6), 2404–2411.
5. Cenci, S., et al. (2000). Estrogen deficiency induces bone loss by enhancing T cell production of TNFa. *Journal of Clinical Investigation, 106*, 1229–1237.
6. Chambliss, K. L., Yuhanna, I. S., Anderson, R. G., Mendelsohn, M. E., & Shaul, P. W. (2002). ER β has non-genomic action in caveolae. *Molecular Endocrinology, 16*(4), 938–946.

7. Chikani, G., Zhu, W., Smart, E. J., et al. (2004). Lipids: Potential regulators of nitric oxide generation. *American Journal of Physiology–Endocrinology and Metabolism, 287*, E386–E389.

8. Chrousos, G. P. (2015). The gonadal hormones & inhibitors. In *Basic and Clinical Pharmacology* (13th ed., pp. 1024–1064).

9. Davey, R. A., & Grossmann, M. (2016). Androgen receptor structure, function, and biology: From bench to bedside. *Clinical Biochemistry Reviews, 37*(1), 3–15.

10. Eisermann, K., & Fraizer, G. (2017). The androgen receptor and VEGF: Mechanisms of androgen-regulated angiogenesis in prostate cancer. *Cancers, 9*(4), E32.

11. English, K. M. J. R., Jones, T. H., Morice, A. H., & Channer, K. S. (2002). Testosterone acts as a coronary vasodilator by a calcium-antagonistic action. *Journal of Endocrinological Investigation, 25*(6), 455–458.

12. Giralt, D., Domingues-Montanari, S., Mendioroz, M., Ortega, L., Maisterra, O., Perea-Gainza, M., & Montaner, J. (2012). The gender gap in stroke: A meta-analysis. *Acta Neurologica Scandinavica, 125*, 83–90.

13. Hayashi, M., Nakashima, T., Yoshimura, N., et al. (2019). Autoregulation of osteocyte Sema3A orchestrates estrogen action and counteracts bone aging. *Cell Metabolism, 29*(3), 627–637.

14. Hergenc, G., Schulte, H., Assmann, G., & Von Eckardstein, A. (1999). Associations of obesity markers, insulin, and sex hormones with HDL-cholesterol levels in Turkish and German individuals. *Atherosclerosis, 145*(1), 147–156.

15. Hodges, Y. K., Tung, L., Yan, X. D., Graham, J. D., Horwitz, K. B., & Horwitz, L. D. (2000). Estrogen receptors alpha and beta: Prevalence of estrogen receptor beta mRNA in human vascular smooth muscle and transcriptional effects. *Circulation, 101*(15), 1792–1798.

16. Hodgin, J. B., Krege, J. H., Reddick, R. L., et al. (2001). Estrogen receptor alpha is a major mediator of 17beta-estradiol's atheroprotective effects on lesion size in Apoe–/– mice. *Journal of Clinical Investigation, 107*, 333–340.

17. Hodis, H. N., Mack, W. J., Azen, S. P., et al. (2003). Hormone therapy and the progression of coronary-artery atherosclerosis in postmenopausal women. *New England Journal of Medicine, 349*(6), 535–545.

18. Hu, Y. C., Wang, P. H., Yeh, S., et al. (2004). Subfertility and defective folliculogenesis in female mice lacking androgen receptors. *Proceedings of the National Academy of Sciences of the United States of America, 101*(31), 11209–11214.

19. Huggins, C., & Hodges, C. V. (1941). Studies on prostatic cancer: I. The effect of castration, estrogen, and androgen injection on serum phosphatases in metastatic carcinoma of the prostate. *Journal of Urology, 168*(1), 9–12.

20. Isidori, A. M., Giannetta, E., Greco, E. A., et al. (2005). Effects of testosterone on body composition, bone metabolism, and serum lipid profile in middle-aged men: A meta-analysis. *Clinical Endocrinology, 63*, 280–293.

21. Jaaskelainen, J. (2012). Molecular biology of androgen insensitivity. *Molecular and Cellular Endocrinology, 352*(1–2), 4–12.

22. Jacobsen, B. M., & Horwitz, K. B. (2012). Progesterone receptors, their isoforms, and progesterone-regulated transcription. *Molecular and Cellular Endocrinology, 357*(1–2), 18–29.

23. Jones, R. D., Hugh Jones, T., & Channer, K. S. (2004). The influence of testosterone upon vascular reactivity. *European Journal of Endocrinology, 151*, 29–37.

24. Kanashiro, C. A., & Khalil, R. A. (2001). Gender-related distinctions in protein kinase C activity in rat vascular smooth muscle. *American Journal of Physiology–Cell Physiology, 280*, C34–C45.

25. Kapoor, D., Malkin, C. J., Channer, K. S., & Jones, T. H. (2005). Androgens, insulin resistance and vascular disease in men. *Clinical Endocrinology, 63*, 239--250.

26. Kneale, B. J., Chowienczyk, P. J., Brett, S. E., Coltart, D. J., & Ritter, J. M. (2000). Gender differences in sensitivity to adrenergic agonists of forearm resistance vasculature. *Journal of the American College of Cardiology, 36*, 1233–1238.

27. Lakoski, S. G., Brosnihan, B., & Herrington, D. M. (2005). Hormone therapy, C-reactive protein, and progression of atherosclerosis: Data from the estrogen replacement on progression of coronary artery atherosclerosis (ERA) trial. *American Heart Journal, 150*, 907–911.

28. Lawrence Riggs, B. (2000). The mechanisms of estrogen regulation of bone resorption. *The Journal of Clinical Investigation, 106*(10), 1203–1204.

29. Lew, R., Komesaroff, P., Williams, M., Dawood, T., & Sudhir, K. (2003). Endogenous estrogens influence endothelial function in young men. *Circulation Research, 93*, 1127–1133.

30. Lloyd-Jones, D. M., Evans, J. C., & Levy, D. (2005). Hypertension in adults across the age spectrum: Current outcomes and control in the community. *JAMA, 294*, 466–472.

31. Manolagas, S. C. (2000). Birth and death of bone cells: Basic regulatory mechanisms and implications for the pathogenesis and treatment of osteoporosis. *Endocrine Reviews, 21*, 115–137.

32. Manson, J. E., Allison, M. A., Rossouw, J. E., et al. (2007). Estrogen therapy and coronary-artery calcification. *New England Journal of Medicine, 356*, 2591–2602.

33. McCrohon, J. A., Death, A. K., Nakhla, S., et al. (2000). Androgen receptor expression is greater in macrophages from male than from female donors. A sex difference with implications for atherogenesis. *Circulation, 101*, 224–226.

34. Mendelsohn, M. E. (2002). Genomic and nongenomic effects of estrogen in the vasculature. *American Journal of Cardiology, 90*(10A), 3F–6F.

35. Mendelsohn, M. E. (2002). Protective effects of estrogen on the cardiovascular system. *American Journal of Cardiology, 89*(12A), 12E–18E.

36. Mendelsohn, M. E., & Karas, R. H. (2005). Molecular and cellular basis of cardiovascular gender differences. *Science, 308*, 1583–1587.

37. Mendelsohn, M. E., & Rosano, G. M. (2003). Hormonal regulation of normal vascular tone in males. *Circulation Research, 93*, 1142–1145.

38. Mikkola, T. S., & Clarkson, T. B. (2002). Estrogen replacement therapy, atherosclerosis, and vascular function. *Cardiovascular Research, 53*, 605–619.

39. Morris, E. (2017). The menopause and post-reproductive health. In *Gynecology by Ten Teachers* (20th ed., chap. 8, pp. 171–194).

40. Nakamura, Y., Suzuki, T., & Sasano, H. (2005). Estrogen actions and in situ synthesis in smooth muscle cells and their correlation with atherosclerosis. *Journal of Steroid Biochemistry and Molecular Biology, 93*, 263–268.

41. Orshal, J. M., & Khalil, R. A. (2004). Gender, sex hormones, and vascular tone. *American Journal of Physiology-Regulatory, Integrative and Comparative Physiology, 286*, R233–R249.

42. Panda, B., Rao, L., Tosh, D., et al. (2011). Germline study of AR gene of Indian women with ovarian failure. *Gynecological Endocrinology, 27*(8), 572–578.

43. Pare, G., Krust, A., Karas, R. H., et al. (2002). Estrogen receptor-α mediates the protective effects of estrogen against vascular injury. *Circulation Research, 90*(11), 1087–1092.

44. Poehlman, E. T., Toth, M. J., & Gardner, A. W. (1995). Changes in energy balance and body composition at menopause: A controlled longitudinal study [Retraction in Sox, H. C. *Annals of Internal Medicine, 123*, 673–675].

45. Raychaudhuri, S. P., Navare, T., Gross, J., et al. (2003). The clinical course of psoriasis during pregnancy. *International Journal of Dermatology, 42*, 518–520.

46. Regitz-Zagrosek, V., Oertelt-Prigione, S., Prescott, E., Franconi, F., Gerdts, E., Foryst-Ludwig, A., & Stangl, V. (2016). Gender in cardiovascular diseases: Impact on clinical manifestations, management, and outcomes. *European Heart Journal, 37*, 24–34.

47. Riggs, B. L., Khosla, S., & Melton, L. J., III. (1998). A unitary model for involutional osteoporosis: Estrogen deficiency causes both type I and type II osteoporosis in postmenopausal women and contributes to bone loss in aging men. *Journal of Bone and Mineral Research, 13*, 763–773.

48. Rosano, G. M., Gebara, O., Sheiban, I., et al. (2006). Acute administration of 17beta-estradiol reduces endothelin-1 release during pacing-induced ischemia. *International Journal of Cardiology, 116*, 34–39.

49. Schweizer, M. T., & Yu, E. Y. (2017). AR-signaling in human malignancies: Prostate cancer and beyond. *Cancers (Basel), 9*(1), 7.

50. Shiina, H., Matsumoto, T., Sato, T., et al. (2006). Premature ovarian failure in androgen receptor-deficient mice. *Proceedings of the National Academy of Sciences of the United States of America, 103*(1), 224–229.

51. Stevenson, S., & Thornton, J. (2007). Effect of estrogens on skin aging and the potential role of SERMs. *Clinical Interventions in Aging, 2*(3), 283–297.

52. Tchernof, A., Poehlman, E. T., & Despres, J. P. (2000). Body fat distribution, the menopause transition, and hormone replacement therapy. *Diabetes and Metabolism, 26*, 12–20.

53. Thornton, M. J. (2002). The biological actions of estrogens on skin. *Experimental Dermatology, 11*, 487–502.

54. Thornton, M. J. (2005). Oestrogen functions in skin and skin appendages. *Expert Opinion on Therapeutic Targets, 9*, 617–629.

55. Tikkanen, M. J., Vihma, V., Jauhiainen, M., et al. (2002). Lipoprotein-associated estrogens. *Cardiovascular Research, 56*, 184–188.

56. Tsai, E. C., Boyko, E. J., Leonetti, D. L., & Fujimoto, W. Y. (2000). Low serum testosterone level as a predictor of increased visceral fat in Japanese American men. *International Journal of Obesity and Related Metabolic Disorders, 24*, 485–491.

57. Tsukahara, K., Moriwaki, S., Ohuchi, A., et al. (2001). Ovariectomy accelerates the photoaging of rat skin. *Photochemistry and Photobiology, 73*, 525–531.

58. Tsukahara, K., Nakagawa, H., Moriwaki, S., et al. (2004). Ovariectomy is sufficient to accelerate

spontaneous skin aging and to stimulate ultraviolet irradiation-induced photoaging of murine skin. *British Journal of Dermatology, 151*, 984–994.

59. Vitale, C., Mercuro, G., Cerquetani, E., et al. (2008). Time since menopause influences the acute and chronic effect of estrogens on endothelial function. *Arteriosclerosis, Thrombosis, and Vascular Biology, 28*, 348–352.
60. von Eckardstein, A., & Wu, F. C. W. (2003). Testosterone and atherosclerosis. *Growth Hormone & IGF Research, 13*, S72–S84.
61. Whirledge, S., & Cidlowski, J. A. (2019). Steroid hormone action. In Yen & Jaffe's *Reproductive Endocrinology* (8th ed., Chapter 5, pp. 115–131). Elsevier.
62. White, B. A. (2013). Introduction to the endocrine system. In *Endocrine and Reproductive Physiology* (4th ed., pp. 1–25e2).
63. Wild, S., Pierpoint, T., McKeigue, P., & Jacobs, H. S. (2000). Cardiovascular disease in women with polycystic ovary syndrome at long-term follow-up: A retrospective cohort study. *Clinical Endocrinology, 52*, 595–600.
64. Worboys, S., Kotsopoulos, D., Teede, H., McGrath, B., & Davis, S. R. (2001). Evidence that parenteral testosterone therapy may improve endothelium-dependent and -independent vasodilation in postmenopausal women already receiving estrogen. *Journal of Clinical Endocrinology & Metabolism, 86*, 158–161.
65. Wu, F. C., & von Eckardstein, A. (2003). Androgens and coronary artery disease. *Endocrine Reviews, 24*, 183–217.
66. Yildiz, O., & Seyrek, M. (2007). Vasodilating mechanisms of testosterone. *Experimental and Clinical Endocrinology & Diabetes, 115*, 1–6.
67. Zhou, Y., Bolton, E. C., & Jones, J. O. (2015). Androgens and androgen receptor signaling in prostate tumorigenesis. *Journal of Molecular Endocrinology, 54*(1), R15–R29.
68. Zhu, Y., Bian, Z., Lu, P., et al. (2002). Abnormal vascular function and hypertension in mice deficient in estrogen receptor β. *Science, 295*, 505–508.

Chapter

MENSTRUAL CYCLE

6

Contents

Unit Introduction

The menstrual cycle, which lasts roughly 28 days on average but can vary from person to person, is a complicated but essential process in the female reproductive system. It is controlled by a complex interaction of hormones and has multiple phases, each with a specific function in getting the body ready for a possible pregnancy. Menstruation, also referred to as a period, is the start of the cycle and signifies the shedding of the uterine lining that had accumulated in preparation for pregnancy during the previous cycle. Hormonal fluctuations cause mood swings and physical symptoms like bloating and cramping, which usually last for three to seven days. The follicular phase, which lasts roughly from day 1 to day 14 of the cycle, comes after menstruation. Follicle-stimulating hormone (FSH) causes multiple ovarian follicles to mature during this phase, each of which contains an immature egg. These follicles produce estrogen as they grow, which encourages the uterine lining to thicken in anticipation of the possible implantation of a fertilized egg. Ovulation is triggered by an increase in luteinizing hormone (LH) around day 14, which is the middle of the cycle. This is the mature egg being released from one of the ovarian follicles into the uterine tube, where should sexual activity take place, it may be fertilized by sperm. A significant event in the menstrual cycle, ovulation is frequently accompanied by changes in vaginal discharge and, in certain cases, mittelschmerz, a mild form of pelvic pain. The luteal phase, which occurs from roughly days 15 to 28 of the cycle, comes after ovulation. The ruptured ovarian follicle develops into the corpus luteum, a structure that secretes progesterone, during this phase. To prepare the uterine lining to support a fertilized egg, progesterone aids in maintaining its thickness. The menstrual cycle restarts if fertilization is unsuccessful because the body sheds the uterine lining again due to a drop in hormone levels.

The primary purpose of the menstrual cycle is reproduction, but other aspects of physical and mental health may also be impacted by hormonal fluctuations. Some people get symptoms at different stages of their cycle, like headaches, breast tenderness, and mood swings. People who are aware of and monitor their menstrual cycle are better able to anticipate these changes and alleviate any discomfort that may be related. For those who have ovaries, the menstrual cycle is a fascinating and complex process that is essential to their reproductive health. Every stage of the menstrual cycle, from ovulation to uterine lining preparation, is critical to fertility and general health. Although it could present difficulties for some, this is an essential and normal part of human biology.

Orientation and Directional Terms:

Terms	Definition	Illustration
Menstrual cycle	The menstrual cycle is counted from the first day of one period to the first day of the next. The cycle isn't the same for everyone.	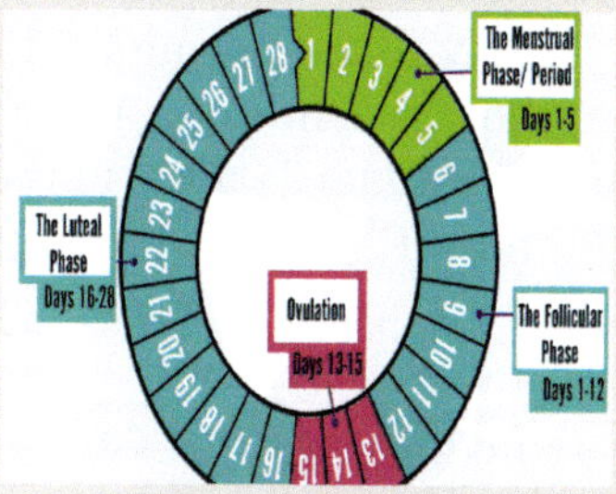
Corpus luteum	The corpus luteum is a temporary collection of cells that forms on your ovary each menstrual cycle if you're still getting a menstrual period.	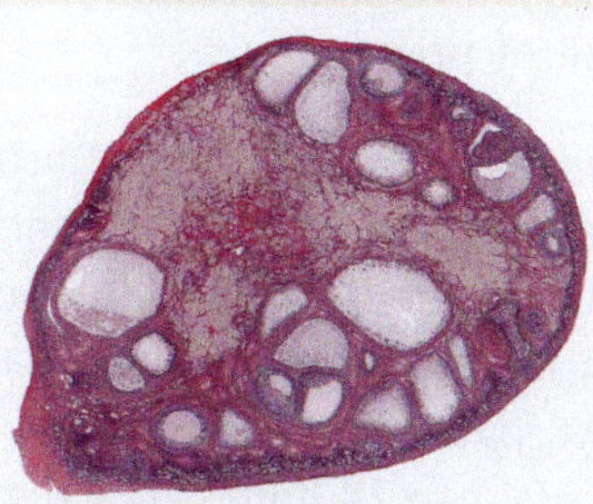
Zygote	A zygote is the first diploid cell that is formed by the fusion of male and female gametes resulting in the formation of an embryo.	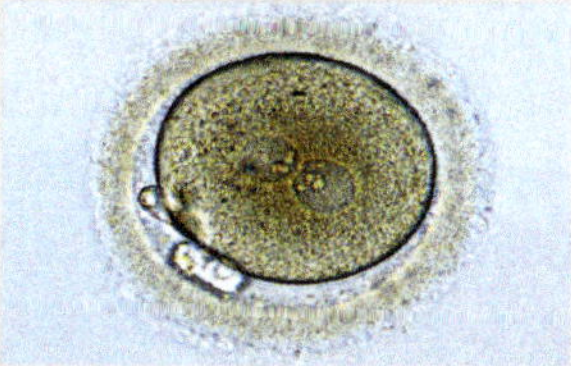
Breast	The breast is one of two prominences located on the upper ventral region of the torso among humans and other primates.	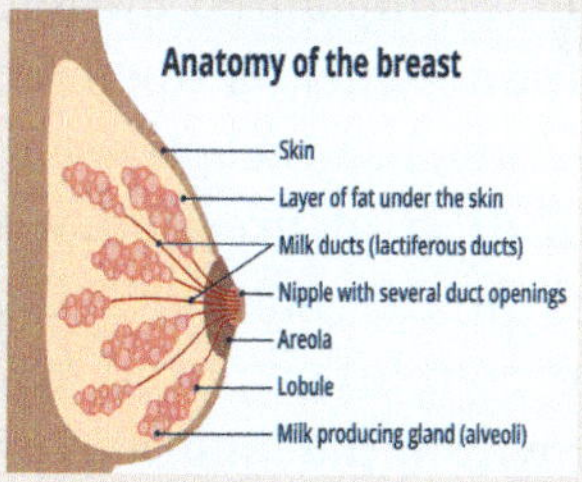
Follicular Phase	The follicular phase is the first half of the menstrual cycle, and is also known as the preovulatory or proliferative phase.	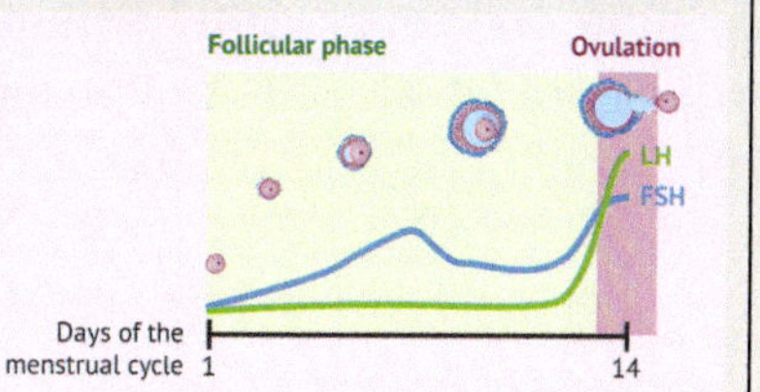

6.1. Normal Menstrual Cycle

The normal menstrual cycle is a recurring process that occurs month after month, with the hypothalamus, pituitary gland, and ovary all playing key roles. Hormones like GnRH, FSH, LH, estradiol, and inhibin A are secreted in a coordinated manner, leading to the development of a dominant follicle, ovulation, and the production of progesterone by the corpus luteum. This cycle typically lasts 28 days, with a normal fluctuation of ±2 days. A regular cycle is crucial for successful embryo implantation in the case of pregnancy.

This requires that, during the ovulatory stage, a capacitated spermatozoon reach an adequate ovule to be fertilized. While spermatozoa can remain in the feminine genital tract for up to five days, ovum fecundation can only occur for a period of 12 to 24 hours. The distal third of the uterine tube is where fertilization takes place, and four days later, the fertilized zygote arrives in the form of a morula to be implanted at the endometrium. When a blastocyst reaches the stage of hatching, it separates from its shaggy region and is implanted during the window of implantation, which is open from days 7 to 9, postovulation, in a receptive endometrium. The first indication of pregnancy is the presence of β-hCG in the mother's blood. Only 25% of fertile couples exposed to pregnancy can conceive within the month of exposure (Wilcox et al., 2000; Hale et al., 2007; Mihm et al., 2011; Skorupskaite et al., 2014; Patricio & Sergio, 2019).

6.1.1. Definition of Normality

Around 28 ± 7 days make up a menstrual cycle. Only 33 patients have cycled every 28 days, and 80% fluctuate between 22 and 32 days. When a cycle's frequency fluctuates by no more than two days, it is referred to as regular. Every cycle's duration is computed from the first day of menstruation to the day before the subsequent menstrual cycle begins. The hypothalamus-pituitary-gonadal axis controls the frequency of the cycle; hormones like luteinizing hormone (LH) and follicle-stimulating hormone (FSH) must reach their effectors at the ovarian level, where a dominant follicle must be developed and recruited. This follicle must secrete enough estradiol to obtain endometrial receptivity while also actively participating in a feedback-regulated control of the cycle.

In the first two years following menarche and during the transition to perimenopause, cycles exhibit greater irregularity. These are the extremes of the reproductive lifespan. The ovarian cycle consists of two phases that are separated by ovulation. The first phase is known as the follicular or proliferative phase and lasts from the start of the cycle to ovulation. The second is known as the luteal phase or secretory phase and occurs between ovulation and the subsequent menstrual cycle.

The maturation of the follicle, which contains an ovule and a retinue of follicular cells, is what defines the follicular phase. These cells oversee converting androstenedione into estradiol, which is then released and, among many other things, promotes endometrial renewal. The follicular cavity that emerges from the ovule after release is called the luteal phase. It is during this phase that the ovule transforms into a corpus luteum, which not only produces significant amounts of estrogen but also releases progesterone. The luteal phase lasts ±14 constant days when comparing different women; it begins with ovulation, which is preceded by a significant increase in LH. Women's average body temperature is continuously 0.5°C higher during this phase than it was during the follicular phase.

The endometrium separates in the absence of embryo implantation, resulting in menstrual flow with normal volume parameters up to 80 mL, duration of 3–8 days, content, lack of clots and symptoms, and absence of pain. It is believed that the hypothalamic-pituitary-gonadal axis is in good health as expressed by the conserved cyclicity.

6.1.2. Important Concepts

1. **Ovarian Reserve:** It is determined during fetal life and represents the number of follicles that a woman has. After that, the number of follicles gradually decreases. Each woman has a set number of ova when she is born, which are lost over time (atresia). Postponing pregnancy is not advised because there is a higher chance that she won't have high-quality ovum when it is time to get pregnant. Fertility in women is lower in the 38–40 age range than in the 25–30 age range. Oocyte atresia is an ongoing process that does not halt, not even during anovulatory or gestational phases.
2. **Oocyte Atresia:** The process of follicular apoptosis appears to have a role in the selection of ideal ovules. In the ovary, roughly 7,000,000 oocytes are formed during the early fetal stage. Apoptotic (programmed death) mechanisms have reduced the ovular reserve to one-third before birth.

   Just 1–2 million oocytes are left in the ovary at birth, and during puberty, 3,00,000 oocytes are typically accessible for ovulation. Throughout their life, they will only ovulate between 400 and 500 times. Then, during a woman's reproductive life, between puberty and menopause, roughly 2,50,000 follicles will eventually die, with perimenopause seeing fewer than 1,000 of them survive (Figure 6.1).

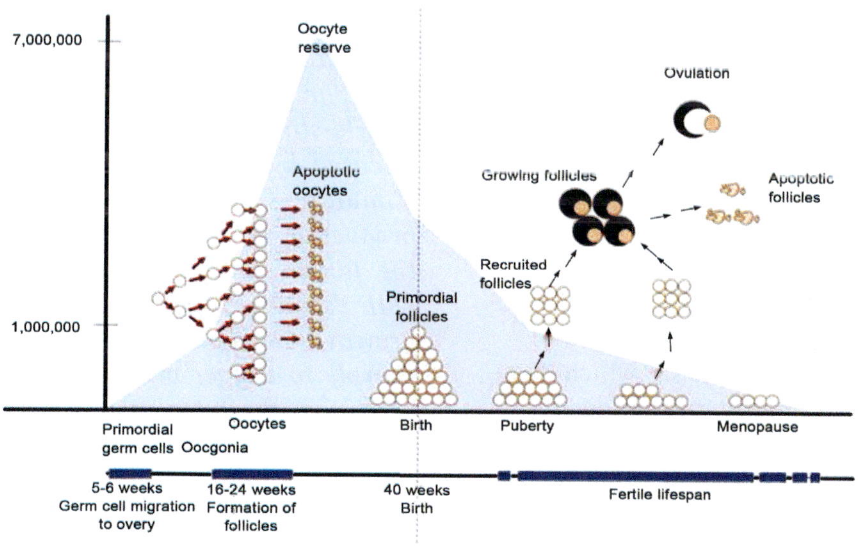

Figure 6.1. *The number of oocytes in any woman is defined now of birth and slows down inevitably during her life from 1 to 2 million at the moment of birth at 3,00,000 to decreasing through her life to 25,000 at 37–38 years and nearly 500 during the post-menopause.*

Source: Patricio, B. P., & Sergio, B. G., (2019). Normal menstrual cycle. IntechOpen. doi: 10.5772/intechopen.79876.

3. **Sex Steroids – Estrogens and Progesterone:** The corpus luteum, the placenta, and the granulosa follicle (if a pregnancy is present) all produce estrogens, which are steroid hormones. Its synthesis is derived from molecules of cholesterol. If a pregnancy is present, the placenta and corpus luteum synthesize progesterone.

The estrogens, the most potent is estradiol. The actions they develop are:

i. **Female Genital Apparatus:** they stimulate the growth and development of the female sexual organs and the proliferation of the endometrium during the sexual cycle.
ii. **Breast:** They favor the growth of the mammary ducts and are, in part, responsible for the development of the mammary gland during puberty.
iii. **Bone:** They regulate the osteoclastic activity and stimulate the osteoblastic activity, in such a way that they are essential to maintain adequate bone mineralization.
iv. **Cardiometabolic:** Estrogen relaxes the smooth muscle of arterioles, increases HDL cholesterol, and lowers LDL cholesterol, which has been associated with the lower incidence of cardiovascular disease that women have in relation to men, especially before menopause.

Another steroid hormone is progesterone. It oversees the endometrial progestational changes. Progesterone acts as a complement to estrogens by stimulating the growth of the lobes on the breasts. Some women experience an increase in basal temperature following ovulation, which is partially attributed to the thermogenic properties of progesterone.

6.1.3. Follicular Phase

On the very first day of menstruation, the follicular phase starts. Before the mature follicle is released during ovulation, the process known as folliculogenesis, or the development of ovarian follicles, starts in the final days of the menstrual cycle (Figure 6.2).

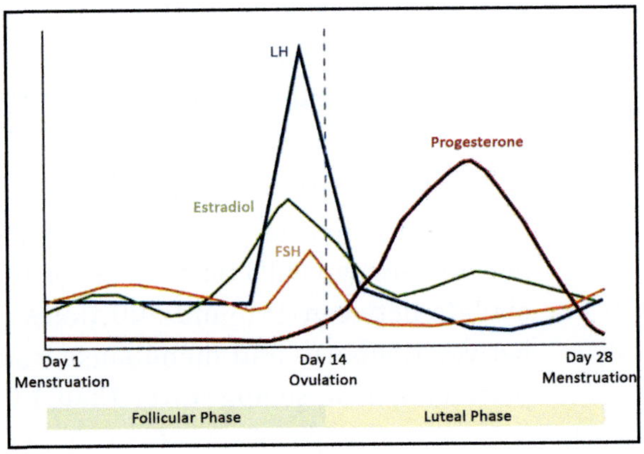

Figure 6.2. *The menstrual cycle has two phases – the follicular phase and luteal phase. The follicular phase begins with menstruation. The follicle-stimulating hormone (FSH) increases released by the anterior pituitary gland and stimulates follicular growth and estradiol production. The 17 beta-estradiol produced by the follicles exerts negative feedback on the FSH. Estradiol continues to increase due to the growth of the dominant follicle. The LH increases sharply to trigger ovulation. Immediately after ovulation, the luteal phase begins. The corpus luteum produces progesterone and 17 beta-estradiol concentrations of progesterone and estradiol decrease, and menstruation begins a new cycle unless pregnancy has been established.*

Source: Patricio, B. P., & Sergio, B. G., (2019). Normal menstrual cycle. IntechOpen. doi: 10.5772/intechopen.79876.

By the time, the corpus Luteum's functional period ends, there is a decrease in the release of sex steroids and inhibin A in cases where a pregnancy did not occur. Both declines lessen the central feedback mechanism's release of FSH, which is reliant on the hypothalamic GnRH's pulsatility. This is how the final few days of the menstrual cycle see an increase in FSH (Figures 6.3 and 6.4).

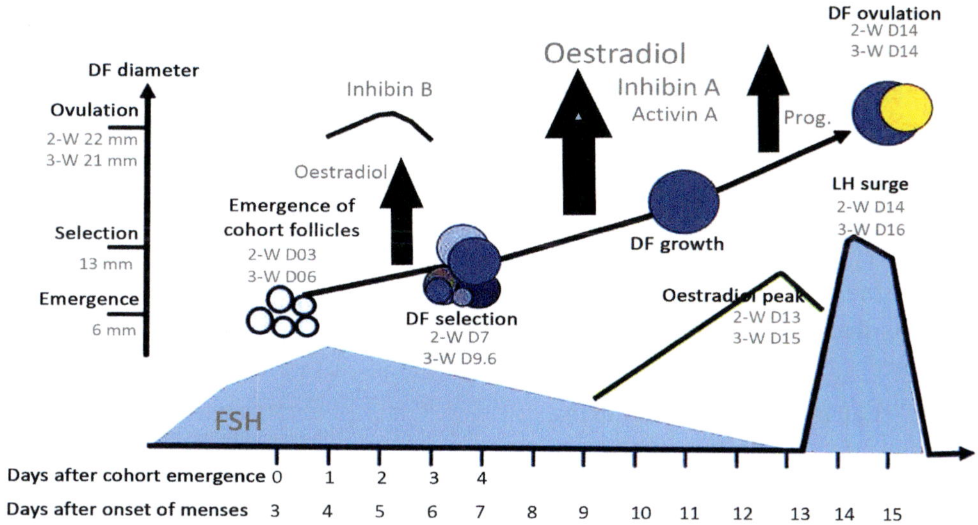

Figure 6.3. *Dynamic scheme of follicular activity and the changes in gonadotropins, steroids, and inhibins during the follicular phase of the menstrual cycle.*

Source: Patricio, B. P., & Sergio, B. G., (2019). Normal menstrual cycle. IntechOpen. doi: 10.5772/intechopen.79876.

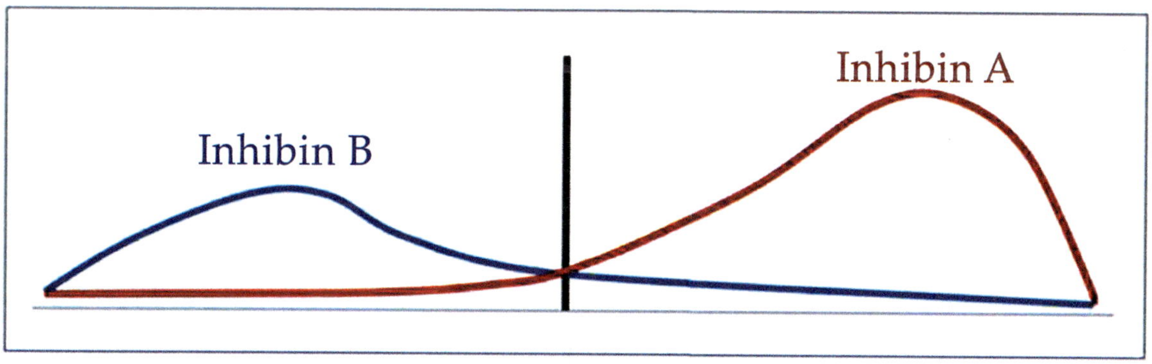

Figure 6.4. *The level of inhibin changes through the menstrual cycle. Inhibin B dominates the follicular phase during the cycle while inhibin A dominates the luteal phase.*

Source: Patricio, B. P., & Sergio, B. G., (2019). Normal menstrual cycle. IntechOpen. doi: 10.5772/intechopen.79876.

It is possible to recruit numerous follicles at once due to the gradual increase in FSH. However, only a small percentage endure to the point where, in about 99% of cycles, only a dominant follicle will be expected to ovulate in the ensuing menstrual cycle. Around 1% of women have codominance, or two dominant follicles, which may eventually result in double ovulation and increase the chance of multiple pregnancies.

In women from 19 to 42 years, the follicular phase has an average duration of 14.6 days, however, to be precise for each woman what step of the cycle is very difficult because of the following reasons:

- The duration of the menstrual cycle is very changing, even among young women of similar ages, with variations described from 25 to 34 days.
- Changes that normally occur during the fertile lifespan, between the menarche to menopause. Some women may have long and irregular cycles, many times associated with abundant uterine bleeding, in the first 2 years after menarche and 4–6 years that precede menopause.
- Besides, there is a wide range of presentation for both phases of the cycle, the follicular phase may last from 10 to 23 days and the luteal phases could last between 7 and 19 days. Only 10% of women with a cycle of 28 days show follicular and luteal phases of 14 days. The variability depends more on the follicular phase, which varies ±3–7 days with time, depending on the estrogen take-off (ETO), at the beginning of the middle follicular phase on each cycle, which is the main explanation for the duration of cycles.
- Finally, despite the normal length of their cycles, 7% of women of 25–39 years may show anovulation, even though is more frequent to observe shorter cycles or longer ones, especially in early post-menarche and pre-menopause (60% between 10 and 14 years and 34% older than 50 years) as seen in Figure 6.5.
- Other environmental, ethnic, or even socioeconomic factors may affect the duration of the cycle and bleeding.

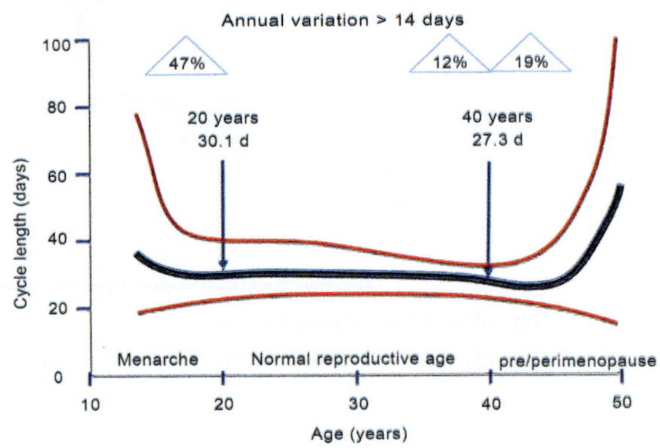

Figure 6.5. *Menstrual cycle lasting variation according to age. The graphic shows the average time of the cycle and the range (percentiles 95 and 5) [yrs.: years; and d: days]. Triangles indicate the group of age in the percentage of women with more than 14 days of variation of a cycle during a year.*

Source: Patricio, B. P., & Sergio, B. G., (2019). Normal menstrual cycle. IntechOpen. doi: 10.5772/intechopen.79876.

In the development of a dominant follicle (DF), three steps have been described namely, recruiting, selection, and dominance (Figure 6.6). The recruiting stage is developed during the days 1–4 of the menstrual cycle.

FSH oversees attracting new follicles to join the pool during the follicular phase. Follicle selection typically takes place between days 5 and 7 of the cycle, allowing only one follicle—the dominant follicle (FD)—to ovulate while the others undergo atresia. The granular layer secretes anti-Müllerian hormone (AMH), which also plays a role in FD selection. On the eighth day of the cycle, the FD suppresses the maturation of the other ovarian follicles by promoting its growth.

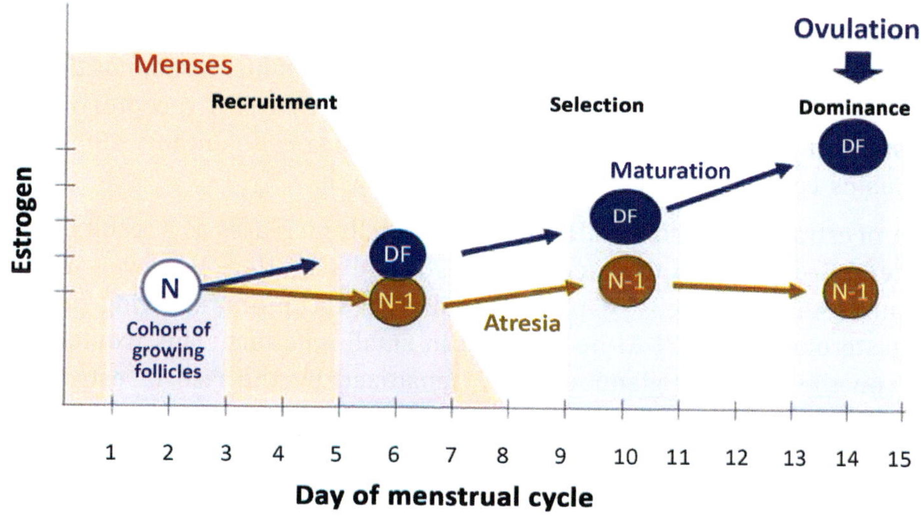

Figure 6.6. *Time-lapse of recruiting, selection, and ovulation of dominant follicle (DF) with the beginning of atresia in the other follicles of the group.*

Source: Patricio, B. P., & Sergio, B. G., (2019). Normal menstrual cycle. IntechOpen. doi: 10.5772/intechopen.79876.

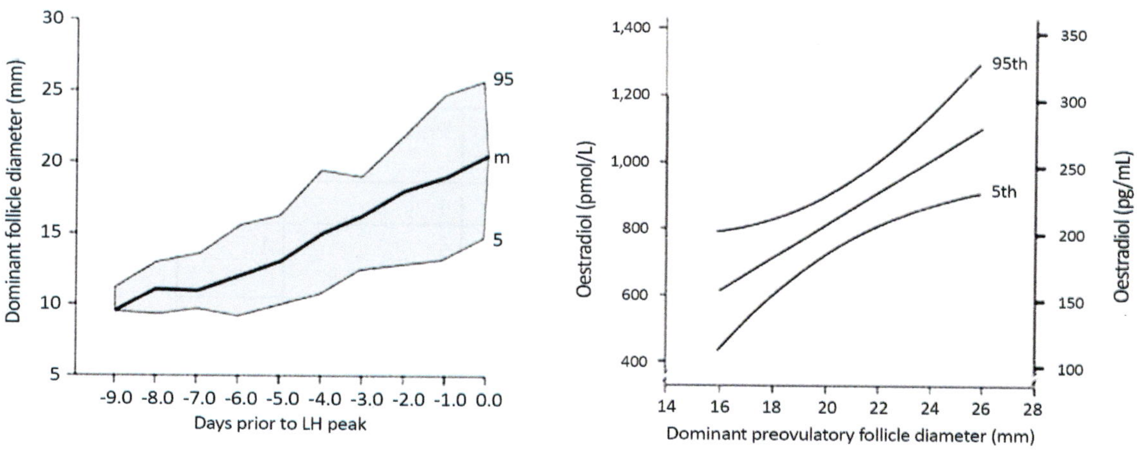

Figure 6.7. *Diameter of dominant follicle (DF) days before LH peak and plasma concentration of estradiol per follicle diameter (curved lines are 95th and 5th percentiles).*

Source: Patricio, B. P., & Sergio, B. G., (2019). Normal menstrual cycle. IntechOpen. doi: 10.5772/intechopen.79876.

Estradiol plasma levels rise during the follicular phase in tandem with the expansion of the DF and granulosa cell population. Granulosa cells only have FSH receptors in their cell membrane. By converting androstenedione, which diffuses from the theca cells, the increase in FSH during the late luteal phase stimulates its own FSH receptors and ultimately increases the secretion of estradiol by the granulosa cells (Figure 6.7).

It is crucial to note that the population of granulosa cells has increased, not the concentration of FSH receptors on them, which is the cause of the increase in FSH receptor numbers. During the secondary stage of follicular development, each granulosa cell contains 1500 FSH receptors; this number remains constant for the duration of DF growth.

The number of estradiol receptors (ER) in granulosa cells increases as a result of their receptors being upregulated in response to the increase in estradiol secretion. However, when estradiol is present, FSH causes the same cells to produce more LH receptors, allowing progesterone and 17-hydroxyprogesterone (17 OHP) to be secreted in small amounts. This would have a positive feedback effect on the pituitary gland. Already sensitized by the rise in estrogen, luteinizing hormone (LH) can be released and reach its peak. Numerous steroidogenic enzymes, including aromatase and 3β-hydroxysteroid dehydrogenase (3β-HSD), are also stimulated by FSH.

Other signaling pathways influence the differentiation of theca cells, in addition to LH. These pathways include insulin-like 3 (INSL3), which seems to regulate LH-mediated androgen biosynthesis and increased luteal regression and apoptosis in follicle cells, bone morphogenetic proteins (BMPs) generated by granulosa cells, and/or oocytes that counteracted the effects of LH and INSL3, the circadian clock genes, androgens, and estrogens, and (2) theca-associated vascular, immune, and fibroblast cells.

In Table 6.1, production rates are presented for sexual steroids during the follicular phase, and luteal phase at the moment of ovulation.

Table 6.1. *Production Rate of Sex Steroids in Women at Different Stages of the Menstrual Cycle*

Sex Steroids	Early Follicular	Preovulatory	Mid-Luteal
Progesterone (mg)	1	4	25
17α-Hydroxyprogesterone (mg)	0.5	4	4
17α-Hydroxyprogesterone (mg)	7	7	7
Androstenedione (mg)	2.6	4.7	3.4
Testosterone (μg)	144	171	126
Estrone (μg)	50	350	250
Estradiol (μg)	36	380	250

Source: Patricio, B. P., & Sergio, B. G., (2019). Normal menstrual cycle. IntechOpen. doi: 10.5772/intechopen.79876.

LH receptors are located at theca cells throughout the whole menstrual cycle, in contrast to granulose cells. Granuloma cells are stimulated by LH receptors. At the theca cells, LH increases the synthesis of androstenedione and, to a lesser extent, testosterone. After androstenedione is transferred to granulosa cells, it undergoes aromatization and ultimately transforms into type I estradiol 17-β-hydroxysteroid dehydrogenase. This is referred to as the "two cells, two gonadotropins, regulation of ovarian synthesis hypothesis" (Figure 6.8).

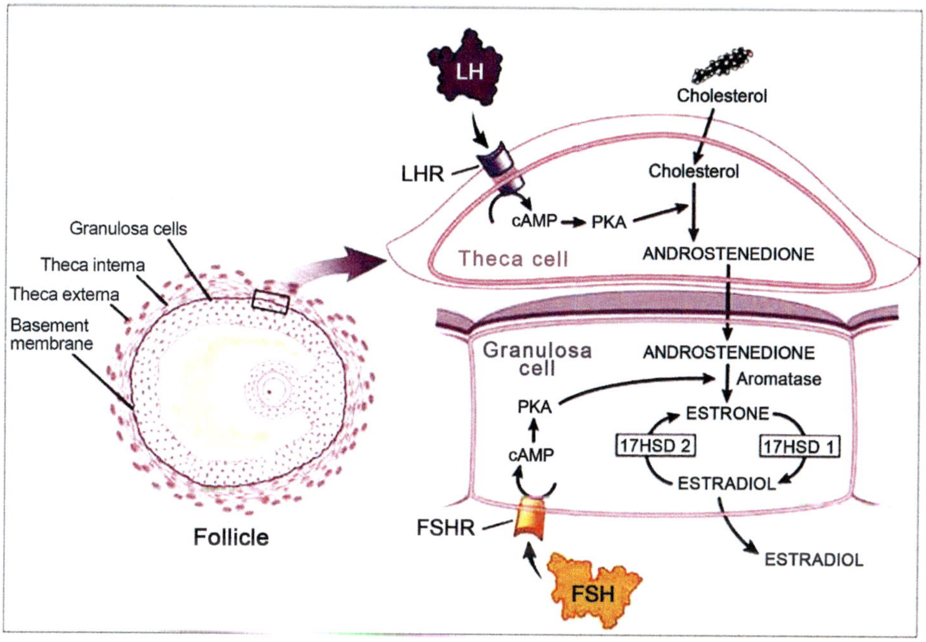

Figure 6.8. *Two cells and two gonadotropins, on the regulation and the synthesis of estrogens at the ovary.*

Source: Patricio, B. P., & Sergio, B. G., (2019). Normal menstrual cycle. IntechOpen. doi: 10.5772/intechopen.79876.

The normal follicular phase has been divided into three stages: (a) early; (b) middle; and (c) late, to allow a better comprehension of the endocrine events that will be finally responsible for ovulation.

1. **Early Follicular Phase (Days 1–4):** It begins with the first day of menstruation. Follicular recruitment occurs due to the elevation of FSH, as a consequence of the decrease in estradiol, progesterone, and inhibin A released by the corpus luteum of the previous cycle, allowing the number of LH receptors to increase in the cells of the teak and the granulosa. The plasma levels of estradiol tend to remain low at this stage (Figure 6.1).
2. **Medium Follicular Phase (Days 5–7):** As the recruitment and growth of follicles induced by FSH progress, estradiol increases slowly in a progressive manner thanks to the increased activity of CYP19, an FSH-dependent aromatase that is present in granulosa cells.

The follicle with the greatest number of FSH receptors has the potential to become the dominant follicle by aromatizing more estradiol. The other follicles experience atresia because they have fewer FSH receptors. Under the influence of LH, thecal cells must produce androgens, which must then diffuse to the granulosa cells to initiate the process of estrogen synthesis. In the theca and granulose, two glycoproteins with local effects—activin and inhibin—are produced concurrently. By inhibiting the synthesis and release of FSH and amplifying the effects of estradiol, inhibitor B produces a negative hypophyseal feedback effect. This would be a strategy to establish dominance, providing the more developed follicle an advantage. A follicle's ability to successfully establish its dominance is indicated by the estrogen take-off (ETO).

The development of the FD's internal theca and increased receptivity to LH stimulates the breakdown of cholesterol molecules into progesterone, which in turn produces testosterone, dehydroepiandrosterone, androstenedione, and other androgens. The granulosa-theca complex of the FD has nearly full functionality to enter the late follicular phase at the end of this phase.

3. **Late Follicular Phase (Days 8–12):** This period is characterized by the elevation of estrogens that come from the DF, reaching its maximum values between 40 and 50 hours, before an elevation of FSH that precedes the ovulatory peak of LH. This preovulatory follicle reaches an average diameter of 15–20 mm (Wilcox et al., 2000; Hale et al., 2007; Mihm et al., 2011; Skorupskaite et al., 2014; Patricio & Sergio, 2019).

6.1.4. Follicular Phase and Fertility

The day before ovulation is when there is the highest chance of successful fertilization. On the other hand, the potentially fertile period can last longer than five days before ovulation, depending on sperm survival. Pregnancies obtained after day 14 are linked to later ovulation, which is characterized by a normal variation in the follicular phase duration based on the time of the embryo's release from the womb.

It is thought that cycles lasting 30–31 days and involving five days of bleeding would have a higher chance of becoming pregnant, possibly as a result of improved DF quality, healthy corpus luteum function, and ideal endometrial receptivity. The timing of the fertile window varies greatly. Many women who have regular menstrual cycles have been reported to be in their fertile window either before or after day 17 of their cycle. However, it appears that when the cycles are short—less than 25 days—the likelihood of getting pregnant is low.

Indirect methods, also known as methods, based on symptoms, are employed in clinical practice to assess the potential for conception. These methods entail monitoring at least one of the three main indicators of fertility—cervical mucus, basal body temperature, and cervix position. Ovulation predictor kits (OPK) are devices that measure the rise in LH that happens 24–36 hours before ovulation. Standard, digital, and advanced digital OPK versions of those urine-based ovulation test kits are available, as are some saliva-based ovulation tests. There are three types of fertility monitors: urine-based, perspiration-based, and saliva-based. Fertility monitors are computerized devices that interpret changes in saliva, urine test results, or basal body temperature. Ultrasonography is the preferred method for effective follicular follow-up in the monitoring of assisted reproductive procedures.

Ovulation inducers, which raise endogenous levels of FSH, or parenterally administered FSH, which rescues multiple follicles from atresia, are employed in infertility treatments. Thus, there is a greater chance of multiple ovulations in this patient. Fascinatingly, the follicular endowment does not decrease when rescuing follicles from atresia, preventing follicles from being depleted more quickly.

6.1.5. Follicle Types

Women are born with primordial follicles (PF), which are held during the prophase of the first meiotic division and are encircled by a single layer of granulosa cells. A woman has antral follicles during adolescence that are dependent on FSH. This follicle matures to preovulatory FD in an average of 14 days. They originate from an FSH-independent recruitment process primarily controlled by anti-Müllerian hormone (AMH), which is secreted by the follicles' granulosa cells during early development and prevents the follicles from moving from the primordiaSl to the primary follicular stage. The follicular reserve can be determined by measuring serum AMH levels (Figures 6.9 and 6.10).

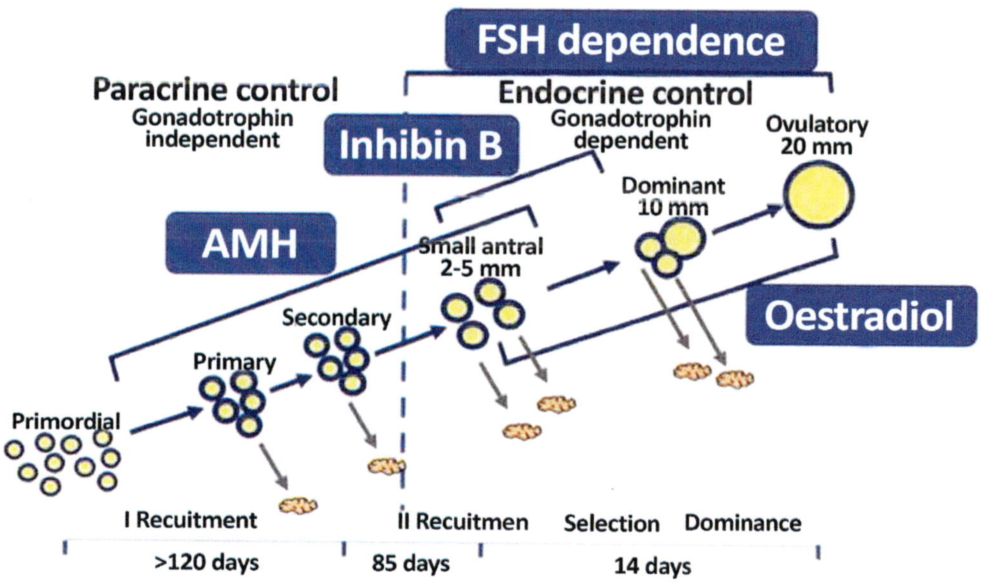

Figure 6.9. *AMH participates in the paracrine control of recruitment in the first stage when the process is still independent of gonadotropins. AMH can not only the number of early antral follicles in the process of development but also those in earlier stages.*

Source: Patricio, B. P., & Sergio, B. G., (2019). Normal menstrual cycle. IntechOpen. doi: 10.5772/intechopen.79876.

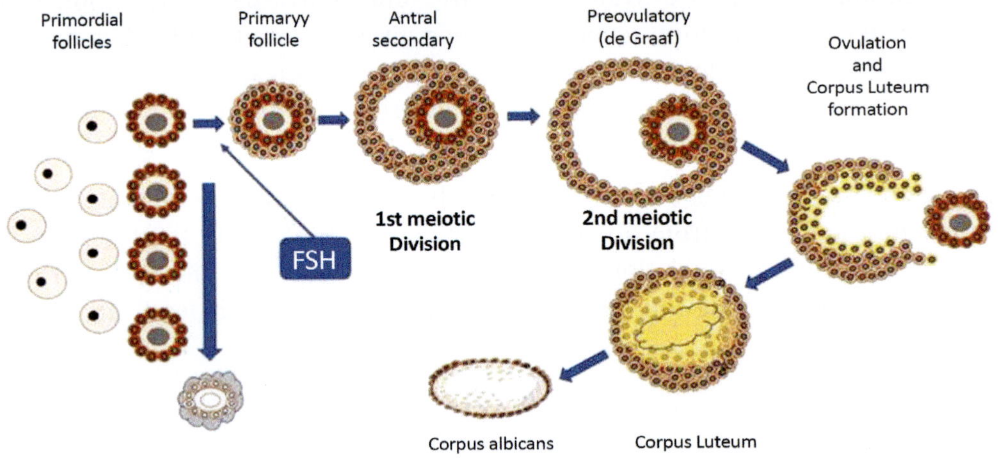

Figure 6.10. *Clinical witnesses of the follicular development in stage pre- and post-dependence of FSH: AMH and ultrasound, respectively.*

Source: Patricio, B. P., & Sergio, B. G., (2019). Normal menstrual cycle. IntechOpen. doi: 10.5772/intechopen.79876.

PF, or primordial follicles, function without FSH. After an average of 60–65 days, they transform preantral follicles (PAF), which are likewise not dependent on FSH and are encircled by theca and granulosa cells in multiple layers. Numerous primordial follicles experience atresia during this process (Figure 6.11).

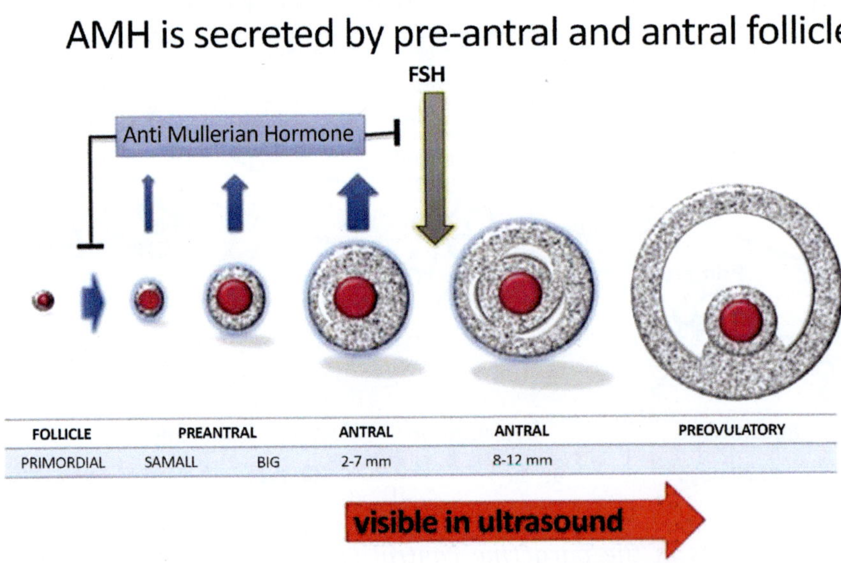

Figure 6.11. *Follicular dynamics and illustration of folliculogenesis process.*

Source: Patricio, B. P., & Sergio, B. G., (2019). Normal menstrual cycle. IntechOpen. doi: 10.5772/intechopen.79876.

The early preantral and antral follicles produce more testosterone and androstenedione than the estrogen rate because they have 5α-reductase. The enzyme 5α-reductase is in charge of changing testosterone into dihydrotestosterone (DHT). A 5α reduction in testosterone prevents DHT from aromatizing. The involution of granulosa cells lowers the levels of inhibin production in women as they age. As a result, the FSH levels rise as she gets closer to menopause, indicating a decline in her ovarian reserve. Conversely, half of the perimenopausal follicles have chromosomal abnormalities, making them the lowest-quality follicles.

Any follicle that develops past this stage will need an interaction because, as previously mentioned, the preantral follicle develops independently of FSH. The releasing hormone of gonadotropin (GnRH), steroidal hormones, and various peptides secreted by dominant follicles all control the secretion of gonadotropin.

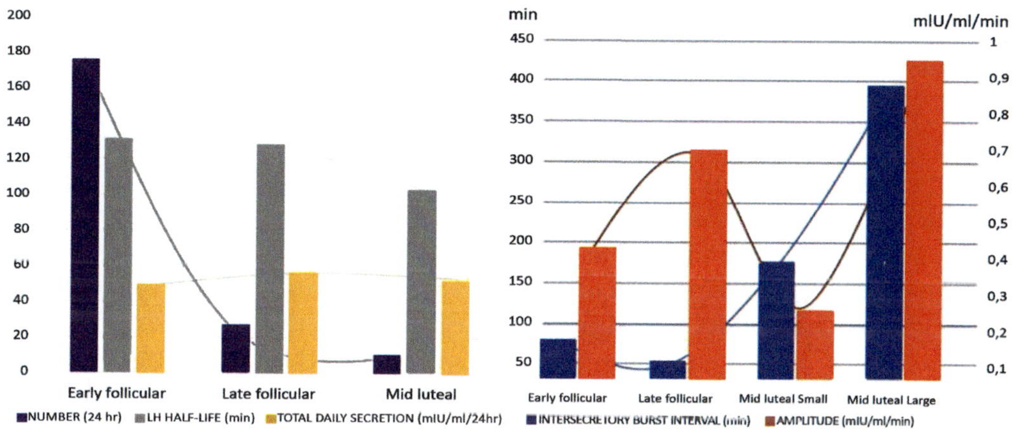

Figure 6.12. *Pulses of LH throughout a normal cycle. The number of pulses per 24 h decreases, but total daily secretion and LH half-life are stable. The inter-secretory burst interval becomes longer as the cycle progresses, being very long in the luteal phase, whereas the pulse amplitude of LH shows a dichotomous behavior, with small and high waves.*

Source: Patricio, B. P., & Sergio, B. G., (2019). Normal menstrual cycle. IntechOpen. doi: 10.5772/intechopen.79876.

Steroids, pituitary hormones, plasmatic proteins, proteoglycans, and non-steroidal ovarian factors are among the substances present in the follicular liquid and are responsible for regulating the ovary's microenvironment and granulosa steroidogenesis. Growth-promoting factors like epidermal growth factor (EGF) and insulin growth factors 1 and 2 (IGF1, IGF2) would be crucial to the development and maturity of oocytes. The liquid has a higher concentration of ovarian steroids than plasmatic concentrations do.

Antral follicles are divided into two populations: large follicles, with a diameter of more than 6 mm, and small follicles, with a diameter of less than 8 mm. FSH concentrations are higher in large follicles. Prolactin concentration is lower, and levels of estrogen, progesterone, and other hormones are higher. Prolactin and androgen levels are higher in small follicles than in large antral follicles.

Furthermore, as previously indicated, FSH rises in the early follicular phase and subsequently starts to fall until the ovulation phase, except for the brief preovulatory peak. On the other hand, because of the positive feedback from rising estrogen levels, LH is low during the early follicular phase and starts to rise during the middle follicular phase.

For a minimum of 48 hours, plasma estradiol levels must be higher than 200 pg/ml to produce positive feedback of LH release. According to the menstrual cycle phase, the anterior pituitary secretes gonadotropins in a pulsatile manner, with varying pulse width and frequency (Figure 6.12).

LH is secreted at a frequency of 60 to 90 minutes during the early follicular phase. The pulse constant widens but the number of pulses, intersecretory burst interval, and pulse amplitude vary. The late follicular phase, which precedes ovulation, is characterized by an increase in pulse frequency and possible widening. After ovulation, most women experience a widening of their LH pulse that increases. Because developing follicles produce inhibin B through negative retroalimentation, FSH levels start to decline once menstruation is produced (Wilcox et al., 2000; Hale et al., 2007; Mihm et al., 2011; Skorupskaite et al., 2014; Patricio & Sergio, 2019).

6.1.6. Ovulation

Around 10 to 12 hours after LH peaks, hatching takes place (Figure 6.8). Estradiol, which is produced at the preovulatory follicle and has levels between 200 and 450 pg/mL, significantly increases to produce an increase in LH. The dominant follicle must grow to a diameter of at least 15 mm to reach the critical concentration of estradiol required to start positive feedback. The rise in LH happens 34–36 hours before ovulation and is a highly accurate indicator of when ovulation will occur (Figure 6.9). The luteinization of granulosa cells, which triggers the production of progesterone and estradiol, is brought on by this elevation in LH. Additionally, with the release of the first polar corpuscle, the LH increase initiates the second meiotic division and the oocyte's chromosomal reduction.

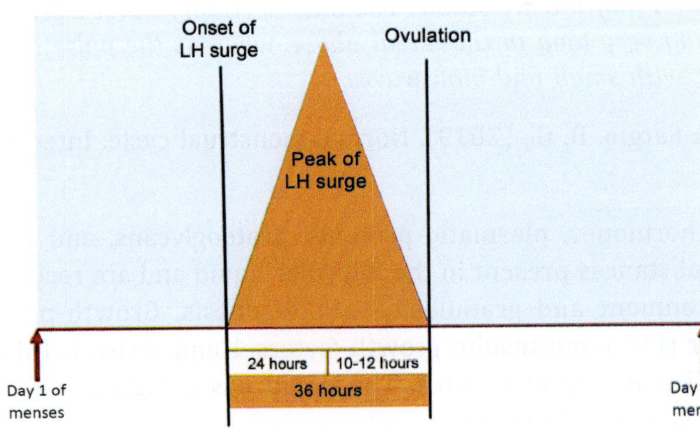

Figure 6.13. *An increase of LH precedes ovulation in 36 hours. Peak, on the other side, precedes ovulation in 10–12 hours.*

Source: Patricio, B. P., & Sergio, B. G., (2019). Normal menstrual cycle. IntechOpen. doi: 10.5772/intechopen.79876.

The sharp decline in estradiol levels occurs right before the peak of LH. This may be the result of progesterone directly inhibiting the synthesis of estradiol or the regulation of LH from its receptor. In the middle of the cycle, progesterone also contributes to the stimulation of an increase in FSH (Figure 6.13).

The release of oocytes from their follicular junctions caused by this increase in FSH would activate the plasminogen activator and boost the number of LH receptors in the granulosa. Unknown is the precise mechanism causing the post-ovulatory fall. The loss of progesterone's inhibitory retroalimentation and the positive retroalimentation of estrogens would result in a decrease in LH (Figure 6.14).

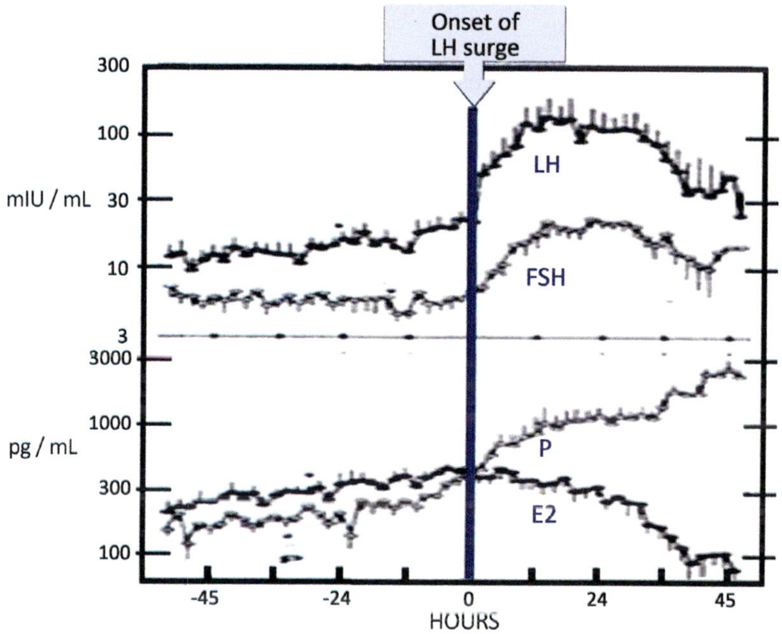

Figure 6.14. *Changes in ovarian gonadotropins and steroids in the middle of the cycle, just before ovulation. The beginning of the increase of LH is at time. 0 time [E2: estrogen; and P: progesterone]. It takes 36 hours from the peak of estrogen until ovulation occurs. The time to ovulation measured from the peak of LH is 12 hours; considering the time of detection in urine, ovulation will take place at 24 hours since LH is measured in the urine. The hormone hCG is similar to LH and can be used as an exogenous hormone to trigger ovulation, which will occur 36 hours after administration.*

Source: Patricio, B. P., & Sergio, B. G., (2019). Normal menstrual cycle. IntechOpen. doi: 10.5772/intechopen.79876.

Progesterone, prostaglandins, and proteolytic enzymes are secreted inside the follicle during the ovulatory phase. This leads to digestion and follicular wall rupture, which permits hatching, also known as ovulation. In response to LH and progesterone, proteolytic enzymes and prostaglandins break down collagen in the follicular wall, causing the cumulus-oocyte complex to burst into an explosive release. Prostaglandins can increase oocyte release, which in turn increases ovarian smooth muscle.

A "stigma" is the location of the rupture in the dominant follicle that is closest to the ovarian surface. Not all the mechanisms have been fully understood. Just before ovulation, the levels of hydroxyeicosatetraenoic acid (HETE), prostaglandins E and F, and other chemicals reach their peak at the follicular level. Proteolytic enzymes are stimulated by prostaglandins, while angiogenesis and hyperemia are stimulated by HETE. Both fertile and infertile women may experience luteinized unruptured follicle syndrome as a result of high doses of prostaglandin inhibitors obstructing follicular rupture.

Therefore, it is advised that women who are trying to conceive, and especially those who are experiencing infertility, refrain from taking inhibitors of prostaglandin synthesis. In fact, inhibitors of cyclooxygenase (COX) are currently being researched as a potential emergency contraceptive substitute for the morning-after pill.

A number of intricate molecular processes that start after the gonadotrophin surge must be given for ovulation to happen. The processes involved are as follows: (a) ovulatory mediators that act through the cumulus cell complex; (b) convergence of ovulatory signals through the cumulus complex coordinates the mechanistic processes that control oocyte maturation and ovulation; and (c) other multiple inputs, such as endocrine hormones, immune and metabolic signals, as well as intrafollicular paracrine factors from the theca, mural, and cumulus granulosa cells, and the oocyte itself. Thus, control over oocyte maturation, development, and ovulation process is exerted by both healthy and meiotically competent oocytes and the coordination and synchronization of endocrine, paracrine, immune, and metabolic signals acting primarily through the cumulus compartment. The mechanisms implied in the rupture of follicles are depicted in Figure 6.15.

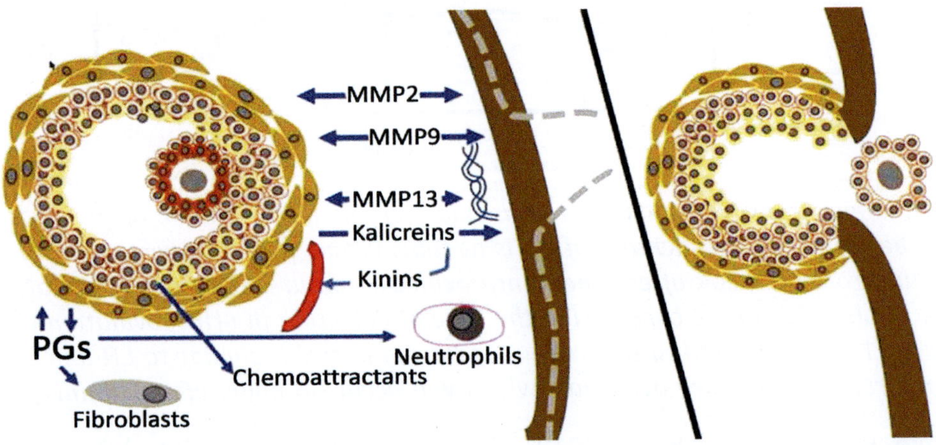

Figure 6.15. *Proposed mechanisms at follicular rupture. LH stimulates the expression of genes in granulosa cells (PR, PGS-2) that control the activation of matrix metalloproteinases (MMPs), leading to the breakdown and remodeling of extracellular matrices and the surface epithelium to allow rupture of the follicle and extrusion of the oocyte (ovulation).*

Source: Patricio, B. P., & Sergio, B. G., (2019). Normal menstrual cycle. IntechOpen. doi: 10.5772/intechopen.79876.

6.1.7. Luteal Phase

Most women go through this phase 14 days after ovulation. The concentration of lutein, a carotenoid, and the incorporation of fat droplets give the granulosa cells that are not released with the oocyte a vacuolated appearance and a distinctive yellow color. Its role as a potent antioxidant has been the only one identified.

The corpus luteum, a transitory endocrine organ that secretes progesterone and whose primary purpose is to prepare the endometrium—which has already been proliferated by the action of follicular phase estrogens—for the implantation of the fertilized egg—is created when the luteinized cells combine with the newly formed theca-lutein cells and the surrounding stroma.

The endometrium expresses molecules of adhesion that render it receptive to the blastocyst. The window of implantation, which occurs between days 7 and 9 after ovulation, is a period of maximum efficiency; implantation cannot occur after day 9, which is why it is referred to as the refractory phase. Maximum vascularization is reached, the basal lamina dissolves, and the capillaries invade the granulosa cell layers eight or nine days after ovulation when implantation is expected. This is in response to the secretion of angiogenic factors, which come from both the granulosa and theca cells, in harmony with the maximum levels of plasma progesterone and estradiol.

LH stimulation is necessary for the corpus luteum to survive, but angiogenesis and LH-mediated processes are also impacted by estradiol metabolites, which function through paracrine-autocrine pathways. At the end of the luteal phase, the corpus luteum loses function unless chorionic gonadotropin is released as a result of an impending pregnancy. If there is no pregnancy, luteolysis takes place in the corpus luteum. Estradiol and prostaglandins cause it to form corpus albicans, a type of scar tissue. As mentioned, during the menstrual cycle, estrogen levels rise and fall twice, peaking in the middle follicular phase, and then dropping sharply after ovulation. They then rise again during the middle luteal phase, coinciding with an increase in progesterone and 17α-hydroxyprogesterone serum levels, which all peak at the end of the cycle (Figure 6.1). It is unclear exactly how the corpus luteum controls the release of steroids. It could be influenced by the way that LH is secreted, modifications to its receptor, or shifts in the amounts of the enzymes that control the synthesis of steroid hormones. The corpus luteum's ability to regulate steroid synthesis may also be influenced by the number of granulosa cells that are generated during the follicular phase and the levels of LDL cholesterol that surround them.

Large and small luteal cells are the two types that exist at least. Progesterone is produced by both but in different ways. Large cells originate from granulosa, are more active in steroidogenesis, secrete a lot of progesterone, and do not increase progesterone secretion in response to cAMP or LH despite having many LH receptors. Rather, they have PGF2a receptors, and when this hormone is present, at least two-second messengers are activated. The secretion of progesterone is reduced upon activation of protein kinase C (PKC).

The concentration of free intracellular calcium rises when PGF2a binds to its receptor; this phenomenon appears to be connected to the induction of cell death and apoptosis. Other autocrine and paracrine factors that affect the large cells include relaxin, oxytocin, and inhibin (Figure 6.16). The small cells are derived from the theca, have LH receptors, and secrete progesterone 5 to 15 times more when exposed to LH or cAMP.

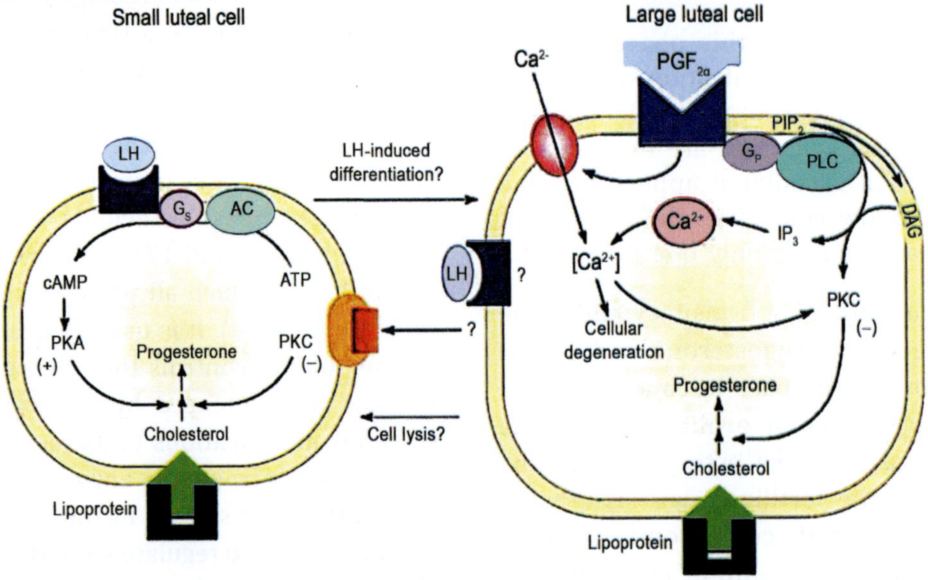

Figure 6.16. *Regulation of small luteal cells (left) and large (right). In small luteal cells, the binding of LH to its receptor activates the second messenger protein kinase A (PKA) pathway, which stimulates the synthesis of progesterone. In large cells, the LH that binds to its receptor does not increase the intracellular concentrations of cAMP nor the synthesis of progesterone, but the binding of PGF2a to its receptor activates PKC, which inhibits the synthesis of progesterone and causes an influx of calcium that leads to cell degeneration. [AC: adenylate cyclase; DAG: diacylglycerol; IP3: inositol 1,4,5-trisphosphate; PIP2: phosphatidylinositol 4,5-bisphosphate; and PLC: phospholipase C]. From Niswender.*

Source: Patricio, B. P., & Sergio, B. G., (2019). Normal menstrual cycle. IntechOpen. doi: 10.5772/intechopen.79876.

The development and maintenance of pregnancy depend on the corpus luteum's production of progesterone. To maintain pregnancy, there are additional mechanisms of luteal maintenance and rescue in addition to luteinization, which is the transformation of an ovulatory follicle into the corpus luteum, and luteal regression to permit a new cycle. Although the corpus luteum can synthesize cholesterol on its own, albeit in smaller amounts, humans prefer to use circulating LDL cholesterol for steroidogenesis.

Lipid steroid precursors are found inside the cells as free cholesterol. Additionally, esterified cholesterol can build up as lipoprotein particles or cytoplasmic lipid droplets within the rough endoplasmic reticulum. These cholesterol fatty acid esters cannot function as direct substrates for the synthesis of steroids or take the place of free cholesterol as a structural component of the plasma membrane. The neutral cholesterol ester hydrolase (NCEH), also referred to as hormone-sensitive lipase, hydrolyzes them because FSH, LH, and hCG tightly regulate their activity in steroidogenic tissues. The pulses of LH secretion are closely linked to progesterone and estradiol secretion during the luteal phase (Figure 6.12). The regulation of the posterior luteal phase and its concordance with the luteal phase function are both influenced by the frequency and widening of LH secretion during the follicular phase.

Progesterone and estradiol secretion during the luteal phase are influenced by the frequency and broadening of pituitary LH pulses (Figure 6.12). Continuous luteal or follicular hormone administration can shorten the half-life of the corpus luteum by lowering the hormone's concentration or reducing its pulses. If FSH levels are insufficient or low during the follicular phase, the luteal phase may also shorten, which will condition the development of a smaller corpus luteum.

The corpus luteum starts to decline 9–11 days after ovulation. The process of involution, or luteolysis, of the corpus luteum is somewhat understood. Prostaglandin F2α has been shown to play a role in luteolysis by stimulating the production of endothelin-1, which inhibits steroid hormone production and promotes the release of growth factors like tumor necrosis factor-alpha (TNFα), oxytocin, and vasopressin. At the same time, prostaglandin F2α also has a luteotropic effect through a self-regulating mechanism.

At the end of the luteal phase, LH's capacity to negatively regulate its own receptor may also be involved. As a result, rather than pulsatile LH secretion, the involution of the corpus luteum must be due to a decrease in LH receptor sensitivity. Lastly, luteolysis and the subsequent decline in progesterone levels would be influenced by the matrix metalloproteinases (Wilcox et al., 2000; Hale et al., 2007; Mihm et al., 2011; Skorupskaite et al., 2014; Patricio & Sergio, 2019).

6.2. Menstruation

Progesterone and estradiol levels start to drop when there is no pregnancy because the corpus luteum shrinks. The degree of coiling and constriction of spiraled arterioles increases with a decrease in progesterone. Because of the reduced blood flow from the superficial, spongy, and compact endometrial layers, this ultimately results in tissue ischemia. Matrix metalloproteinases are important in the initiation of menstrual bleeding in the human endometrium by causing the extracellular matrix of this mucosa to degrade after the drop in serum concentrations of ovarian steroids. Uterine smooth muscle contractions and the separation of deteriorated tissue are brought on by endometrial prostaglandins.

The instability of the lysosomal membranes in the endometrial cells may result in the release of prostaglandins. Because of the extent of this effect, women who experience excessive uterine bleeding may benefit from treatment with prostaglandin synthesis inhibitors. Red blood cells, proteolytic enzymes, endometrial tissue separation, and inflammatory exudates make up menstrual flow.

The estrogen generated by the newly formed follicles starts to encourage the regeneration of the endometrial superficial layers two days after the onset of menstruation, even though the endometrium is still being shed. A veil covering the denuded endometrial vessels forms more easily as a result of the long constriction of the vessel caused by the estrogen secreted by the developing follicles.

Menstruation typically lasts between four and six days, although it can sometimes last up to eight days. As previously stated, 30 milliliters is the average bleeding loss, and anything over 80 milliliters is deemed abnormal. A few years back, the International Federation of Gynecology and Obstetrics proposed a generalized classification to characterize bleeding abnormalities.

6.2.1. Types of Endometrium

Depending on the menstrual cycle, the endometrial characteristics in gynecological ultrasound vary, displaying varying thicknesses based on the stage of the cycle (Figure 6.17).

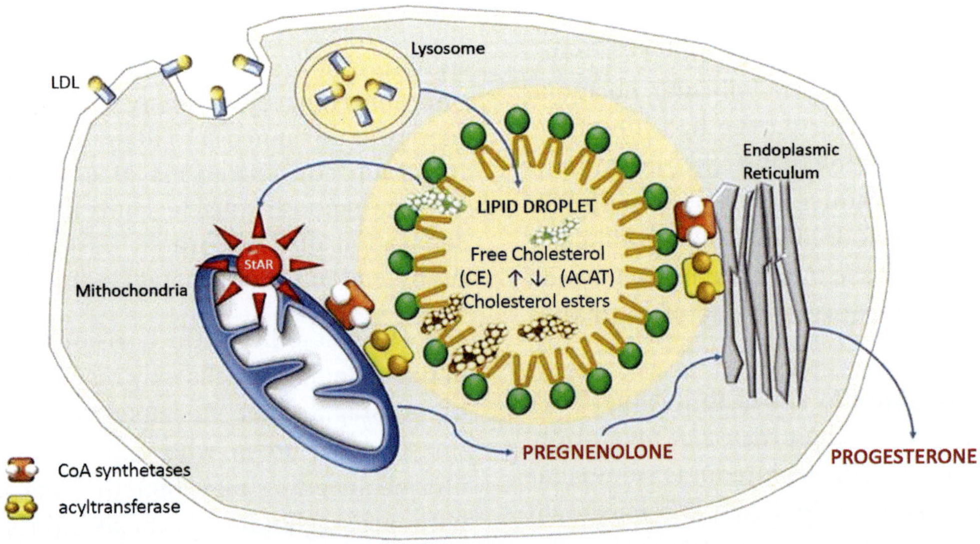

Figure 6.17. *The main substrate for human steroidogenesis is LDL cholesterol: it is incorporated by endocytosis and stored as free cholesterol or as an ester. Esterified cholesterol is hydrolyzed cholesterol esterases (CE) and transported as free cholesterol to the mitochondria. It passes from the outer mitochondrial membrane to the internal membrane, with the concurrence of the steroidogenic acute regulatory protein (StAR), peripheral type benzodiazepine receptors, and endozepine. In mitochondria, cholesterol is converted to pregnenolone by cytochrome P450scc, which is transported out of the mitochondria and converted to progesterone by 3β-hydroxysteroid dehydrogenase, D5, D4 isomerase (3β-HSD), which is present in the smooth endoplasmic reticulum.*

Source: Patricio, B. P., & Sergio, B. G., (2019). Normal menstrual cycle. IntechOpen. doi: 10.5772/intechopen.79876.

1. **Endometrium Type 0, Postmenstrual:** It is characterized because only a fine refractive line can be seen. It is the endometrium typical of postmenopause, postpartum, or after a uterine scraping. Most postmenopausal women are between 3 and 5 mm thick, but it is normal up to 8 mm if there has been no unexpected bleeding.
2. **Endometrium Type 1, Preovulatory:** It is called trilaminar endometrium, and refers to the observation of three refractive lines. This stage corresponds to the proliferative or estrogenic phase. In an early follicular stage, the size of the endometrium is between 3 and 4 mm thick, while in the stage close to ovulation, it can reach 9–11 mm.
3. **Endometrium Type 2,**

Postovulatory: In this stage, the progesterone matures the already proliferated endometrium, especially in its glandular and vascular structures, thickening the endometrium. The ultrasound image becomes whiter to the extent that it contains more water and glycogen. This layer of reflectivity represents most of the endometrium toward the end of the luteal phase.

4. **Endometrium Type 3, Premenstrual:** In this stage, there is only one large refractive line that corresponds to the late secretory phase (Wilcox et al., 2000; Hale et al., 2007; Mihm et al., 2011; Skorupskaite et al., 2014; Patricio & Sergio, 2019).

6.2.2. Endocrine Regulation of the Menstrual Cycle

Following gonadal axis maturity, GnRh is secreted pulsatile to the pituitary portal system every 60–90 minutes by neurons located in the preoptic area as well as the infundibular and arcuate nuclei in the hypothalamus.

To produce and sustain the effect of releasing both FSH and LH on the gonadotropic cells of the anterior part of the pituitary gland, frequency, and amplitude are necessary. The pulsatility of GnRH as well as the positive and negative feedback mechanisms of sex steroids will determine the amounts of each that are secreted.

Estrogen selectively modulates FSH at both the hypothalamus and the adenohypophysis levels, sensitizing, and counter-regulating it in response to other factors like inhibins A and B. While there are estrogens in the luteal and late follicular phases, LH is sensitive to positive feedback. However, when estrogen levels drop at the end of the cycle, the feedback turns negative. The LH surge is not prevented by progesterone administration in the late well-estrogenized follicular phase, according to recent evidence. This is significant because progesterone would not interfere with ovulation.

In contrast, kisspeptin expression is downregulated by low levels of estradiol during the early follicular and luteal phases, which lowers the amplitude of GnRH pulses. Conversely, progesterone would raise dynorphin expression, which lowers kisspeptin expression. The luteal phase's lower frequency of GnRH pulses has been linked to these alterations. GABA and endogenous opioids inhibit the pulsatile secretion of GnRH, whereas glutamate and norepinephrine are other modulators that promote it.

The arcuate/infundibular nucleus is the site of auto-synaptic action for neurokinin B and dynorphin neuropeptides. Specifically, an increase in neurokinin B (NKB) expression stimulates GnRH secretion and kisspeptin secretion by inhibiting the pulsatility of GnRH. Conversely, an increase in dynorphin (Dyn) expression decreases kisspeptin secretion. We call this system KNDy. Estradiol levels are low and FSH levels are slightly elevated at the start of the menstrual cycle. This ratio can attract follicles, and when that occurs, it causes an increase in inhibin A as well as estradiol, which in turn causes a persistent drop in FSH during the follicular phase.

The day the FD is defined marks the peak of FSH concentrations, which are then steadily reduced from day 5 to day 13 of the follicular phase, peaking right before ovulation (Figure 6.14). There comes a point at which the peak of FSH and LH, which results in ovulation, is triggered by estradiol levels. Progesterone, estradiol, and inhibin A decrease in tandem with the rise in activin A as the luteal phase progresses. Four days before menstruation, during the luteal phase to the subsequent follicular phase, FSH rises. This is the time when follicular recruitment takes place and inhibin B rises.

In the second half of the luteal phase (Figure 6.18), the concentration of activin A secreted by the follicles increases; at the beginning of the luteal phase, it decreases; during the early luteal phase, it increases; and finally, in parallel with estradiol and inhibin A, it increases during the middle luteal phase (Figure 6.19).

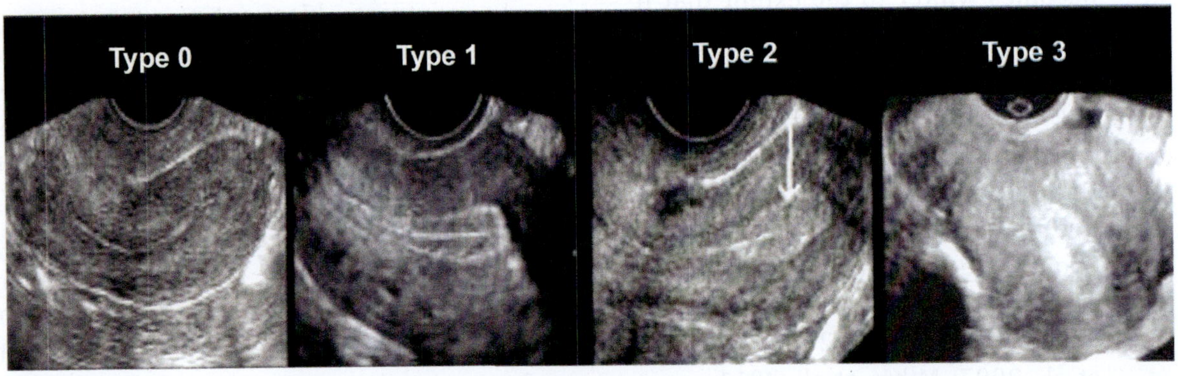

Figure 6.18. *Types of endometrium in transvaginal ultrasound. The endometrium was classified into four types (0, 1, 2, and 3) according to the appearance of the myometrium-endometrium and endometrium-endometrium interfaces, the texture, and the thickness of the functional layer. Type 0: Smooth, thin as a pencil line; Type 1: trilaminar structure with an iso- or hypoechoic functional layer; Type 2: also trilaminar, but the myometrium-endometrium interfaces are thicker than those of type 1; and Type 3: thick and homogeneous echogenic image. The type of endometrium correlates with the day of the menstrual cycle. Ultrasound is defined on day 0 as the day of the follicle break. Type 0 is usually found on day −11, during and immediately after menstruation. Type 1 is observed during the middle follicular phase and until day +2. Types 2 and 3 are observed after the ovulatory days. The endometrium increases more thickness during the preovulatory phase (average +5.5 mm), and in the luteal phase, the average is +2.6 mm.*

Source: Patricio, B. P., & Sergio, B. G., (2019). Normal menstrual cycle. IntechOpen. doi: 10.5772/intechopen.79876.

Even at the nadir, older women have higher FSH levels, and this increase happens early in the luteal phase. A group of follicles is recruited early on, but the selection of DF is different and can proceed or lag. As a result, the cycle becomes more variable at the expense of a fluctuating follicular phase known as the "lag phase," which ends when the ETO is generated.

When the estradiol overt elevation is reached, the FD is selected, and this is known as the ETO. The endometrial level of the cycle is hormonally monophasic if an FD capable of ovulating is not achieved, as the woman may experience a hyperestrogenic state without establishing a corpus luteum. The monophasic hyperestrogenism that affects about one-third of women in perimenopause can be explained by the pathophysiological basis shown in Figure 6.20.

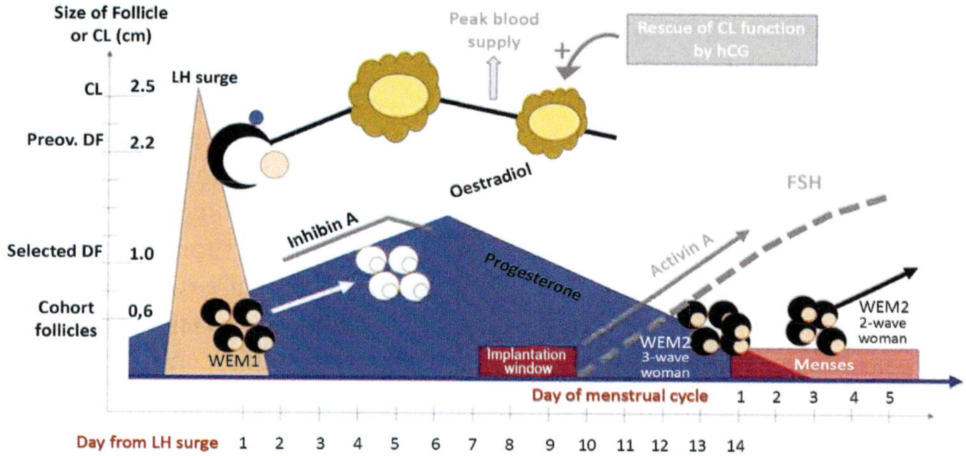

Figure 6.19. *The scheme shows luteal events, follicular changes, and hormones during the luteal phase in a woman; CL: corpus luteum; DF: dominant follicle; WEM1–3: wave emergency 1, 2, or 3 at the cycle; the waves of the follicle of light gray color indicates the low frequency of the principal waves (selection of DF) during luteal phase or early follicular ones in women of 2 or 3 waves. The estradiol rise in the follicular phase begins after the emergence of the ovulatory DF and becomes more rapid following DF selection and occurs earlier in women with 2 versus 3 follicle waves per cycle. After ovulation, estradiol concentrations increase to the mid-luteal phase (days 7–9 after ovulation) and then decline, and this is due to luteal estradiol secretion and is unaffected by minor or major anovulatory waves.*

Source: Patricio, B. P., & Sergio, B. G., (2019). Normal menstrual cycle. IntechOpen. doi: 10.5772/intechopen.79876.

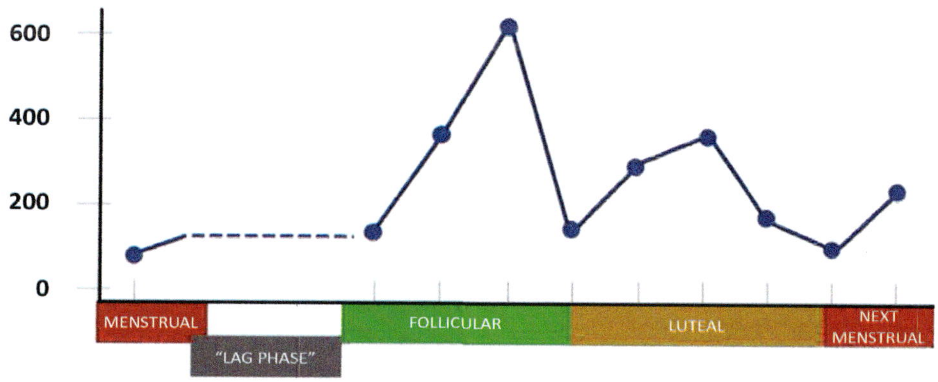

Figure 6.20. *The variability in perimenopause depends on the lag phase, a delayed recruitment process.*

Source: Patricio, B. P., & Sergio, B. G., (2019). Normal menstrual cycle. IntechOpen. doi: 10.5772/intechopen.79876.

An ongoing negative energy imbalance causes atresia of FD, which in turn causes anovulation and amenorrhea. It also decreases the pulsatility of LH. Losing weight is linked to a decrease in LH pulses, which causes hypothalamic amenorrhea that is reversible and functional. Conversely, women with polycystic ovary syndrome or adolescents with irregular cycles experience an increase in LH pulsatility, which is also linked to anovulation; however, in these cases, DF selection is absent (Wilcox et al., 2000; Hale et al., 2007; Mihm et al., 2011; Skorupskaite et al., 2014; Patricio & Sergio, 2019).

6.3. Hormonal Regulation of the Menstrual Cycle

The intricate and precisely calibrated process of hormone regulation of the menstrual cycle serves as the foundation for the periodic alterations that take place in the female reproductive system. The complex interaction between these hormones helps the body get ready for a possible pregnancy by coordinating a sequence of physiological processes that either lead to menstruation or conception.

Several important hormones produced by various body glands, such as the pituitary, ovaries, and hypothalamus, are at the core of hormonal regulation. Together, these hormones control both the thickening and shedding of the uterine lining (menstruation) and the development and release of an egg (ovulation).

Usually, there are multiple phases to the menstrual cycle, each of which is distinguished by unique hormonal fluctuations and physiological processes. Gonadotropin-releasing hormone (GnRH), which is released from the hypothalamus, signals the start of the follicular phase. Follicle-stimulating hormone (FSH) and luteinizing hormone (LH) are released into the bloodstream by the anterior pituitary gland in response to stimulation by GnRH. The growth and maturation of ovarian follicles, each of which contains an immature egg, are significantly aided by the hormone FSH. The follicles generate a growing amount of estrogen as they grow, a hormone that encourages the endometrium, the lining of the uterus, to thicken in anticipation of possible implantation. To preserve hormonal equilibrium, estrogen also has a negative feedback loop on the pituitary and hypothalamus, controlling the release of GnRH, FSH, and LH.

The midpoint of the menstrual cycle is usually when a surge in LH occurs, which is eventually triggered by rising estrogen levels. The release of a mature egg from the ovary is known as ovulation, and it is initiated by this spike in LH. Important events in the menstrual cycle, such as the size of the dominant follicle and the levels of LH and estrogen, affect ovulation.

The rupturing follicle becomes the corpus luteum, a transitory endocrine structure, after ovulation. Progesterone is a hormone secreted by the corpus luteum that is essential for lining the uterus in preparation for possible implantation. Progesterone facilitates endometrial growth and vascularization, which makes the environment conducive to the implantation and development of a fertilized egg. Progesterone also prevents the release of FSH and LH, which in turn stops the luteal phase's development of new follicles and ovulation.

The corpus luteum starts to degenerate if fertilization and implantation are unsuccessful, which lowers progesterone and estrogen levels. Menstruation, in which the thicker uterine lining is shed, and the unfertilized egg is expelled from the body, is brought on by this decline. One menstrual cycle ends, and a new one begins with the onset of menstruation. Menstrual cycle regulation is a complicated and dynamic process that is impacted by many variables, such as stress, diet, and underlying medical disorders. Menstrual cycle abnormalities like oligomenorrhea (infrequent menstruation) or amenorrhea (absence of menstruation) can be caused by disruptions in hormone production or signaling. Instances that affect fertility and reproductive health, such as endometriosis and polycystic ovary syndrome (PCOS), can also be attributed to hormonal imbalances.

It is crucial to comprehend how hormones control the menstrual cycle to diagnose, treat, and maximize fertility problems related to reproductive health. Research has advanced our knowledge of the intricate relationships between hormones and the reproductive system, which has resulted in the creation of novel therapies for infertility and menstrual problems. Through deciphering the enigmas surrounding hormone regulation, researchers and medical professionals persistently enhance the well-being of those impacted by reproductive health concerns.

6.3.1. Hormonal Effects on the Reproductive Tract

6.3.1.1. Endometrium

The varying concentrations of estrogen and progesterone during the menstrual cycle have specific effects on the endometrium. These changes can be seen using sonography and can be dated histologically. The most accurate way to histologically date the endometrium is by performing a biopsy 2–3 days before expected menstruation.

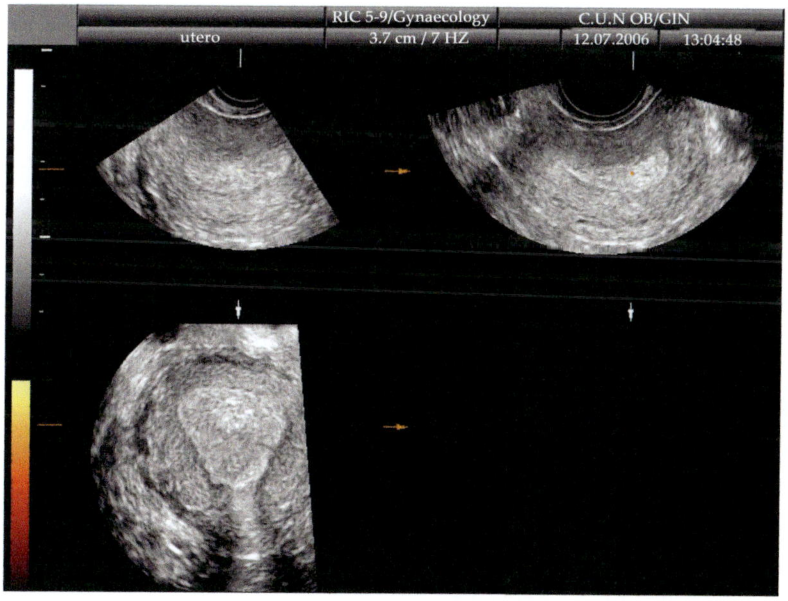

Figure 6.21. *Characteristic sonographic endometrial changes are seen throughout the menstrual cycle.*

Source: Alcázar, J. L., (2006). Three-dimensional ultrasound assessment of endometrial receptivity: A review. Reprod. Biol. Endocrinol., 4, 56. https://doi.org/10.1186/1477-7827-4-56.

The proliferative phase is harder to date accurately compared to the luteal phase, with narrow, tubular glands and some mitosis and pseudostratification present. During the luteal phase, on cycle day 16, the glands show a pseudostratified appearance with glycogen accumulating at the base and some nuclei displaced towards the center. This confirms the formation of a functional, progesterone-producing corpus luteum. Progesterone in the luteal phase decreases the biologic activity of estradiol on the endometrium by reducing estradiol receptors, increasing the enzymatic activity of 17β-hydroxysteroid dehydrogenase type II, and boosting the activity of estrone sulfotransferase (Figure 6.21).

The endometrial glands enlarge and become more twisted on cycle day 17. On cycle day 18, the epithelium's vacuoles shrink in size and are usually found close to the nuclei. Furthermore, the apex of the endometrial cells now contains glycogen. By cycle day 19, intraluminal secretions start to appear and the pseudostratification and vacuolation almost entirely vanish. The endometrial stroma starts to swell on cycle days 21 or 22. Cycle Day 23 marks the appearance of stromal mitoses and the enlargement of stromal cells surrounding spiral arterioles. On cycle day 24, stromal mitoses become more noticeable, and predecidual cells start to form around the spiral arterioles. The predecidual cells start to differentiate beneath the surface epithelium on cycle day 25. On cycle day 27, the upper endometrial stroma is visible as a solid sheet of fully developed decidua-like cells with a noticeable lymphocytic infiltration. Cycle day 28 marks the start of menstruation.

Further studies have focused on identifying various endometrial stem cell subtypes. Notably, menstrual fluid could potentially serve as a convenient source for specific types of these stem cells. This discovery could pave the way for advancements in treating various gynecologic conditions like endometriosis and Asherman syndrome, as well as non-gynecologic disorders such as neurological and cardiac ailments.

6.3.1.2. Cervix

The secretion of mucous glands in the endocervix is influenced by changes in steroid hormone levels. Following menstruation, the cervical mucous is minimal and thick. In the late follicular phase, as estradiol levels increase, the cervical mucous becomes clear, abundant, and stretchy. The amount of cervical mucous produced during this phase is significantly higher compared to earlier in the cycle. The elasticity of the mucous can be measured using a method called spinnbarkeit, where it is spread between two glass slides. When viewed under a microscope, the cervical mucous will exhibit a unique ferning or palm-leaf pattern. After ovulation, when progesterone levels rise, the cervical mucous returns to being thick, dense, and less in quantity.

6.3.1.3. Vagina

The vaginal epithelium is likewise uniquely affected by variations in progesterone and estrogen levels. Exfoliated vaginal epithelial cells are basophilic and have vesicular nuclei in the early follicular phase. The late follicular phase and the rising estradiol level cause the vaginal epithelial cells to become acidophilic and have pyknotic nuclei. During the luteal phase, progesterone increases, causing a decrease in acidophilic cells and an increase in leukocytes (Wilcox et al., 2000; Hale et al., 2007; Mihm et al., 2011; Skorupskaite et al., 2014; Patricio & Sergio, 2019).

6.3.2. Hormonal Control of the Menstrual Cycle

The ovarian hormones are secreted in the urine in altered forms and circulate in the blood. Chemical methods for estimating urinary output provide information on blood levels and the total production of these substances. Numerous synthetic variations of progesterone and various natural estrogens have been developed; many of these are effective when taken orally and are used as oral contraceptives and treatments for hormonal imbalances.

The anterior lobe of the pituitary gland, located in a tiny slit at the base of the skull, secretes gonadotropic hormones, which are necessary for the ovarian cyclic events previously discussed. Follicle-stimulating hormone (FSH), luteinizing hormone (LH), and possibly luteotropic hormone (LTH) are the two, and possibly three, gonadotropic hormones.

The first half of the menstrual cycle is when the most FSH is secreted, and the middle of the cycle is when the most LH is secreted. It is thought that ovulation and follicle ripening are caused by the successive actions of FSH and LH. While ovulation can be successfully induced with FSH and LH alone in women undergoing infertility treatment, LTH is required in certain animals to maintain the corpus luteum. Administering excessive doses of FSH has resulted in multiple births due to multiple ovulations.

The ovary is stimulated by the pituitary gland to produce progesterone and estrogens, but there is a "negative feedback" mechanism whereby the estrogens block the pituitary gland's release of FSH (and likely increase the release of LH). Progesterone is also thought to prevent LH from being produced further. The hypothalamus regulates the basic rhythm of this process, which involves the pituitary stimulating the ovary and the ovary inhibiting the pituitary. However, oral contraceptives, which contain progestogens (which are modified forms of progesterone) and estrogens, can prevent ovulation.

The brain's hypothalamus is connected to the anterior lobe of the pituitary gland via its stalk. Numerous significant hormones, such as growth hormones, gonadotropic hormones, and those regulating the function of the thyroid and adrenal glands, are secreted by the anterior lobe. The pituitary stalk's veins carry substances from the hypothalamus that trigger the release of hormones from the pituitary, such as FSH and LH, as well as a substance that prevents the release of LTH. Undoubtedly, the hypothalamus is impacted by higher brain centers, which explains why menstrual irregularities can occasionally occur after emotional stress (Wilcox et al., 2000; Hale et al., 2007; Mihm et al., 2011; Skorupskaite et al., 2014; Patricio & Sergio, 2019).

A Closer Look

Folliculogenesis

Folliculogenesis is the intricate process by which ovarian follicles mature, essential for female fertility. It begins with the activation of primordial follicles, a pool of dormant follicles present from birth, characterized by a single layer of granulosa cells surrounding the oocyte. Activation transitions these two primary follicles, where granulosa cells proliferate and form a cuboidal shape. As follicles progress to the secondary stage, the granulosa cells further proliferate and theca cells, recruited from the surrounding stroma, differentiate into an internal and external layer, contributing to estrogen production. The tertiary or antral follicle stage is marked by the formation of a fluid-filled cavity called the antrum, which enlarges as the follicle grows. This stage is dependent on the interplay of hormonal signals, particularly Follicle-Stimulating Hormone (FSH) and Luteinizing Hormone (LH). FSH promotes granulosa cell proliferation and antral expansion, while LH induces theca cells to produce androgens, which granulosa cells convert to estrogen.

A crucial aspect of folliculogenesis is atresia, where a significant number of follicles undergo programmed cell death at various stages, ensuring only the most viable follicles reach maturity. Ultimately, a dominant follicle is selected for ovulation. This dominant follicle responds robustly to FSH and LH, culminating in the pre-ovulatory surge of LH, which triggers the resumption of meiosis in the oocyte and the breakdown of the follicular wall, allowing the mature oocyte to be released.

Following ovulation, the remnants of the follicle transform into the corpus luteum, which secretes progesterone to maintain the endometrium for potential implantation. If fertilization does not occur, the corpus luteum degenerates, leading to a drop in progesterone and the onset of menstruation. Folliculogenesis, therefore, is a continuous and highly regulated process, essential for reproductive health and the menstrual cycle (Wilcox et al., 2000; Hale et al., 2007; Mihm et al., 2011; Skorupskaite et al., 2014; Patricio & Sergio, 2019).

Summary

- The menstrual cycle is a complex, yet vital, process that occurs in the female reproductive system, typically lasting around 28 days, though it can vary from person to person.
- The moment of greatest likelihood of successful fertilization is intercourse on the day before ovulation. However, the potentially fertile period, which depends on sperm survival, can extend from 5 days before ovulation.
- At born, woman count with primordial follicles (PF), each surrounded by one layer of cells of granulosa and are detained at the pro phase of the first meiotic division. During adolescence, the woman has antral follicles that depend on FSH.
- The hormonal regulation of the menstrual cycle is a sophisticated and finely tuned process that underpins the cyclic changes occurring within the female reproductive system.
- The ovarian hormones circulate in the blood and are excreted in modified forms in the urine. Estimation of the urinary output by chemical methods gives an indication of the blood levels and of the total production of these substances.

References

1. Bilezikjian, L. M., Blount, A. L., Leal, A. M., Donaldson, C. J., Fischer, W. H., & Vale, W. W. (2004). Autocrine/paracrine regulation of pituitary function by activin, inhibin, and follistatin. *Molecular and Cellular Endocrinology, 225*(1–2), 29–36.
2. Broekmans, F. J., Visser, J. A., Laven, J. S., Broer, S. L., Themmen, A. P., & Fauser, B. C. (2008). Anti-Müllerian hormone and ovarian dysfunction. *Trends in Endocrinology and Metabolism, 19*(9), 340–347.
3. Christenson, L. K., & Devoto, L. (2003). Cholesterol transport and steroidogenesis by the corpus luteum. *Reproductive Biology and Endocrinology, 1*, 90.
4. Devoto, L., Henríquez, S., Kohen, P., & Strauss, J. F. 3rd. (2017). The significance of estradiol metabolites in human corpus luteum physiology. *Steroids, 123*, 50–54.
5. Doshi, S. B., & Agarwal, A. (2013). The role of oxidative stress in menopause. *Journal of Midlife Health, 4*(3), 140–146.
6. Duffy, D. M. (2015). Novel contraceptive targets to inhibit ovulation: The prostaglandin E2 pathway. *Human Reproduction Update, 21*(5), 652–670.
7. Hale, G. E., Zhao, X., Hughes, C. L., Burger, H. G., Robertson, D. M., & Fraser, I. S. (2007). Endocrine features of menstrual cycles in middle and late reproductive age and the menopausal transition are classified according to the staging of the reproductive aging workshop (STRAW) staging system. *The Journal of Clinical Endocrinology and Metabolism, 92*(8), 3060–3067.
8. Henriet, P., Cornet, P. B., Lemoine, P., Galant, C., Singer, C. F., Courtoy, P. J., & Marbaix, E. (2002). Circulating ovarian steroids and endometrial matrix metalloproteinases (MMPs). *Annals of the New York Academy of Sciences, 955*, 119–138.
9. Hutchens, E. G., Ramsey, K. A., Howard, L. C., Abshire, M. Y., Patrie, J. T., & McCartney, C. R. (2016). Progesterone has rapid positive feedback actions on LH release but fails to reduce LH pulse frequency within 12 hours in estradiol-pretreated women. *Physiological Reports, 4*(16), e12891.

10. Jesam, C., Salvatierra, A. M., Schwartz, J. L., & Croxatto, H. B. (2010). Suppression of follicular rupture with meloxicam, a cyclooxygenase-2 inhibitor: Potential for emergency contraception. *Human Reproduction, 25*(2), 368–373.
11. Kim, S. H., Burt Solorzano, C. M., & McCartney, C. R. (2018). Progesterone administration does not acutely alter LH pulse secretion in the mid-follicular phase in women. *Physiological Reports, 6*(8), e13680.
12. La Marca, A., Broekmans, F. J., Volpe, A., Fauser, B. C., Macklon, N. S., & ESHRE Special Interest Group for Reproductive Endocrinology–AMH Round Table. (2009). Anti-Mullerian hormone (AMH): What do we still need to know? *Human Reproduction, 24*(9), 2264–2275.
13. Lehman, M. N., Coolen, L. M., & Goodman, R. L. (2010). Minireview: Kisspeptin/neurokinin B/dynorphin (KNDy) cells of the arcuate nucleus: A central node in the control of gonadotropin-releasing hormone secretion. *Endocrinology, 151*(8), 3479–3489.
14. Mihm, M., Gangooly, S., & Muttukrishna, S. (2011). The normal menstrual cycle in women. *Animal Reproduction Science, 124*(3–4), 229–236.
15. Munro, M. G., Critchley, H. O., Broder, M. S., Fraser, I. S., & FIGO Working Group on Menstrual Disorders. (2011). FIGO classification system (PALM-COEIN) for causes of abnormal uterine bleeding in nongravid women of reproductive age. *International Journal of Gynaecology and Obstetrics, 113*(1), 3–13.
16. Niswender, G. D. (2002). Molecular control of luteal secretion of progesterone. *Reproduction, 123*(3), 333–339.
17. Niswender, G. D., Juengel, J. L., Silva, P. J., Rollyson, M. K., & McIntush, E. W. (2000). Mechanisms controlling the function and life span of the corpus luteum. *Physiological Reviews, 80*(1), 1–29.
18. Patricio, B.-P., & Sergio, B.-G. (2019). Normal menstrual cycle. *IntechOpen*. doi: 10.5772/intechopen.79876.
19. Reed, B. G., & Carr, B. R. (2018). The normal menstrual cycle and the control of ovulation. In L. J. De Groot, G. Chrousos, K. Dungan, K. R. Feingold, A. Grossman, J. M. Hershman, & A. K. Gupta (Eds.), *Endotext*. South Dartmouth, MA: MDText.com, Inc.
20. Richards, J. S., Ren, Y. A., Candelaria, N., Adams, J. E., & Rajkovic, A. (2018). Ovarian follicular theca cell recruitment, differentiation, and impact on fertility: 2017 update. *Endocrine Reviews, 39*(1), 1–20.
21. Russell, D. L., & Robker, R. L. (2007). Molecular mechanisms of ovulation: Coordination through the cumulus complex. *Human Reproduction Update, 13*(3), 289–312.
22. Skorupskaite, K., George, J. T., & Anderson, R. A. (2014). The kisspeptin-GnRH pathway in human reproductive health and disease. *Human Reproduction Update, 20*(4), 485–500.
23. Small, C. M., Manatunga, A. K., Klein, M., Feigelson, H. S., Dominguez, C. E., McChesney, R., & Marcus, M. (2006). Menstrual cycle characteristics: Associations with fertility and spontaneous abortion. *Epidemiology, 17*(1), 52–60.
24. Stocco, C., Telleria, C., & Gibori, G. (2007). The molecular control of corpus luteum formation, function, and regression. *Endocrine Reviews, 28*(1), 117–149.
25. Welt, C. K., Pagan, Y. L., Smith, P. C., Rado, K. B., & Hall, J. E. (2003). Control of follicle-stimulating hormone by estradiol and the inhibin's: Critical role of estradiol at the hypothalamus during

the luteal-follicular transition. *The Journal of Clinical Endocrinology and Metabolism, 88*(4), 1766–1771.

26. Wilcox, A. J., Dunson, D., & Baird, D. D. (2000). The timing of the "fertile window" in the menstrual cycle: Day-specific estimates from a prospective study. *BMJ, 321*(7271), 1259–1262.

27. Wise, L. A., Mikkelsen, E. M., Rothman, K. J., Riis, A. H., Sørensen, H. T., Huybrechts, K. F., & Hatch, E. E. (2011). A prospective cohort study of menstrual characteristics and time to pregnancy. *American Journal of Epidemiology, 174*(6), 701–709.

Chapter

FERTILIZATION AND EARLY DEVELOPMENT

7

Contents

Unit Introduction

The process of fertilization is the beginning of a wonderful journey, the growth of the reproductive system, and the creation of new life. The union of a sperm and an egg starts a complicated process that eventually results in the formation of a zygote, which is the first stage of embryonic development. Human fertilization normally takes place in the uterine tube, which is where sperm cells travel through the female reproductive tract after ejaculating. Sperm cells are propelled by their flagella. During ovulation, the ovary releases the egg, or ovum, which is then caught by the uterine tube's fimbriae. It is waiting for sperm to arrive here. When a sperm can pass through the egg's outer layers and fuse with its membrane to form a zygote, this is known as fertilization.

After fertilization, a sequence of events takes place to stop more sperm from entering and to start the embryogenesis process. To ensure that only one sperm fertilizes the egg, the zona pellucida, a glycoprotein-rich matrix surrounding the egg, changes to become impenetrable to other sperm. The genetic material from the egg and sperm combines simultaneously to form a diploid cell with a full complement of chromosomes, which symbolizes the genetic blueprint of the newly formed individual. The zygote divides rapidly into new cells through a process known as cleavage after fertilization. These divisions start quickly and produce smaller, undifferentiated cells called blastomeres. The zygote undergoes cleavage to become a solid ball of cells called the morula, which matures into the hollow, fluid-filled structure known as the blastocyst as it continues. The inner cell mass and the outer layer of trophoblast cells make up the two different cell populations that make up the blastocyst. The inner cell mass will eventually develop into the embryo proper, while the trophoblast cells will eventually give rise to the placenta. The process of implantation, which occurs as soon as the blastocyst enters the uterus, is essential to establishing pregnancy. To facilitate the establishment of blood flow between the embryo and the mother, the blastocyst attaches itself to the uterine wall during implantation and starts to invade the maternal tissues.

Many different chemical and cellular processes work together to tightly control and orchestrate the process of fertilization and the early development of reproductive anatomy. Any anomalies or disturbances during this crucial time could have a significant impact on the development of the embryo and the health of the reproductive system. Comprehending the complexities of these mechanisms not only illuminates the genesis of life but also bears possible consequences for assisted reproductive technologies, contraception, and infertility management (Wassarman, 1999; WHO Laboratory Manual for the Examination of Human Semen and Sperm-cervical Mucus Interaction, 2010).

Orientation and Directional Terms:

Terms	Definition	Illustration
Embryonic development	Human embryonic development or human embryogenesis is the development and formation of the human embryo.	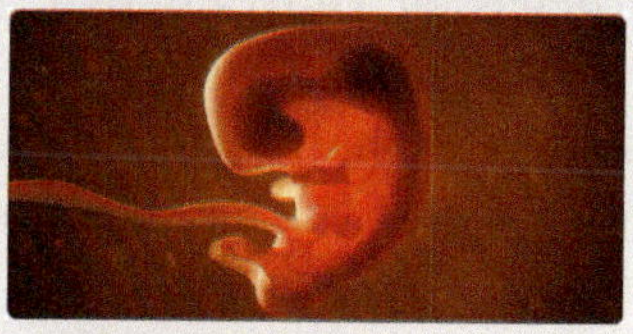
Zona pellucida	The zona pellucida is the specialized area surrounding mammalian oocytes (eggs).	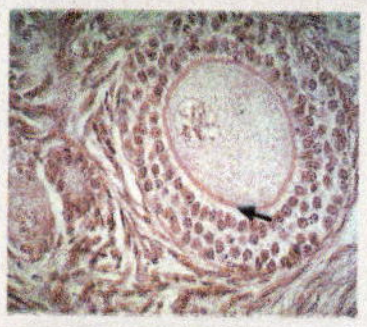
Enzymes	Enzymes are proteins that help speed up chemical reactions in our bodies. Enzymes are essential for digestion, liver function and much more.	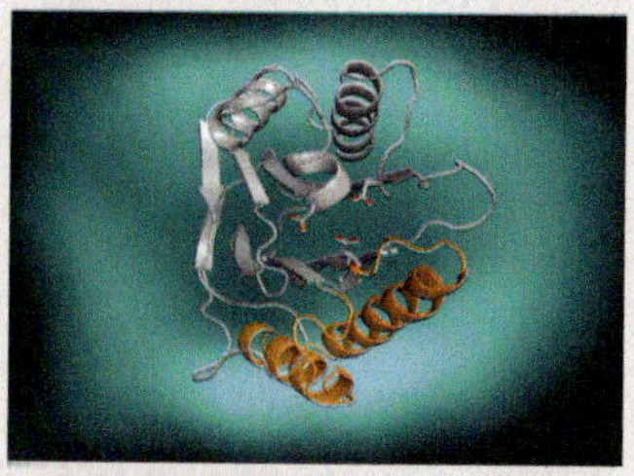
Trophoblast cells	Trophoblasts are the cells constituting fetal components in the placenta and fetal membrane.	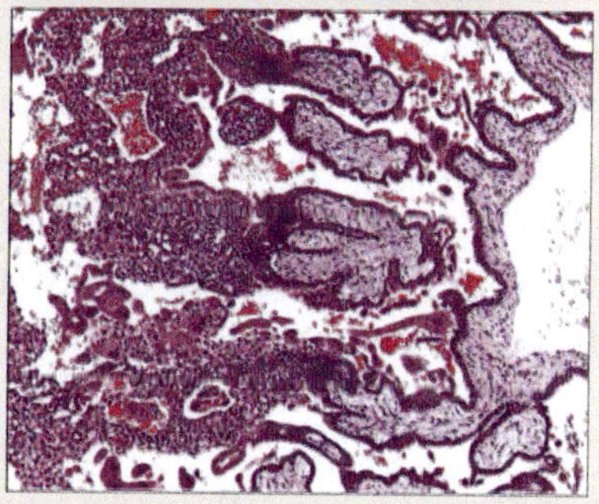

7.1. Process of Fertilization

The union of an egg cell and a sperm cell during fertilization is the start of an amazing journey in the process of reproductive anatomy. The process is intricate and expertly planned, and it results in the creation of a new person. The uterine tube, where the egg, or ovum, is released from the ovary during ovulation and awaits the arrival of sperm, is where fertilization normally takes place. After ejaculation, sperm cells travel through the female reproductive tract in search of an egg. They do this by contracting rhythmically and moving their flagella. Only a small percentage of the sperm cells released during ejaculation make it through the cervix, uterus, and uterine tube, where fertilization occurs.

Sperm must get past many obstacles as they approach the egg to reach their target. The cervical mucus serves as the first barrier, acting as a filter to only let the healthiest and most motile sperm through. Once inside the uterus, sperm must navigate a narrow passageway to pass through the uterine tube, the site of fertilization. They have to deal with the vaginal acidic environment and the female reproductive tract's immune system along the way.

Sperm go through a process known as capacitation when they get to the uterine tube. This process modifies their motility and membrane characteristics and makes them ready to fertilize an egg. The zona pellucida, a glycoprotein-rich matrix encircling the egg, is then bound to the fertilized sperm by interactions with specific proteins on their surface.

Sperm undergo the acrosome reaction, which releases enzymes from the acrosome, a specialized vesicle at the tip of the sperm head once they are bound to the zona pellucida. The sperm can pass through the zona pellucida and get to the plasma membrane of the egg thanks to these enzymes. The process of fertilization begins when a single sperm successfully penetrates the zona pellucida.

The sperm and egg fuse when they come into contact with the egg's plasma membrane, creating a fertilization cone. The completion of meiosis, the process by which the egg's nucleus divides to form a mature egg cell, and the release of calcium ions are among the biochemical reactions that are set off by this fusion event.

A zygote is created when the nuclei of an egg and sperm combine to form the first cell of a new person. The zygote, which represents the genetic code of the new organism, has a full complement of chromosomes, half from the sperm and half from the egg. The zygote divides rapidly as it passes through the uterine tube and moves toward the uterus, forming the solid ball known as the morula.

After that, the morula divides and rearranges its cells one more time, eventually creating the hollow, fluid-filled structure known as the blastocyst. The inner cell mass and the outer layer of trophoblast cells make up the two different cell populations that make up the blastocyst. The placenta will develop from the trophoblast cells, and the embryo proper will grow from the inner cell mass. The blastocyst adheres to the uterine wall and forms connections with the mother's blood supply during the implantation process, which occurs as it enters the uterus. Interactions between the blastocyst and the maternal tissues enable implantation, an essential stage in the establishment of pregnancy.

A new person is created through the intricate process of fertilization, which unites an egg and sperm. It is a highly controlled and synchronized sequence of events that starts with the sperm traveling in the direction of the egg and ends with the blastocyst being implanted in the uterus. The advancement of reproductive biology, the creation of assisted reproductive technologies, and the development of infertility treatments all depend on our ability to comprehend the complexities of fertilization.

7.1.1. Sperm-Egg Interaction and Formation of Zygote

Important stages in the reproduction process, the sperm-egg contact and the subsequent zygote formation signify the beginning of new life. This complex process entails a sequence of precisely timed molecular and cellular events that combine the genetic material of two gametes to form a single diploid cell that can differentiate into a new organism.

Millions of sperm cells are released into the female reproductive tract during ejaculation, marking the beginning of the sperm's journey toward the egg. These sperm cells go through a difficult process known as capacitation, which modifies their motility and membrane characteristics and makes them able to fertilize an egg. The fertilized sperm then follow chemical cues and mechanical forces through the cervix and uterus to reach the uterine tube, where fertilization occurs. An egg cell matures inside the ovary in the meantime, and it is released during ovulation. The zona pellucida, or protective layer, envelops the ovum, or egg, and is lined with cumulus cells. The egg waits for sperm to arrive in order to be fertilized as it passes through the uterine tube.

Sperm engage in a variety of interactions with the zona pellucida, the glycoprotein-rich matrix encircling the egg, as soon as they get close to the egg. Specialized proteins on the sperm surface attach to receptors on the zona pellucida to mediate these interactions. The acrosome reaction, which is initiated by binding to the zona pellucida, releases the enzymes that are housed in the acrosome, a specialized vesicle located at the tip of the sperm head. The sperm can pass through the zona pellucida and get to the plasma membrane of the egg thanks to these enzymes.

A single sperm undergoes fusion with the egg upon coming into contact with the egg's plasma membrane, creating a fertilization cone. The completion of meiosis, the process by which the egg's nucleus divides to form a mature egg cell, and the release of calcium ions are among the biochemical reactions that are set off by this fusion event. A zygote is created when the nuclei of an egg and sperm combine to form the first cell of a new person.

The zygote, which represents the genetic code of the new organism, has a full complement of chromosomes, half from the sperm and half from the egg. This historic moment initiates the process of embryonic development and initiates a series of cellular events that culminate in the formation of a fully developed organism.

The process of cleavage causes the zygote to divide rapidly into multiple cells after fertilization. Blastomers, which are smaller, undifferentiated cells, are produced as a result of these divisions. The zygote undergoes cleavage to become a solid ball of cells called the morula, which matures into the hollow, fluid-filled structure known as the blastocyst as it continues. The inner cell mass and the outer layer of trophoblast cells are the two different cell populations that make up the blastocyst. The placenta will develop from the trophoblast cells, and the embryo proper will grow from the inner cell mass. An essential stage in establishing pregnancy is implantation, which the blastocyst goes through as it passes through the uterine tube and approaches the uterus.

The development of the zygote and the interaction between the sperm and the egg are fundamental processes in reproduction that are necessary for life to continue. With the help of mechanical forces and chemical cues, sperm and egg perform a complex dance that eventually creates a new person with the capacity for growth, development, and eventual birth. Comprehending the complexities of this procedure is essential for progressing the field of reproductive biology, as well as for creating assisted reproductive technologies and infertility treatments.

7.1.1.1. Fertilization

The process of fertilization involves the union of a maternal egg nucleus and a paternal sperm nucleus to create the primary nucleus of an embryo. The fusion of the genetic material of two distinct sex cells, or gametes, which each carry half the number of chromosomes typical of the species, is the essence of fertilization in all organisms. In microorganisms and protozoans, the simplest type of fertilization is the exchange of genetic material between two cells.

The merging of the two gametes' membranes, which creates a channel that permits material to move from one cell to the other, is the first important step in fertilization. In more developed plants, pollination occurs before fertilization. During pollination, pollen is transferred to and makes contact with the female gamete or macrospore. In most advanced animals, fusion is followed by a single spermatozoon penetrating the egg. After fertilization, a cell known as a zygote is created that can divide into multiple cells to create an adult (Wassarman, 1999; WHO Laboratory Manual for the Examination of Human Semen and Sperm-cervical Mucus Interaction, 2010) (Figure 7.1).

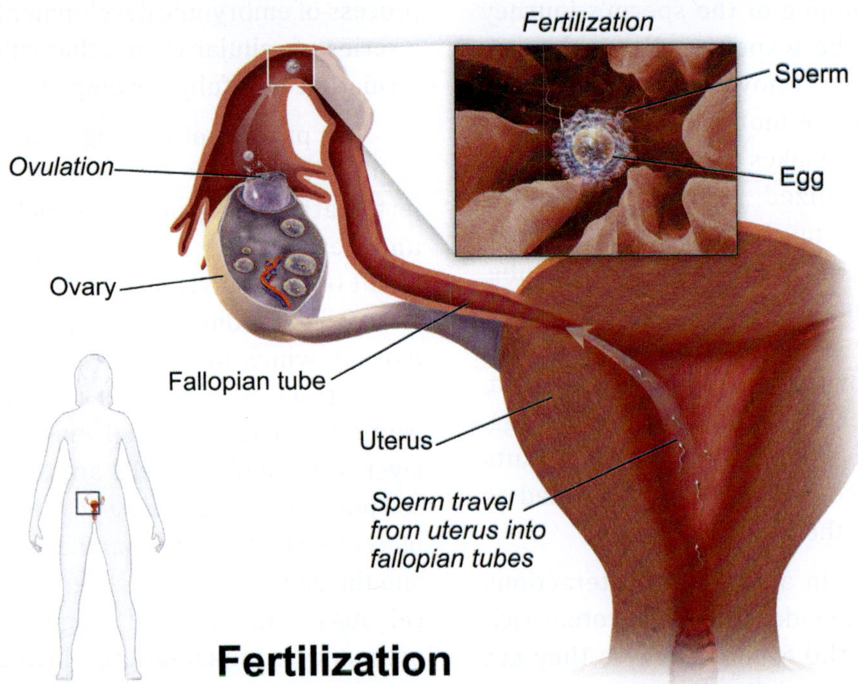

Figure 7.1. *In mammals, eggs are released by the ovaries. If an egg meets a sperm cell, it may become fertilized. The fertilized egg travels to the uterus, where it grows and develops into a new individual.*

Source: By BruceBlaus. When using this image in external sources it can be cited as: Blausen.com staff (2014). "Medical Gallery of Blausen Medical 2014." WikiJournal of Medicine, 1(2). doi: 10.15347/wjm/2014.010. ISSN 2002-4436. Own work, CC BY 3.0, https://commons.wikimedia.org/w/index.php?curid=29738545.

Multiple reactions in the egg are triggered by the union of two gametes. One of these modifies the egg membrane or membranes, preventing multiple spermatozoa from attaching and penetrating. Only one spermatozoal nucleus truly fuses with the egg nucleus in species where multiple spermatozoons typically enter an egg (polyspermy). The most significant outcome of fertilization is the activation of the egg, which permits cell division. It is possible to activate an egg using chemical and physical agents during parthenogenesis, a process in which fertilization does not take place. Spermatozoon intervention is not always necessary, though. Aphids, bees, and rotifers are examples of invertebrates that typically reproduce through parthenogenesis.

Spermatozoa may be attracted to specific chemicals produced by the egg in plants. With the probable exception of some cnidarians (coelenterates), it seems likely that random collisions are the basis for egg-spermatozoa contact in animals. However, many animals' gelatinous coats around their eggs act as a trap for spermatozoa, improving the likelihood of a successful sperm-egg interaction.

Marine invertebrate eggs, particularly those of echinoderms, are traditional study subjects for fertilization. These transparent eggs are useful for biochemical and molecular research as well as studies observing living cells because the fertilization time can be precisely controlled, many eggs develop at roughly the same rate under the right circumstances, and large quantities of the eggs are available. Some teleost and amphibian eggs have also been employed with good outcomes.

7.1.1.2. Maturation of the Egg

The process of maturation is the last stage of oogenesis, the development of functional eggs that can attach to spermatozoa and produce a response that stops multiple spermatozoa from entering. Furthermore, a mature egg's cytoplasm can facilitate the modifications that result in the fusion of the nuclei of the spermatozoa and the egg, starting the process of embryonic development.

7.1.1.3. Egg Surface

Certain components of an egg's surface, specifically cortical granules, indicate a mature state. Cortical granules found in sea urchin eggs are located beneath the plasma membrane of mature eggs and have a size of 0.8–1.0 microns, surrounded by a membrane resembling the egg's plasma membrane. These granules are produced in the Golgi complex within the cell and then move to the surface of the developing egg.

The ability of a sea urchin egg's surface to affect light passage unevenly in various directions is known as birefringence, and it is a sign that the molecules that make up the surface layers are arranged in a specific way. Given that birefringence develops with egg maturity, particular molecular configurations are probably linked to the characteristics of an adult egg membrane. An adult egg can sustain the development of a zygote nucleus; that is, i.e., the outcome of the nuclei of the egg and spermatozoa fusing. Meiosis, the process of reducing the number of chromosomes in eggs, is typically not finished in eggs before fertilization. In these situations, the fertilizing spermatozoon stays below the surface of the egg until the egg has finished going through meiosis, at which point it undergoes modifications and movements that cause the egg to fuse and form a zygote.

7.1.1.4. Egg Coats

Most animal eggs have envelopes covering their surfaces. These envelopes can be thick membranes in fish, insects, and mammals, or soft, gelatinous coats in echinoderms and some amphibians. Therefore, spermatozoa must break through these envelopes to reach the egg surface; in fact, they are broken down by the enzymes (organic catalysts) found in spermatozoa. In certain circumstances (e.g., fishes, and insects) have an opening in the envelope called a micropyle that allows a spermatozoon to enter and reach the egg.

Eggs from echinoderms and amphibians have jelly coats made of complex carbohydrates known as sulfated mucopolysaccharides. Mammalian eggs have an envelope that is more intricate. A thick layer of zona pellucida, a complex of carbohydrates and proteins, envelops the egg. An outer layer known as the corona radiata, is made up of numerous cell layers and is formed by follicle cells adhering to the oocyte before it leaves the ovarian follicle, enveloping the zona.

While it was previously believed that the jelly coat of an echinoderm egg contained a substance called fertilizin that played a key role in sperm-egg interaction and egg activation, it has since been discovered that fertilizin is the same as the jelly-coat material itself. However, there is evidence to suggest that the egg envelopes still have a role in fertilization, as contact with the egg coat triggers the acrosome reaction in sperm.

7.1.2. Events of Fertilization: Sperm–Egg Association

The spermatozoon-egg association happens when their plasma membranes fuse together, and it requires the spermatozoa to undergo the acrosome reaction. The acrosome, a protrusion at the front tip of the spermatozoa, experiences several distinct structural alterations following contact between a spermatozoon and an egg. The plasma membrane of the sperm fuses with the acrosomal vesicle's surrounding membrane at the acrosomal tip to form an opening when the acrosomal vesicle, a structure inside the acrosome, bursts. The acrosomal granule, which is contained within the acrosomal vesicle, vanishes as the opening forms (Figure 7.2).

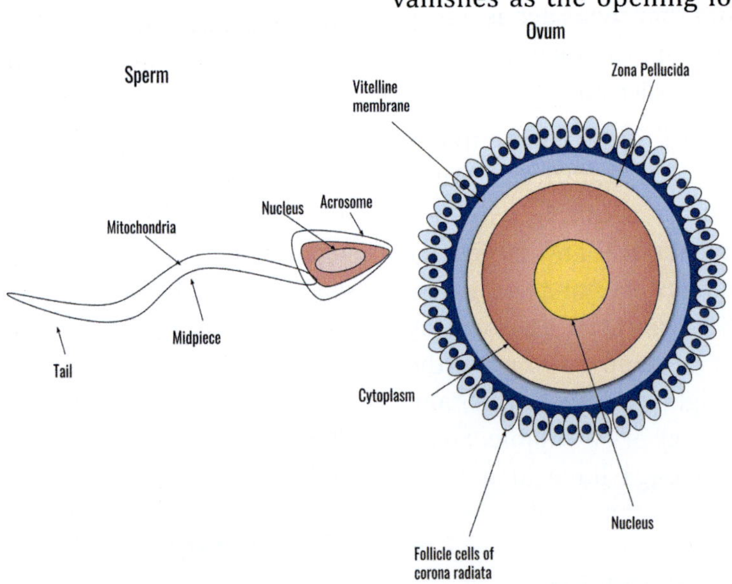

Figure 7.2. *These a sperm cell comes in contact with the outer layers of an egg cell, the acrosome, which is a prominence at the anterior tip of the spermatozoa, undergoes a series of well-defined structural changes that open a path for the sperm nucleus.*

Source: By Atdoan0 – Own work, CC BY-SA 4.0, https://commons.wikimedia.org/w/index.php?curid=69565828.

The lysin that is released when the granule dissolves breaks down the vitelline coat of the egg, enabling the spermatozoon to enter the egg. The area of the acrosomal membrane opposite the aperture clings to the spermatozoon's nuclear envelope, creating a shallow outpocketing that quickly lengthens into the acrosomal tubule, a thin tube that reaches the egg surface and unites with the egg plasma membrane. The spermatozoal nucleus can enter the egg through the tubule that is thereby formed, which also maintains continuity between the spermatozoon and the egg. The acrosomal membrane and spermatozoal plasma membrane, on the other hand, do not penetrate the interior of the egg. Other spermatozoal structures that may be carried within the egg include the midpiece and a portion of the tail. Whole spermatozoa cannot fuse with the egg nucleus or cause an activation response when injected into unfertilized eggs. The spermatozoal plasma membrane degrades as the spermatozoal nucleus is drawn into the egg; after the process, the continuity of the egg plasma membrane is restored. This description of the sperm-egg association process, initially reported for the acorn worm Saccoglossus (Phylum Enteropneusta), is generally applicable to most eggs that have been investigated to date.

Spermatozoa must experience a physiological change known as capacitation during their passage through the female genital tract of mammals to participate in fertilization. Once in the interior of the egg, they can traverse the egg envelopes and undergo the acrosome reaction. Hyaluronidase, an enzyme, breaks down hyaluronic acid, a substance that binds corona radiata cells together, causing the cells in the outer egg envelope (corona radiata) to disperse. When the spermatozoon passes through the corona radiata, the enzyme may be inside the acrosome and released as a consequence of the acrosome reaction. By the time a spermatozoon comes into contact with the dense layer encasing the egg (zona pellucida), the reaction has already progressed significantly. Its passage through the zona pellucida resembles an oblique slit that is formed by the sperm's head oscillation close to the zona pellucida attachment site.

In mammals, the spermatozoon attaches to the egg surface on its side rather than at the tip like in other animals, allowing the spermatozoon to rest flat on the egg surface. This attachment involves multiple points of fusion between the plasma membranes of the two gametes, which occurs through the formation of numerous small vesicles (Wassarman, 1999; WHO Laboratory Manual for the Examination of Human Semen and Sperm-cervical Mucus Interaction, 2010).

7.1.3. Specificity of Sperm–Egg Interaction

The process of fertilization is unique to each species, and the zona pellucida, which coats the egg, is crucial to the sperm egg binding process. Generally speaking, the zona pellucida only matches and binds with sperm of the same species because the biochemistry (zona pellucid) of each species varies. For instance, only the spermatozoa of the same species are clumped together, or agglutinate, in solutions of the jelly coat among echinoderms. However, modest damage to an egg surface in both echinoderms and amphibians allows for heterologous fertilization—fertilization with spermatozoa from different species—a process that has been used to produce some hybrid larvae. In addition, when the egg's zona pellucida is removed, binding between sperm and egg of different species may happen.

Members of the chordate subphylum Tunicata, ascidians, also known as sea squirts, lay their eggs on thick membranes called chorions. Test cells are found in the space between the chorion and the egg. Ascidians are animals that possess both male and female reproductive organs in their gametes. Although their gametes mature simultaneously, self-fertilization does not take place. However, if the test cells and the chorion are removed, self-fertilization as well as fertilization with spermatozoa of different species are both possible outcomes.

7.1.3.1. Prevention of Polyspermy

Most animal eggs are monospermic, i.e., a single spermatozoon is allowed entry into an egg. Certain characteristics of the egg surface protect in certain cases against multiple sperms penetrating the egg (polyspermy); in other cases, however, the egg envelopes play the role. During the process of egg maturation, known as oogenesis, certain eggs undergo a molecular rearrangement that affects their ability to develop a polyspermy-preventing reaction. Despite their capacity to attach themselves to spermatozoa, immature sea urchin eggs also permit multiple penetration, i.e., they are not able to produce a response that would stop polyspermy. Specific features of the egg surface must be differentiated by the time meiosis stops, which is when the egg is ready to be fertilized since mature eggs of most animals are fertilized before completion of meiosis and can develop a polyspermy-preventing reaction.

In certain mammalian eggs, the zona pellucida's characteristics determine the defense against polyspermy, i.e., spermatozoa that have begun to pass through the zona do not permit more spermatozoa to enter (zona reaction). However, in other mammals, as evidenced by the abundance of spermatozoa in the area between the zona and egg surface, the zona reaction either does not occur or occurs weakly. In these circumstances, the egg surface contains the polyspermy-preventing response. While some animal species' eggs (e.g., certain birds, reptiles, amphibians, and sharks) are inherently polyspermic; all other spermatozoa degenerate. Only one spermatozoal nucleus unites with an egg nucleus to form a zygote nucleus (Wassarman, 1999; WHO Laboratory Manual for the Examination of Human Semen and Sperm-cervical Mucus Interaction, 2010).

7.1.3.2. Formation of the Fertilization Membrane

At the surface of the egg, the most striking changes occur after fertilization. The sea urchin egg is the most well-known example, and it is explained below. The vitelline membrane, which rises from the egg surface immediately after fertilization, is one reaction. The membrane is extremely thin at first, but it quickly thickens, forms a well-organized molecular structure, and is given the name fertilization membrane. Concurrently, there is a significant rearrangement of the molecular structure of the egg surface. It takes roughly one minute for the processes that result in the formation of the fertilization membrane.

The thin vitelline membrane separates at the location on the sea urchin egg's outer surface where a spermatozoan attaches. The granules open and their contents are extruded into the perivitelline space as a result of the cortical granules' membranes coming into contact with and fusing with the inner aspect of the egg's plasma membrane, i.e., the gap that exists between the raised vitelline membrane and the egg surface. The formation of the fertilization membrane occurs when a portion of the granules' contents fuse with the vitelline membrane; if this process is not allowed to occur, the membrane stays thin and pliable. The hyaline layer, a transparent layer that forms on the egg's surface and is also derived from the cortical granules, is crucial for maintaining the integrity of the blastomeres—the cells created during the egg's division or cleavage. As a result, the plasma membrane surrounding a fertilized egg is a mosaic structure made up of regions made from cortical granule membranes and patches of the original plasma membrane of the unfertilized egg. The processes that lead to the formation of the fertilization membrane include the outflow of potassium ions (charged particles) and a change in the electric charge across the plasma membrane, known as the fertilization potential. These processes are comparable to those that take place in a stimulated nerve fiber. The permeability of the egg's plasma membrane to different molecules increases several times as a result of fertilization. The activation of a membrane transport mechanism located on the surface could be the cause of this alteration.

7.1.3.3. Formation of the Zygote Nucleus

The spermatozoal nucleus, now known as the male pronucleus, expands and disperses its chromosomal material, taking on an appearance resembling that of the female pronucleus after it enters the egg cytoplasm. The male pronucleus in the egg undergoes rapid disintegration of its membrane envelope, but it is quickly replaced by a new one. Two structures known as centrioles, which aid in cell division, initially accompany the male pronucleus as it rotates 180° and advances in the direction of the egg nucleus. The first cleavage spindle is produced by the spermatozoal centrioles following contact between the male and female pronuclei. This process occurs before the fertilized egg divides. A process known as membrane fusion, in which two adjacent membranes fuse at their point of contact to create the continuous nuclear envelope that envelops the zygote nucleus, may occasionally result in the fusion of the two pronuclei.

7.1.3.4. Zygote

The fertilized egg cell known as a zygote is the product of the union of a male gamete (sperm) and a female gamete (egg, or ovum). The zygote stage, which is short in the embryonic development of humans and other animals, is followed by cleavage, in which the single cell divides into smaller cells. An organism with its genetic makeup begins its development with the zygote. The zygote is diploid (carries two sets of chromosomes) because it is endowed with genes from two parents. Every organism—aside from bacteria—reproduces diploid zygotes through the joining of haploid gametes. This process is known as sexual reproduction.

All the necessary components for development are present in the zygote, but they only exist as an encoded set of instructions that are in the genes of chromosomes. The new zygote's genes are not activated to produce proteins until multiple cell divisions leading up to cleavage. Through the process of mitosis, the relatively large zygote directly divides into numerous smaller cells of conventional size during cleavage (ordinary cell proliferation by division). These smaller cells, known as blastomeres, are appropriate for serving as the organism's initial building blocks.

Humans have identical twins that arise from a zygote that divides into two distinct cell masses relatively early in the process of growth. These two masses develop into embryos despite having the same genetic makeup. Contrarily, fraternal twins are created from two distinct zygotes, which are two distinct eggs fertilized by two distinct sperm (Wassarman, 1999; WHO Laboratory Manual for the Examination of Human Semen and Sperm-cervical Mucus Interaction, 2010).

7.1.4. Biochemical Analysis of Fertilization

Early research on the biochemical changes during fertilization primarily focused on the respiratory metabolism of the egg. Initial findings suggested that sea urchin eggs exhibited a higher rate of oxygen consumption immediately following fertilization or parthenogenetic activation, leading to the belief that fertilization involved overcoming a metabolic barrier in the unfertilized egg. However, further studies have demonstrated that this increased oxygen consumption is not a consistent occurrence in all animal eggs during fertilization, with some even showing a temporary decrease in oxygen consumption.

The egg has all the necessary components at fertilization to carry out protein synthesis and, consequently, development through the blastula, an early stage of embryogenesis. Most messenger RNA molecules, which are ribonucleic acid molecules formed during oogenesis and stored in the egg, direct the majority of immediate post-fertilization protein synthesis. Furthermore, the unfertilized egg contains components of the cell called ribosomes, which control protein synthesis up to the blastula stage (a much earlier stage in the mammalian embryo). New ribosomes and molecules of a different type of RNA involved in protein synthesis, known as transfer RNA, are synthesized at a later stage in embryonic development (gastrulation). In addition to reaching the blastula stage, fertilized eggs grown in the presence of the antibiotic actinomycin—which inhibits RNA synthesis—also exhibit an identical rate of protein synthesis to untreated embryos.

The extremely low rate of protein synthesis observed in unfertilized sea urchin eggs and those of other marine animals investigated thus far indicates that the machinery for synthesizing proteins in the unfertilized egg may be inhibited by something. Since the rate of protein synthesis rises right after fertilization, it might be influenced by an inhibitor's modification or elimination. For instance, the low efficiency of the protein synthesizing machinery in the sea urchin egg appears to be dependent on specific ribosome characteristics. In an unfertilized sea urchin egg, most of the ribosomes are single ribosomes or so-called monosomes; however, shortly after fertilization, the single ribosomes interact with messenger RNA molecules to form polyribosomes, which are the active units in protein synthesis. This process has also been observed in the eggs of a few other studied marine animals. An inhibitor that is linked to unfertilized sea urchin egg ribosomes prevents messenger RNA molecules from binding to the ribosomes, which results in inefficiency in protein synthesis. The inhibitor is eliminated nearly immediately after fertilization, possibly through enzymatic breakdown.

Thus, the ribosome level controls the overall rate of protein synthesis, at least in sea urchin eggs, and the activation of protein synthesis after fertilization begins with the ribosomes being "turned on." In vertebrates, including amphibians, meiosis, and ovulation of the egg result in the activation of protein synthesis. The messenger RNAs in the oocyte attach to the ribosomes to start the process of protein synthesis (Wassarman, 1999; WHO Laboratory Manual for the Examination of Human Semen and Sperm-cervical Mucus Interaction, 2010).

7.2. Early Embryonic Development

A single fertilized egg can develop into a multicellular organism, but early embryonic development is a crucial stage in this process. The process starts with fertilization, in which an egg and sperm cell combine to form a zygote, which restores the diploid chromosome number and starts development. After that comes cleavage, a sequence of quick mitotic divisions that result in the production of smaller cells called blastomeres and eventually form a solid ball of cells called a morula. Following blastulation, the morula develops into a blastocyst, which will eventually give rise to the embryo. It is distinguished by an inner cell mass (ICM), an outer cell layer (trophoblast), and a fluid-filled cavity (blastocoel). After implantation, the blastocyst connects to the mother's blood supply by embedding itself in the uterine wall.

The single-layered blastula becomes a multi-layered gastrula during the critical reorganization stage known as gastrulation, which creates the three main germ layers—the ectoderm, mesoderm, and endoderm. The skin and nervous system are developed by the ectoderm, the muscles, bones, and circulatory system by the mesoderm, and the respiratory and digestive systems by the endoderm.

The body plan is then determined during the process of organogenesis. Neurulation, the development of the neural tube (the future central nervous system), and the somites' segmentation—which results in the vertebrae and related musculature—are important events. The development of major organs and limb buds occurs during this stage as well. Cell signaling pathways, gene expression, and other factors control these processes (e.g., Wnt, BMP, and Notch), morphogen gradients, and cell migration, which guarantee accurate tissue and organ development in both space and time. Gaining knowledge of these mechanisms is essential to comprehending both normal development and congenital anomalies.

1. **Cleavage and Blastulation:** These are crucial stages in early embryonic development that transform a single-cell zygote into a structured, multicellular embryo.
2. **Cleavage:** It is the series of rapid mitotic cell divisions that the zygote undergoes immediately after fertilization. Key features of this stage include:
    i. **Rapid Divisions:** The zygote divides into smaller cells called blastomeres without increasing in overall size. These divisions are rapid and synchronous initially.

    ii. **Formation of the Morula:** After several rounds of division, the embryo forms a solid ball of cells known as the morula, typically by the 16-cell stage.

    iii. **Reduction in Cell Size:** With each division, the blastomeres become smaller as they share the cytoplasm of the original zygote, ensuring that the overall size of the embryo does not increase.
3. **Blastulation:** It follows cleavage and marks the formation of a fluid-filled cavity within the morula, transforming it into a blastocyst. Key features of this stage include:
    i. **Blastocoel Formation:** A cavity called the blastocoel forms within the cell mass, leading to the differentiation of cells.

    ii. **Trophoblast and Inner Cell Mass (ICM):** Cells begin to differentiate into two main types:
        a. **Trophoblast:** The outer layer of cells that will eventually contribute to the formation of the placenta, providing nutrients and support to the developing embryo.

        b. **Inner Cell Mass (ICM):** A cluster of cells inside the blastocyst that will develop into the embryo proper.

    iii. **Hatching and Implantation:** The blastocyst eventually hatches from the zona pellucida (a protective glycoprotein layer) and prepares for implantation into the uterine wall, a critical step for establishing a connection with the maternal blood supply.

These stages are orchestrated by a tightly regulated sequence of genetic and molecular events, ensuring the successful transition from a single cell to a structured, multicellular organism ready for further development.

7.2.1. Sperm Flow Cytometry: Beyond Human Fertilization and Embryo Development

Since the introduction of assisted reproductive technology (ART), there has been a renewed focus on understanding human reproductive processes. New information from cellular and molecular diagnostic methods is crucial in the reproductive field in the 21st century. Not only in early reproductive processes like gametogenesis, but also in peri-implantation processes involving the sperm-oocyte interaction, cellular changes observed during fertilization, and the early and late embryo development, ART has been involved in the description of alternative pathways in basic cellular functions. The application of flow cytometry (FC) in this field has aided in the standardization of an increasing number of diagnostic and therapeutic approaches, as well as the comprehension of all these processes.

Various processes are involved in the early stages of human gametogenesis, with the spermatozoon playing a crucial role in fertilization. It not only serves as a carrier of genetic material but also interacts with other internal components such as RNAm and mitochondrial organelles. Spermatogenesis is influenced by programmed cell death pathways, particularly during packaging and cytoplasmic structure elongation. Flow cytometry has become a valuable tool for diagnosing and treating infertility by allowing for the precise selection and differentiation of spermatozoa from subfertile individuals. In modern *in-vitro* fertilization techniques, such as intracytoplasmic sperm injection (ICSI), these advances in discrimination tools have resulted in improved embryo outcomes.

The introduction of multiple enzymes into the cytoplasm of the egg occurs in the first stage of the sperm/oocyte interaction, known as the acrosome reaction. Acromegalyser-reacted human sperm scoring enables a faster, easier, and more precise FC method. When a spermatozoon enters an ovum, the process of sperm chromatin decondensation takes place. During the early stages of embryo development, the interaction between the male and female pronuclei has been demonstrated to be predictive. Thanks to FC, we now know that the quality of the embryo is affected by the early distribution of organelles such as mitochondria before genetic activation in stage eight cells takes place. Furthermore, during the peri-implantation phase, the condition of the egg and sperm may have an impact on polarity and blastocyst development.

Over many generations, people have entertained fantasies about the possibility of having children of a specific sex. Predetermination of sex is typically motivated by social norms or a desire to prevent the possible conception of a child who may have an X-linked recessive disorder. The use of FC in spermatozoa selection has made this possible (Wassarman, 1999; WHO Laboratory Manual for the Examination of Human Semen and Sperm-cervical Mucus Interaction, 2010).

7.2.2. Flow Cytometry to Explore Human Spermatozoa: Reproductive Impact

Negative male reproductive health conditions have been linked in recent years to an increase in testicular cancer, hypospadias, anatomical dysfunction, and abnormal semen parameters, as well as an increase in the need for antiretroviral therapy (ART). The World Health Organization's guidelines for diagnosing male infertility include a visual evaluation of semen analysis, which is not standardized and has shown variation among technicians and laboratories globally. Furthermore, no molecular or functional tests are used regularly, and the subjective assessment of sperm morphology, viability, motility, and number does not assess all the biological traits of sperm that may be crucial during the interaction between the egg and spermatozoa. The development of new and improved diagnostic techniques that lessen operator variability reflecting sperm defects not accessible by the conventional microscope scoring becomes crucial because male infertility can account for up to 50% of the dysfunctional reproductive process. In this context, the application of FC offers an automated, quick, sensitive, objective, multiparametric, and repeatable method for evaluating male infertility, particularly in ART candidates. Sperm concentration could be ascertained with a flow cytometer since it can record thousands of events at a constant flow rate in a matter of seconds. To assess spermatogenesis and determine the total number in a known volume, haploid mature cells, haploid round spermatids, and diploid cells are often distinguished using DNA dyes during the cell number assessment process with FC. Spermatozoa numbers can be more reliably obtained by using fluorospheres as an internal control and by properly adjusting the flow.

To test the effects of cell sorting, swim-up, cryopreservation, and efforts to create populations enriched in highly motile spermatozoa, FC has evaluated sperm motility using markers of mitochondrial membrane potential. Numerous essential stains, including ethidium homodimer and propidium iodine (PI), have been used in studies on cell viability. When these dyes attach to nucleic acids, they break through the plasmalemma of the cell and release red fluorescence. Other viability probes that enter metabolically active cells, such as SYBR-14 and fluorescein diacetate, release green fluorescence. To assess sperm viability, PI/SYBR-14 is arguably the most used combination.

7.2.3. Acrosome Reaction: Fertilizing Spermatozoa-Oocyte Binding

It is widely acknowledged that ejaculated spermatozoa must experience capacitation, identify and attach to the zona pellucida, and go through the acrosome reaction to fertilize the egg. The most notable alterations to the sperm during capacitation include modifications to the plasma membrane, an increase in specific intracellular messengers, and an increase in the phosphorylation of a group of proteins by various kinases.

An essential step in the spermatozoa's exocytic process, the acrosome reaction is necessary for fertilization. Only a few of the many sperm plasma membrane candidates for zona pellucida-sperm binding have been demonstrated to be important in the acrosome reaction's induction. A zona pellucida glycoprotein (ZP3) may function as a ligand for one or more sperm plasma membrane receptor(s) to trigger the acrosome reaction *in vivo*. Meanwhile, another protein, ZP2, aids in the secondary binding of spermatozoa that have undergone an acrosome reaction to the zona matrix penetration. According to multiple studies, sperm responsiveness to acrosome reaction inducers was decreased in infertile patients; as a result, assessing acrosome reaction can help determine the best ART technique to use and predict the success of fertilization. The traditional methods for assessing acrosome intactness include phase-contrast, fluorescent, and even electron microscopy. Nevertheless, the FC can be used in place of microscopy to examine large numbers of sperm and determine the temporal occurrence of the acrosome reaction. The fluorescently labeled probes attach to the mannose and galactose components of the acrosomal matrix. Only spermatozoa that have damaged or reacted with the acrosome will stain because probes cannot pass through an intact acrosomal membrane. For both fresh and *in vitro-capacitated* sperm, double staining for membrane integrity and acrosomal integrity is a reasonably reliable method.

Furthermore, several studies have shown the potential of FC to investigate the physiological and molecular alterations that allow sperm to fertilize. For instance, CD46 on the inner acrosomal membranes of human sperm serves to shield the spermatozoa from complement-mediated lysis. Carver and associates showed that a high fertilization prediction using flow cytometric analysis of the CD46 antigen is feasible. Furthermore, a recent study demonstrates that a decrease in Na+ mediated by inhibition of epithelial Na+ channels and regulated by PKA is involved in the capacitation-associated hyperpolarization of the sperm plasma membrane potential (Wassarman, 1999; WHO Laboratory Manual for the Examination of Human Semen and Sperm-cervical Mucus Interaction, 2010).

7.2.4. The Ubiquitin-Proteasome Pathway

All cells with a nucleus contain the protein ubiquitin. With an isopeptide that binds the E-amino group of a lysine residue in substrate proteins and the C-terminal glycine of ubiquitin, this protein forms covalent bonds with other proteins. We refer to this phenomenon as ubiquitination. Numerous fertilization processes have been linked to ubiquitination. For instance, during spermatogenesis, transition proteins and permanent protamines replace the spermatid's nuclear histones. This process, which results in a sharp decrease in the sperm centrosome, is also seen during spermatid elongation. Normally, ubiquitination takes place in the cytosol or nucleus of the cell, but in certain cases, such as when spermatozoa are defective, it happens on their surface during post-testicular sperm maturation in the epididymis. The surface-ubiquitin detection has the potential to be a biomarker for infertility diagnostics and aids in the identification of spermatozoa with defects. Obtaining a single sample of semen can facilitate the detection and measurement of ubiquitin expression.

7.2.5. Human Spermatozoa Related to Abnormal Fertilization and Embryo Development: Evidence From ART

In vitro fertilization (IVF) has been demonstrated to have biological diagnostic properties in the fertilization process in addition to facilitating gamete interaction and helping to resolve fertility dysfunction. Male factor infertility is frequently treated with intracytoplasmic sperm injection (ICSI), a procedure in which a mature spermatozoon is injected into a metaphase II oocyte. By using this method, the effects of the microinjection should be ascertained to assess both the process's safety and any potential long-term repercussions. This is a result of ICSI skipping a lot of the natural fertilization processes. The concept of paternal contribution to faulty fertilization and abnormal embryogenesis has received initial support in the last two decades, even though successful fertilization is unquestionably dependent upon multiple inherent qualities of the oocyte. These lines of evidence have resulted from the use of assisted reproductive technology (ART). In the early stages, the newly formed zygote initiates the cleavage divisions by relying on the endogenous information of the oocyte. The transcription then begins when the embryo reaches the four to eight-cell stage. Because of this, sperm nuclear defects are not often found before the eight-cell stage of embryogenesis, which is when sperm gene expression begins to increase. Deficits in sperm cytoplasm can be identified in the single-cell zygote and later during the preimplantation stage. The early paternal effect is thought to involve aberrations of the centrosome-cytoskeletal apparatus and sperm abnormalities connected to oocyte activation (no sperm delivery or dysfunctional oocyte-activating factor). Furthermore, it is observed that the late paternal effect is associated with abnormalities in sperm mitochondrial or mRNA delivery, as well as changes in sperm DNA chromatin.

Early and late paternal effects are two ways that the anomalies associated with genomic imprinting changes can manifest themselves. There is substantial evidence linking aberrant sperm parameters—most notably teratozoospermia, but also oxidative damage and DNA fragmentation to delayed or unsuccessful fertilization and, crucially, abnormal embryo development.

Ejaculated human spermatozoa may present various degrees of DNA damage. Different theories have been proposed to explain its origin:

- Harm could occur now of DNA packing or can be the result of it during the transition of histone to protamine complex in the spermiogenesis process.
- DNA fragmentation could be the consequence as well of direct oxidative damage that has been associated with xenobiotics, antioxidant depletion, smoking, heat exposure, presence of ions in sperm culture media, and leukocyte contamination of semen.
- DNA damage that could be the consequence of apoptosis.

The presence of apoptosis in ejaculated spermatozoa may result from a variety of wounds. When apoptosis occurs *in vivo*, it can be caused by various factors such as hormone depletion, radiation, heat, chemicals, and toxic agents; epididymal signals from abnormal and/or senescent spermatozoa or leukocytes that release reactive oxygen species and other mediators of inflammation/infection; or seminal levels from reactive oxygen species, antioxidant deficiency, or other sources. Furthermore, elements found in the female tract may cause apoptosis. Apoptosis is brought on *in vitro* by various manipulation techniques or incubation in insufficient culture media. Current techniques do not recognize spermatozoa that undergo apoptosis independently of the stimulus. However, there is a chance that these spermatozoa will transfer an unhealthy genome to the egg, which could lead to poor embryo development, miscarriage, or birth abnormalities.

It has long been known that the mature sperm nucleus's chromatin can be packaged abnormally. Furthermore, there is a clear correlation between nuclear DNA damage in mature spermatozoa and low semen parameters, as well as a possible relationship between aberrant chromatin packaging and nuclear DNA damage. Different animal species have endogenous bases in their DNA that are regularly expressed at specific stages of spermiogenesis; these endogenous bases are present during spermiogenesis but become invisible once chromatin packaging is finished. It is known that during protamination, chromatin rearrangement is fixed, and torsional stress is released by the endogenous nuclease topoisomerase 11 by creating and binding nicks.

Numerous investigations have shown that the quality of sperm DNA has a strong predictive ability for *in vitro* fertilization. Tomlinson and colleagues demonstrate that the amount of

DNA fragmentation measured by *in situ* nick translation was the only factor in IVF that showed a significant difference between the groups of pregnant and nonpregnant patients.

The Sperm Chromatin Structure Assay (SCSA) is a diagnostic tool used to assess DNA stability in sperm and is linked to successful fertilization, blastocyst formation, and ongoing pregnancy in *in-vitro* fertilization and ICSI cycles. This test measures the susceptibility of sperm DNA to denaturation by exposing it to acid for 30 seconds and then staining it with acridine orange, with the addition of flow cytometry (FC) making the results more reliable. FC analysis has shown that methods such as swim-up and percoll gradient centrifugation can improve the percentage of sperm with normal chromatin structure in samples with poor initial quality.

With FC, it is possible to quickly assess the expression of sperm apoptotic-like markers, and variations between people with normal and aberrant sperm parameters have been observed. Sperm annexin V labeling can be used to identify the translocation of phosphatidylserine from the inner to the outer leaflet of the plasma membrane, which is one of the initial stages of apoptosis. To perform sperm FC analysis, annexin V is currently available conjugated with a broad range of fluorochromes. An additional marker of apoptosis is increased membrane permeability, which can be identified in membrane-undamaged spermatozoa using a combination of dyes. When annexin V and PI are combined, it becomes possible to identify spermatozoa with damaged plasma membranes and alterations that resemble apoptosis. By utilizing FC, these two parameters distinguish between four types of sperm: live, live early "apoptotic," dead and late "apoptotic," and late "necrotic" cells. While annexin V/PI measures early sperm apoptosis-like changes, flow cytometric analysis of DNA fragmentation evaluated by terminal deoxynucleotidyl transferase-mediated UTD nick-end labeling (TUNEL) measures changes at the later stage (late apoptosis) (Evenson, 1990; Ferrara et al., 1997; Golan et al., 1997; Garrido et al., 2002).

7.2.6. Gender DNA-Based Spermatozoa Sex Selection

In vivo techniques like timed intercourse, ovulation induction, and artificial insemination do not significantly impact the sex ratio, according to data supporting routine preconceptional gender selection techniques. The sex ratio at birth is dramatically altered by the *in vitro* gradient methods separation of X- and Y-bearing spermatozoa. However, these were uncontrolled trials, and molecular biological methods failed to demonstrate a significant change in the Y-to-X-bearing spermatozoa ratio for clinical use. However, preimplantation diagnosis or sperm separation by FC in conjunction with IVF has been used in recent scientific studies to enable reliable preconceptional sex selection. These techniques serve to prevent disorders associated with sex. Most of them lack a medical or therapeutic indication, and both classify *in vitro* fertilization as an invasive procedure. Since both require the invasive IVF process, most people believe they shouldn't be used for non-medical purposes. In the future, enough selected gametes for artificial insemination may be produced by the increase in the FC output of specific X and Y spermatozoa. This method will offer a workable, non-intrusive way to choose sex for social reasons.

The Hoechst 33342 fluorescent dye, which binds to DNA, exhibits variability in chromatin staining. This allows for the classification of individual cells based on their fluorescence, which is detected by FC. Subsequently, a biopsy of the developing embryo (preimplantation genetic diagnosis, PGD) or the polymerase chain reaction (PCR) or FISH on treated spermatozoa is used to determine the use of specific spermatozoa.

The main safety concern with the sorting technique is the potential hazards it poses to the DNA of the sperm. A chemical compound is used that binds to DNA and emits light energy when exposed to a laser beam. The laser beam transfers energy to the atoms surrounding the DNA, potentially creating molecular species that can damage other molecular junctions and the DNA itself. Mature sperm lack mechanisms to repair damaged DNA, with repair only occurring in the egg after fertilization. Increased DNA disruptions can lead to a higher likelihood of errors.

7.2.6.1. Perspectives for Sperm Flow Cytometry

Over the past 20 years, FC has transformed the understanding of reproductive biology. Not only has sperm-oocyte interaction changed, but many dogmas have also, primarily concerning the fertilization process. To effectively support infertile couples and achieve these reproductive goals, assisted reproductive technology requires our comprehension of the molecular network associated with the human model. Flow cytometry is an amazing tool that can be used to select human gametes to improve reproductive health. Additionally, FC has clarified these processes in terms of molecular understanding, mainly for clinical application. In the coming years, we will see developments in the field of human fertilization and embryo development, with the FC continuing to be a valuable resource despite offspring modulation (Evenson, 1990; Ferrara et al., 1997; Golan et al., 1997; Garrido et al., 2002).

A Closer Look

Zona Pellucida

The zona pellucida is a critical structure found in the reproductive system of mammals, particularly within the ovaries. It surrounds and encases the oocyte, or immature egg cell, serving multiple essential functions throughout the process of fertilization and early embryo development. First and foremost, the zona pellucida acts as a protective barrier for the oocyte. It provides a physical shield, safeguarding the delicate inner contents of the egg from external factors and potential damage. This protective role is vital, as the oocyte undergoes maturation within the follicle of the ovary and awaits fertilization.

Moreover, the zona pellucida plays a pivotal role in facilitating fertilization itself. It serves as a crucial site for sperm recognition and binding. Spermatozoa must first penetrate the zona pellucida to reach and fertilize the oocyte. This process involves specific interactions between molecules on the surface of the sperm and receptors within the zona pellucida, ensuring the successful fusion of the sperm with the egg.

Furthermore, following fertilization, the zona pellucida undergoes structural changes to prevent polyspermy, the fertilization of a single egg by multiple sperm. These modifications, which occur rapidly after sperm penetration, involve alterations in the composition and properties of the zona pellucida, making it impermeable to additional sperm and thus preserving the genetic integrity of the resulting embryo.

Throughout early embryonic development, the zona pellucida continues to play essential roles. It provides support and structural integrity to the developing embryo as it undergoes cleavage divisions and travels through the uterine tube toward the uterus for implantation.

The zona pellucida is a specialized extracellular matrix that surrounds the oocyte, fulfilling crucial functions in protecting the egg, facilitating fertilization, preventing polyspermy, and supporting early embryonic development. Its intricate role highlights its significance in the reproductive process and the establishment of new life in mammals.

Summary

- Fertilization marks the initiation of a remarkable journey, the development of reproductive anatomy, and the onset of new life. It's a complex process that begins with the union of a sperm and an egg, leading to the formation of a zygote, the first step in embryonic development.
- The sperm-egg interaction and the subsequent formation of a zygote represent pivotal moments in the process of reproduction, marking the inception of new life.
- The acrosome reaction of spermatozoa is a prerequisite for the association between a spermatozoon and an egg, which occurs through fusion of their plasma membranes.
- Early embryonic development is a critical phase in the formation of a multicellular organism from a single fertilized egg. It begins with fertilization, where a sperm cell unites with an egg cell to form a zygote, restoring the diploid chromosome number and initiating development.
- In-vitro fertilization (IVF) facilitates the interaction between gametes, but beyond the resolution of fertility dysfunction, it has been shown its biological diagnostic qualities in the fertilization process. Intracytoplasmic sperm injection (ICSI) is a technique where the mature spermatozoon is injected into a metaphase II oocyte, it is regularly used in cases of male factor infertility.

References

1. Aitken, R. J. (2006). Sperm function tests and fertility. *International Journal of Andrology, 29*(1), 69–75.
2. Aitken, R. J., & De Iuliis, G. N. (2007). Value of DNA integrity assays for fertility evaluation. *Society of Reproduction and Fertility Supplement, 65*, 81–92.
3. Auger, J., Leonce, S., Jouannet, P., & Ronot, X. (1993). Flow cytometric sorting of living, highly motile human spermatozoa based on evaluation of their mitochondrial activity. *Journal of Histochemistry & Cytochemistry, 41*(8), 1247–1251.
4. Baarends, W. M., Hoogerbrugge, J. W., Roest, H. P., Ooms, M., Vreeburg, J., Hoeijmakers, J. H., & Grootegoed, J. A. (1999). Histone ubiquitination and chromatin remodeling in mouse spermatogenesis. *Developmental Biology, 207*(2), 322–333.
5. Baldi, E., Luconi, M., Bonaccorsi, L., Krausz, C., & Forti, G. (1996). Human sperm activation during capacitation and acrosome reaction: Role of calcium, protein phosphorylation, and lipid remodeling pathways. *Frontiers in Bioscience, 1*, d189–205.
6. Barroso, G., Mercan, R., Ozgur, K., Morshedi, M., Kolm, P., Coetzee, K., Kruger, T., & Oehninger, S. (1999). Intra- and inter-laboratory variability in the assessment of sperm morphology by strict criteria: Impact of semen preparation, staining techniques and manual versus computerized analysis. *Human Reproduction, 14*(8), 2036–2040.
7. Barroso, G., Morshedi, M., & Oehninger, S. (2000). Analysis of DNA fragmentation, plasma membrane translocation of phosphatidylserine and oxidative stress in human spermatozoa. *Human Reproduction, 15*(6), 1338–1344.

8. Carver-Ward, J. A., Jaroudi, K. A., Hollanders, J. M., & Einspenner, M. (1996). High fertilization prediction by flow cytometric analysis of the CD46 antigen on the inner acrosomal membrane of spermatozoa. *Human Reproduction, 11*(9), 1923–1928.

9. Cayli, S., Sakkas, D., Vigue, L., Demir, R., & Huszar, G. (2004). Cellular maturity and apoptosis in human sperm: Creatine kinase, caspase-3 and Bcl-XL levels in mature and diminished maturity sperm. *Molecular Human Reproduction, 10*(5), 365–372.

10. Chan, P. J., Corselli, J. U., Patton, W. C., Jacobson, J. D., Chan, S. R., & King, A. (2001). A simple comet assay for archived sperm correlates DNA fragmentation to reduced hyperactivation and penetration of zona-free hamster oocytes. *Fertility and Sterility, 75*(1), 186–192.

11. Chen, J. L., & Longo, F. J. (1996). Expression and localization of DNA topoisomerase II during rat spermatogenesis. *Molecular Reproduction and Development, 45*(1), 61–71.

12. Cordelli, E., Eleuteri, P., Leter, G., Rescia, M., & Spanò, M. (2005). Flow cytometry applications in the evaluation of sperm quality: Semen analysis, sperm function, and DNA integrity. *Contraception, 72*(4), 273–279.

13. Cross, N. L., Morales, P., Overstreet, J. W., & Hanson, F. W. (1988). Induction of acrosome reactions by the human zona pellucida. *Biology of Reproduction, 38*(1), 235–244.

14. Duran, E. H., Morshedi, M., Taylor, S., & Oehninger, S. (2002). Sperm DNA quality predicts intrauterine insemination outcome: A prospective cohort study. *Human Reproduction, 17*(12), 3122–3128.

15. Escoffier, J., Krapf, D., Navarrete, F., Darszon, A., & Visconti, P. E. (2012). Flow cytometry analysis reveals a decrease in intracellular sodium during sperm capacitation. *Journal of Cell Science, 125*(Pt 2), 473–485.

16. Eustache, F., Jouannet, P., & Auger, J. (2001). Evaluation of flow cytometric methods to measure human sperm concentration. *Journal of Andrology, 22*(4), 558–567.

17. Evenson, D. P. (1990). Flow cytometric analysis of male germ cell quality. *Methods in Cell Biology, 33*, 401–410.

18. Evenson, D. P., Darzynkiewicz, Z., & Melamed, M. R. (1980). Relation of mammalian sperm chromatin heterogeneity to fertility. *Science, 210*(4474), 1131–1133.

19. Evenson, D., Darzynkiewicz, Z., Jost, L., Janca, F., & Ballachey, B. (1986). Changes in accessibility of DNA to various fluorochromes during spermatogenesis. *Cytometry, 7*(1), 45–53.

20. Ferrara, F., Daverio, R., Mazzini, G., Bonini, P., & Banfi, G. (1997). Automation of human sperm cell analysis by flow cytometry. *Clinical Chemistry, 43*(5), 801–807.

21. Garrido, N., Meseguer, M., Remohi, J., Pellicer, A., & Simón, C. (2002). Flow cytometry in human reproductive biology. *Gynecological Endocrinology, 16*(6), 505–521. https://doi.org/10.1080/gye.16.6.505.521.

22. Golan, R., Shochat, L., Weissenberg, R., Soffer, Y., Marcus, Z., Oschry, Y., & Lewin, L. M. (1997). Evaluation of chromatin condensation in human spermatozoa: A flow cytometric assay using acridine orange staining. *Molecular Human Reproduction, 3*(1), 47–54. https://doi.org/10.1093/molehr/3.1.47.

23. Grunewald, S., Sharma, R., Paasch, U., Glander, H. J., & Agarwal, A. (2009). Impact of caspase activation in human spermatozoa. *Microscopy Research and Technique, 72*(11), 878–888. https://doi.org/10.1002/jemt.20740.

24. Hossain, M. S., Johannisson, A., Wallgren, M., Nagy, S., Siqueira, A. P., & Rodriguez-Martinez, H. (2011). Flow cytometry for the assessment of animal sperm integrity and functionality: State of the art. *Asian Journal of Andrology, 13*(3), 406–419. https://doi.org/10.1038/aja.2010.139.

25. Jensen, T. K., Carlsen, E., Jørgensen, N., Berthelsen, J. G., Keiding, N., Christensen, K., Petersen, J. H., Knudsen, L. B., Skakkebæk, N. E., et al. (2002). Poor semen quality may contribute to the recent decline in fertility rates. *Human Reproduction, 17*(6), 1437–1440. https://doi.org/10.1093/humrep/17.6.1437.

26. Kramer, R. Y., Garner, D. L., Bruns, E. S., Ericsson, S. A., & Prins, G. S. (1993). Comparison of motility and flow cytometric assessments of seminal quality in fresh, 24-hour extended and cryopreserved human spermatozoa. *Journal of Andrology, 14*(5), 374–384. https://doi.org/10.1002/j.1939-4640.1993.tb00533.x.

27. Larson, K. L., DeJonge, C. J., Barnes, A. M., Jost, L. K., & Evenson, D. P. (2000). Sperm chromatin structure assay parameters as predictors of failed pregnancy following assisted reproductive techniques. *Human Reproduction, 15*(8), 1717–1722. https://doi.org/10.1093/humrep/15.8.1717.

28. Levek-Motola, N., Soffer, Y., Shochat, L., Raziel, A., Lewin, L. M., & Golan, R. (2005). Flow cytometry of human semen: A preliminary study of a non-invasive method for the detection of spermatogenetic defects. *Human Reproduction, 20*(12), 3469–3475. https://doi.org/10.1093/humrep/dei233.

29. Martínez-Pastor, F., Mata-Campuzano, M., Alvarez-Rodríguez, M., Alvarez, M., Anel, L., & de Paz, P. (2010). Probes and techniques for sperm evaluation by flow cytometry. *Reproduction in Domestic Animals, 45*(Suppl 2), 67–78. https://doi.org/10.1111/j.1439-0531.2010.01609.x.

30. McPherson, S., & Longo, F. J. (1993). Chromatin structure-function alterations during mammalian spermatogenesis: DNA nicking and repair in elongating spermatids. *European Journal of Histochemistry, 37*(2), 109–128.

31. Oehninger, S., Morshedi, M., Weng, S. L., Taylor, S., Duran, H., & Beebe, S. (2003). Presence and significance of somatic cell apoptosis markers in human ejaculated spermatozoa. *Reproductive Biomedicine Online, 7*(4), 469–476. https://doi.org/10.1016/S1472-6483(10)61937-1.

32. Oosterhuis, G. J., Mulder, A. B., Kalsbeek-Batenburg, E., Lambalk, C. B., Schoemaker, J., & Vermes, I. (2000). Measuring apoptosis in human spermatozoa: A biological assay for semen quality. *Fertility and Sterility, 74*(2), 245–250. https://doi.org/10.1016/S0015-0282(00)00680-6.

33. Patrat, C., Serres, C., & Jouannet, P. (2000). The acrosome reaction in human spermatozoa. *Biology of the Cell, 92*(3–4), 255–266. https://doi.org/10.1016/S0248-4900(00)89050-0.

34. Ricci, G., Perticarari, S., Fragonas, E., Giolo, E., Canova, S., Pozzobon, C., Guaschino, S., & Presani, G. (2002). Apoptosis in human sperm: Its correlation with semen quality and the presence of leukocytes. *Human Reproduction, 17*(10), 2665–2672. https://doi.org/10.1093/humrep/17.10.2665.

35. Sakkas, D., Manicardi, G., Bianchi, P. G., Bizzaro, D., & Bianchi, U. (1995). Relationship between the presence of endogenous nicks and sperm chromatin packaging in maturing and fertilizing

mouse spermatozoa. *Biology of Reproduction, 52*(5), 1149–1155. https://doi.org/10.1095/biolreprod52.5.1149.

36. Sakkas, D., Mariethoz, E., & St John, J. C. (1999). Abnormal sperm parameters in humans are indicative of an abortive apoptotic mechanism linked to the Fas-mediated pathway. *Experimental Cell Research, 251*(2), 350–355. https://doi.org/10.1006/excr.1999.4580.
37. Sakkas, D., Moffatt, O., Manicardi, G. C., Mariethoz, E., Tarozzi, N., & Bizzaro, D. (2002). Nature of DNA damage in ejaculated human spermatozoa and the possible involvement of apoptosis. *Biology of Reproduction, 66*(4), 1061–1067. https://doi.org/10.1095/biolreprod66.4.1061.
38. Storey, B. T. (1995). Interactions between gametes leading to fertilization: The sperm's eye view. *Reproduction, Fertility and Development, 7*(4), 927–942. https://doi.org/10.1071/RD9950927.
39. Sun, J. G., Jurisicova, A., & Casper, R. F. (1997). Detection of deoxyribonucleic acid fragmentation in human sperm: Correlation with fertilization in vitro. *Biology of Reproduction, 56*(3), 602–607. https://doi.org/10.1095/biolreprod56.3.602.
40. Sutovsky, P. (2003). Ubiquitin-dependent proteolysis in mammalian spermatogenesis, fertilization, and sperm quality control: Killing three birds with one stone. *Microscopy Research and Technique, 61*(1), 88–102. https://doi.org/10.1002/jemt.10317.
41. Swain, J. E., & Pool, T. B. (2008). ART failure: Oocyte contributions to unsuccessful fertilization. *Human Reproduction Update, 14*(5), 431–446. https://doi.org/10.1093/humupd/dmn018.
42. Tesarik, J., Greco, E., & Mendoza, C. (2004). Late, but not early, paternal effect on human embryo development is related to sperm DNA fragmentation. *Human Reproduction, 19*(3), 611–615. https://doi.org/10.1093/humrep/deh135.
43. Tomlinson, M. J., Moffatt, O., Manicardi, G. C., Bizzaro, D., Afnan, M., & Sakkas, D. (2001). Interrelationships between seminal parameters and sperm nuclear DNA damage before and after density gradient centrifugation: Implications for assisted conception. *Human Reproduction, 16*(10), 2160–2165. https://doi.org/10.1093/humrep/16.10.2160.
44. Troiano, L., Granata, A. R., Cossarizza, A., Kalashnikova, G., Bianchi, R., Pini, G., Tropea, F., Carani, C., & Franceschi, C. (1998). Mitochondrial membrane potential and DNA stainability in human sperm cells: A flow cytometry analysis with implications for male infertility. *Experimental Cell Research, 241*(2), 384–393. https://doi.org/10.1006/excr.1998.4064.
45. Van Blerkom, J. (2000). Intrafollicular influences on human oocyte developmental competence: Perifollicular vascularity, oocyte metabolism, and mitochondrial function. *Human Reproduction, 15*(Suppl 2), 173–188. https://doi.org/10.1093/humrep/15.suppl_2.173.
46. Virro, M. R., Larson-Cook, K. L., & Evenson, D. P. (2004). Sperm chromatin structure assay (SCSA) parameters are related to fertilization, blastocyst development, and ongoing pregnancy in in vitro fertilization and intracytoplasmic sperm injection cycles. *Fertility and Sterility, 81*(5), 1289–1295. https://doi.org/10.1016/j.fertnstert.2003.10.036.
47. Visconti, P. E., Bailey, J. L., Moore, G. D., Pan, D., Olds-Clarke, P., & Kopf, G. S. (1995). Capacitation of mouse spermatozoa. I. Correlation between the capacitation state and protein tyrosine phosphorylation. *Development, 121*(4), 1129–1137. https://doi.org/10.1242/dev.121.4.1129.
48. Wang, X., Sharma, R. K., Sikka, S. C., Thomas Jr, A. J., Falcone, T., & Agarwal, A. (2003). Oxidative stress is associated with increased apoptosis leading to spermatozoa DNA damage

in patients with male factor infertility. *Fertility and Sterility, 80*(3), 531–535. https://doi.org/10.1016/S0015-0282(03)00729-1.

49. Wassarman, P. M. (1999). Mammalian fertilization: Molecular aspects of gamete adhesion, exocytosis, and fusion. *Cell, 96*(2), 175–183. https://doi.org/10.1016/S0092-8674(00)80559-2.

50. World Health Organization. (2010). *WHO Laboratory Manual for the Examination of Human Semen and Sperm-cervical Mucus Interaction* (4th ed.). Cambridge University Press.

Chapter

PREGNANCY AND PARTURITION

8

Contents

Unit Introduction

Parturition, also referred to as childbirth, is the physiological process that completes pregnancy, which is the process by which a woman carries and cares for a developing fetus. This complex process culminates in the baby's expulsion from the uterus and involves many physiological and hormonal changes in both the mother and the fetus. Fertilization is the first step in the pregnancy process, where a sperm fertilizes an egg to create a zygote. The zygote starts the process of gestation by rapidly dividing its cells as it passes through the uterine tube and inserts itself into the uterine lining. The fetus grows from a tiny cluster of cells into a fully formed infant over the course of about 40 weeks. The mother's body goes through significant changes during pregnancy to support the developing fetus. Hormonal changes, such as elevated estrogen and progesterone, suppress uterine contractions, encourage placenta growth, and get the breasts ready for lactation, all of which contribute to the maintenance of the pregnancy. The mother's circulatory system changes to make room for the extra blood volume required to give the fetus oxygen and nourishment. Her respiratory system improves in the interim to handle the increased oxygen requirements of pregnancy.

The uterus grows larger during pregnancy to make room for the developing fetus, which puts pressure on the tissues and organs around it. The pelvic ligaments' relaxation and the uterine muscles' stretching and thinning both contribute to this expansion. The fetus prepares for delivery by assuming a head-down position toward the end of pregnancy, with the head usually engaging in the pelvis.

Hormonal and mechanical factors interact in a complex way to cause parturition or childbirth. Hormones released by the developing fetus prompt the mother's body to start the labor process. Effacement and dilation, the gradual softening and thinning of the cervix, are usually associated with regular contractions of the uterus. The process known as descent is aided by these contractions as the baby is forced lower through the birth canal. The second stage of labor starts when the baby's head enters the vagina from the cervix. To remove the baby from the birth canal, the mother actively pushes during each contraction during this stage. With one last push, the baby leaves the mother's body, inhaling for the first time and beginning the journey toward an independent life. The third stage of labor is when the placenta and fetal membranes are removed from the uterus after the baby is born. More uterine contractions help to separate the placenta from the uterine wall and expel it through the vagina, which facilitates this stage. Both the mother and the fetus undergo several physiological and hormonal changes during the complicated processes of pregnancy and parturition. Pregnancy is an amazing journey that showcases the human body's adaptability and resilience from conception to delivery (Cunningham et al., 2005).

Orientation and Directional Terms:

Terms	Definition	Illustration
Muscles	Muscles have a range of functions from pumping blood and supporting movement to lifting heavy weights or giving birth.	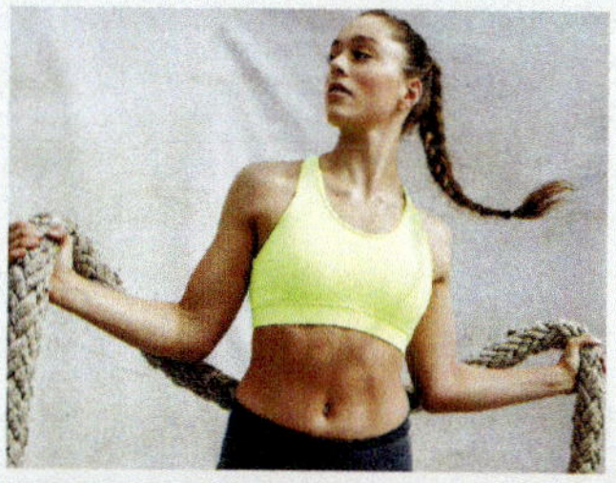
Cervix	The cervix is a dynamic fibromuscular organ of the female reproductive system that connects the vagina with the uterine cavity.	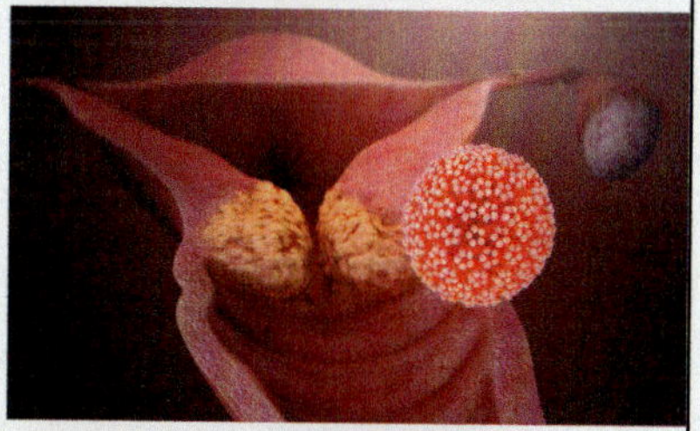
Placenta	The placenta is an organ that forms in the womb, also called the uterus, during pregnancy.	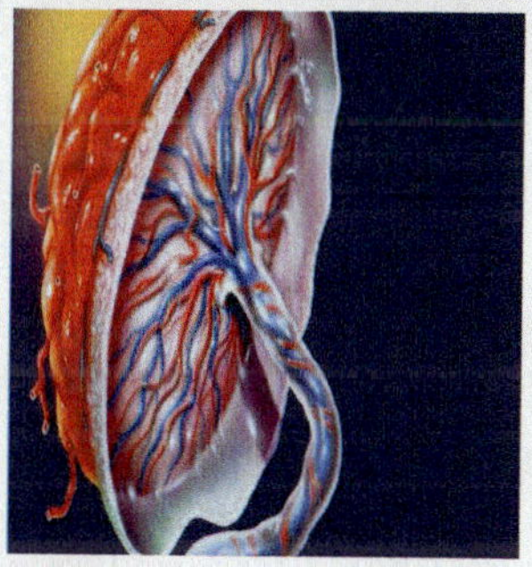
Human chorionic gonadotropin	Human chorionic gonadotrophin (hCG) is a hormone produced by the placenta during pregnancy. It's sometimes called the pregnancy hormone because of its unique role in supporting a pregnancy.	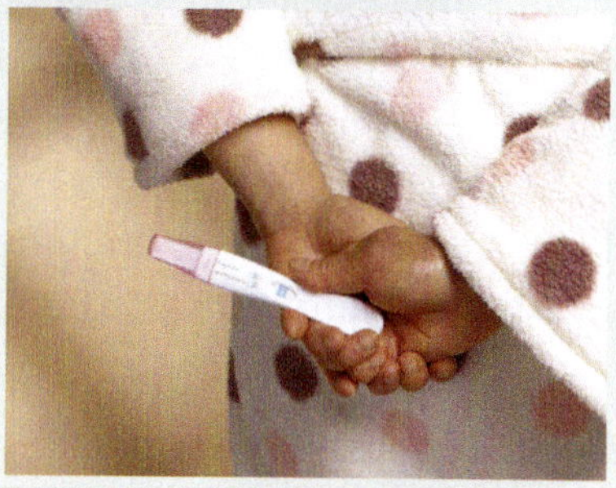
Multigravida	multigravida (plural multigravidas or multigravidae). A pregnant woman who has had at least two previous pregnancies	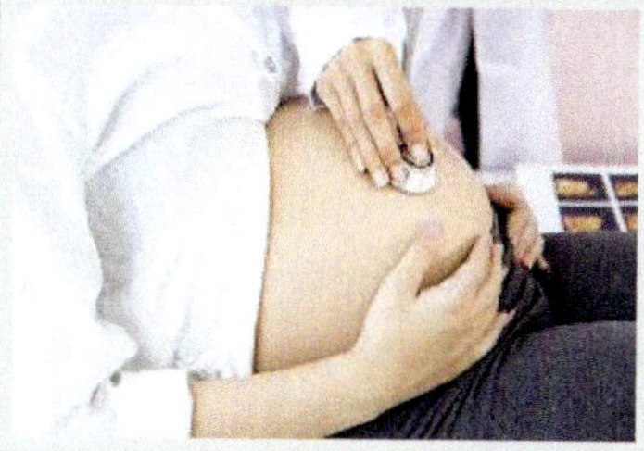

8.1. Anatomy of the Pregnant Uterus and Placenta

The structure and function of the placenta are intimately linked to the remarkable changes that the pregnant uterus goes through to support and accommodate the growing fetus. Comprehending the structure of the placenta and uterus during pregnancy is essential to appreciate the intricacies involved in pregnancy and childbirth.

The uterus, sometimes referred to as the womb, is a pear-shaped, hollow organ that is situated in the pelvis between the rectum and the bladder. The uterus grows considerably during pregnancy to hold the developing fetus. The gradual displacement of surrounding organs and the thinning and stretching of the uterine muscles facilitate this expansion. The uterus can grow to accommodate a fetus weighing several pounds by the end of the pregnancy.

The placenta is one of the most distinguishing characteristics of the pregnant uterus. The placenta is a transient organ that grows throughout pregnancy and is essential for allowing the mother and fetus to exchange nutrients and oxygen. It is joined to the fetus by the umbilical cord and affixed to the uterine wall. The placenta, which is made up of both fetal and maternal tissues, acts as a barrier to keep the blood from mingling while still allowing vital substances to be exchanged.

There are multiple layers in the placenta, and each one serves a specific purpose. The chorion, the outermost layer, is made of many projections that resemble fingers and is derived from fetal tissues. These projections are referred to as chorionic villi. The fetus and mother exchange gases and nutrients through these villi, which are drenched in maternal blood. The decidua basalis, the placenta's innermost layer, is made of maternal tissues and gives the developing placenta support and nutrition.

A sophisticated network of blood vessels within the placenta facilitates the exchange of waste products, nutrients, and oxygen between the circulatory systems of the mother and the fetus. The uterine arteries allow maternal blood to enter the placenta, where it is subsequently delivered to the chorionic villi via a network of smaller vessels. Here, waste products and carbon dioxide travel from the fetal blood into the mother's circulation while nutrients and oxygen diffuse across the placental barrier and into the fetal blood.

In addition, the placenta functions as an endocrine organ, generating hormones necessary for sustaining pregnancy. Human chorionic gonadotropin (hCG), one of these hormones, aids in maintaining the early stages of pregnancy until the placenta fully matures and begins to produce hormones on its own. In addition, the placenta secretes progesterone and estrogen, which are essential for controlling physiological changes in the mother that take place during pregnancy, including the expansion and maturation of the breasts and the relaxation of the uterine muscles.

The placenta and uterus change dynamically during pregnancy to support and maintain the health of the developing fetus. These modifications, which affect both structure and function, enable the fetus and mother to exchange hormones, gases, and nutrients effectively. Healthcare professionals must have a thorough understanding of the anatomy of the placenta and uterus to monitor pregnancy progress and take appropriate action to ensure the health of the mother and unborn child (Cunningham et al., 2005).

8.1.1. Gravidity and Parity

An understanding of the following terms used to describe pregnancy and the pregnant woman is essential to the study of maternity care:

- **Gravida:** A woman who is pregnant.
- **Gravidity:** Pregnancy.
- **Multigravida:** A woman who has had two or more pregnancies.
- **Multipara:** A woman who has completed two or more pregnancies to the stage of fetal viability.
- **Nulligravida:** A woman who has never been pregnant.
- **Nullipara:** A woman who has not completed a pregnancy with a fetus or fetuses who have reached the stage of fetal viability.
- **Parity:** The number of pregnancies in which the fetus or fetuses have reached viability when they are born, not the number of fetuses (e.g., twins) born. Whether the fetus is born alive or is stillborn (a fetus who shows no signs of life at birth) after viability is reached does not affect parity.
- **Postdate or Post-Term:** A pregnancy that goes beyond 42 weeks of gestation.
- **Preterm:** A pregnancy that has reached 20 weeks of gestation but before completion of 37 weeks of gestation.
- **Primigravida:** A woman who is pregnant for the first time.
- **Primipara:** A woman who has completed one pregnancy with a fetus or fetuses who have reached the stage of fetal viability.
- **Term:** A pregnancy from the beginning of week 38 of gestation to the end of week 42 of gestation.
- **Viability:** Capacity to live outside the uterus; about 22 to 24 weeks since last menstrual period, or fetal weight greater than 500 g.

During history-taking interviews, information regarding gravidity and parity is obtained and can be entered into patient records in a variety of ways. One way to represent gravidity and parity is with two numbers. For example, 1/0 signifies that a woman is not yet pregnant and is conceiving her first child. Five digits separated by hyphens is another technique that is commonly used in maternity centers.

This system provides additional precise parity information. The first digit represents the total number of pregnancies, including the current one (gravidity); the second represents the total number of term births; the third indicates the number of preterm births; the fourth represents the total number of abortions (miscarriages or elective terminations of pregnancy before viability); and the fifth represents the total number of children who are currently alive. The acronym GTPAL (gravidity, term, preterm, abortions, living children) can be used to help with memory retention.

For example, if a woman pregnant only once gives birth at week 34 and the infant survives, the abbreviation that represents this information is "1-0-1-0-1." During her next pregnancy, the abbreviation is "2-0-1-0-1" (Table 8.1).

Table 8.1. *Human Fecundity Over the Last Four Centuries*

Population Studied	Publication	Fecundity Index
Canada (Québec), 18th century	Henrypin (1954)	0.31
China 20th century	Wang et al. (2003)	0.40
France, 17th and 18th centuries	Charbonneaux (1970)	0.21
Great Britain, 20th century	Vessey et al. (1976)	0.21

Mexico, 20th century	Balakrishnan (1979)	0.21
Peru, 20th century	Balakrishnan (1979)	0.17
The Netherlands, 20th century*	van Noord Zaadstra et al. (1991)	0.54
USA (Hutterite sect) 20th century	Sheps (1965)	0.28
USA, 20th century	Zinamen et al. (1996)	0.30

* After 2 months at age 31. Modified and reprinted with permission from Benagiano et al.,

Source: Benagiano, G., Mancuso, S., Guo, S. W., & Di Renzo, G. C., (2023). Events leading to the establishment of pregnancy and placental formation: The need to fine-tune the nomenclature of pregnancy and gestation. International Journal of Molecular Sciences, 24(20), 15420. https://doi.org/10.3390/ijms242015420.

8.1.2. Pregnancy Tests

Early pregnancy detection makes it possible to start treatment early. Human chorionic gonadotropin, or hCG, is the first biochemical marker of pregnancy. Pregnancy tests look for either the hCG or its beta (β) subunit. β-hCG production can be seen as early as 7 to 10 days after conception, starting on the day of implantation. About 60 to 70 days into the pregnancy, the amount of hCG peaks and then begins to decline until about 80 days into the pregnancy. It remains that way for about 30 weeks, at which point it gradually increases until term. Above normal hCG levels may indicate an ectopic pregnancy or aberrant gestation. In certain situations, such as when a fetus has Down syndrome or is experiencing multiple gestations, an abnormally slow rise or fall in hCG levels may indicate an impending miscarriage.

Serum and urine pregnancy tests are performed in lab settings, offices, women's health centers, and clinics. Urine tests can also be performed at home. Serum and urine tests can provide accurate results. A 7–10 ml venous blood sample is drawn for serum testing. Urine tests usually require first-voided morning urine because its hCG levels are comparable to those in serum. Randomly selected urine samples usually have lower levels. Urine test costs are lower and produce results more quickly than serum test costs.

There are lots of options for pregnancy tests. The nurse should adhere to the manufacturer's instructions when using a test. Pregnancy tests known as radioimmunoassay (RIA) tests use radioactive techniques to measure the beta subunit of hCG in serum or urine samples. The nurse should adhere to the manufacturer's instructions when using a test. Radioimmunoassay (RIA) tests are pregnancy tests that look for the beta subunit of hCG in serum or urine samples.

The radioreceptor assay (RRA) is a serum test used to measure a blood sample's ability to block the binding of radiolabeled hCG to receptors. The test has a 90–95% accuracy rate in the first six to eight days after conception. The enzyme-linked immunosorbent assay is the most used pregnancy test (ELISA). It binds to hCG in urine using enzymes and a specific monoclonal antibody called anti-hCG. Depending on the specific test, levels of hCG as low as 25 milli-international units/ml may be detected as early as seven days after conception. It can be done at home or in the office and takes less than five minutes to finish. A straightforward color shift signifies a successful test outcome. Most home pregnancy tests that are available over the counter rely on ELISA technology. For these one-step tests, the woman usually applies urine to a strip and reads the results.

The test kits come with instructions on how to collect the specimen, perform the test, and interpret the results. Users with any queries or worries about test methods or outcomes can get in touch with most kit manufacturers at the toll-free number they provide. The most common error made when using home pregnancy tests is to take the test too early in the pregnancy.

Results of pregnancy tests need to be interpreted cautiously. The type of pregnancy test, its level of sensitivity (ability to detect low levels of a substance) and specificity (ability to discern the absence of a substance), as well as the woman's medical history, must all be considered. This information includes the time of her most recent LNMP, the length of her usual cycle, and the results of any previous pregnancy tests. Finding out about the woman's drug history and whether or not she abuses substances is crucial because some drugs can cause false-positive results when taken with anticonvulsants and tranquilizers, while promethazine and diuretics can cause false-negative results. Hormone-producing tumors, incorrect specimen collection, and laboratory errors can also result in false positives. In situations where doubt exists, more testing or evaluation might be required (Cunningham et al., 2005).

8.1.3. Adaptations to Pregnancy

Maternal physiologic adaptations are believed to be caused by pregnancy hormones, growing uterus, and other tissues, which put mechanical pressure on the body. These modifications support the fetus's growth and development, protect the woman's regular physiological processes, and meet the metabolic demands of pregnancy. While pregnancy is a common occurrence, problems can still occur.

8.1.4. Signs of Pregnancy

Certain physiological changes are acknowledged as indicators and manifestations of pregnancy. Presumptive signs and symptoms (those that the woman feels changed) are categorized into three main groups, e.g., breast changes, amenorrhea, exhaustion, nausea, and vomiting); likely (those changes noted by an examiner, e.g., Hegar sign, ballottement, and pregnancy tests); and positive (those indicators that can only be ascribed to the fetus's existence, e.g., palpating fetal movements, visualizing the fetus, and hearing fetal heart tones). These pregnancy symptoms are enumerated in Table 8.2, along with other possible causes and times they may appear.

Table 8.2. *Anthropometric Data of Women: P0: Before Pregnancy; P1: in the First Trimester; P2: in the Second Trimester; and P3: in the Third Trimester [30, 31]*

	Mean ± SD			
	P0	**P1**	**P2**	**P3**
Pregnancy Week	–	12.00 ± 0.78	24.86 ± 1.03	35.46 ± 0.66
Body Height (m)	1.67 ± 0.04	1.67 ± 0.04	1.67 ± 0.04	1.67 ± 0.04
Body Mass (kg)	59.30 ± 7.72	60.42 ± 6.73	66.39 ± 7.96	70.99 ± 9.14
BMI (kg/m^2)	21.31 ± 2.24	21.68 ± 2.01	23.72 ± 2.32	25.57 ± 2.88
Pelvic Tilt (deg)	9.90 ± 2.86	9.85 ± 3.54	12.03 ± 3.69	14.52 ± 3.77
Pelvic width (cm)	24.84 ± 1.27	24.96 ± 1.31	26.61 ± 1.95	27.69 ± 2.23
Pelvic Width in Relation to the Width in P0 (%)	100%	100.5%	107.1%	111.5%

Source: Michnik, R., Zadoń, H., Nowakowska-Lipiec, K., & Forczek-Karkosz, W., (2022). How does the lumbopelvic complex cope with the obstetrical load during standing? Ergonomic aspects of body posture in pregnant women. Applied Sciences, 12(9), 4330. https://doi.org/10.3390/app12094330.

8.1.5. Reproductive System and Breasts

8.1.5.1. Uterus

8.1.5.1.1. Changes in Size, Shape, and Position

The remarkable growth of the uterus is stimulated by elevated progesterone and estrogen levels during the first trimester. Early uterine enlargement is caused by many factors, including increased vascularity and blood vessel dilatation, hyperplasia (the formation of new muscle fibers and fibroelastic tissue), hypertrophy (the enlargement of preexisting muscle fibers and fibroelastic tissue), and decidua development. At 7 weeks of gestation, the uterus is the size of a large hen's egg; at 10 weeks, it doubles in size to an orange; and at 12 weeks, it reaches the largest size of a grapefruit. The mechanical pressure of the developing fetus is the main cause of uterine enlargement after the third month. As the uterus gets bigger, it shifts in position and shape. During conception, the uterus resembles an upside-down pear. The uterine walls thicken and become more elastic during the second trimester, causing the uterus to become spherical or globular. After the fetus lengthens and emerges from the pelvis into the abdominal cavity, the uterus becomes bigger and more ovoid. Pregnancy may become apparent after the 14th week, though this mostly depends on the woman's height and weight. Abdominal enlargement may be less obvious in the nullipara when there is good abdominal muscle tone. Posture also affects the type and degree of abdominal enlargement. During a typical pregnancy, the uterus grows steadily. The uterus can be palpated above the symphysis pubis as it grows between the 12th and 14th weeks of pregnancy (Figure 8.2). The uterus gradually rises to the level of the umbilicus at 22 to 24 weeks of gestation, and at term, it nearly reaches the xiphoid process. When the fetus begins to descend and engage in the pelvis (lightening), the fundal height decreases between weeks 38 and 40 (*see* Figure 8.2, dashed line). Lightning usually occurs in the nullipara about two weeks before labor commences and in the multipara at the start of labor (Figure 8.1).

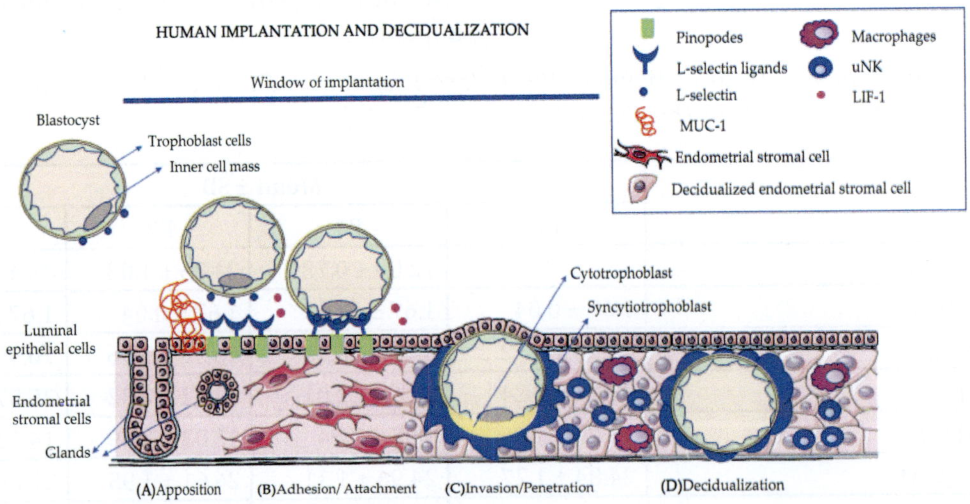

Figure 8.1. *Schematic representation of the main phases of human implantation: apposition, adhesion/ attachment, invasion/penetration, and decidualization. (A) Apposition: The blastocyst expresses L-selectin that reacts with its ligands. The presence of Mucin-1 repels the blastocyst and prevents it from attaching outside of the window of receptivity. (B) Adhesion: The blastocyst promotes cleavage of*

Mucin-1 at the implantation site to ensure successful attachment. (C) Invasion: Blastocyst trophoblast cells penetrate the endometrial epithelium and reach the stroma. As soon as implantation is initiated and the embryo reaches the stromal cells surrounding the embryo, these transform into decidualized cells. And (D) Decidualization: During the decidualization process, immune cells, such as macrophages and uterine natural killer (uNK) cells, play an important role in promoting an environment conducive to successful implantation.

Source: Benagiano, G., Mancuso, S., Guo, S. W., & Di Renzo, G. C., (2023). Events leading to the establishment of pregnancy and placental formation: The need to fine-tune the nomenclature of pregnancy and gestation. International Journal of Molecular Sciences, 24(20), 15420. https://doi.org/10.3390/ijms242015420.

Uterine enlargement is measured using fundal height, which is also commonly used to estimate the duration of pregnancy. However, variations in the position of the fundus or the fetus, variations in the amount of amniotic fluid present, the presence of multiple fetuses, maternal obesity, and variations in examiner techniques can all affect how accurate this estimation of the length of pregnancy is (Figure 8.2).

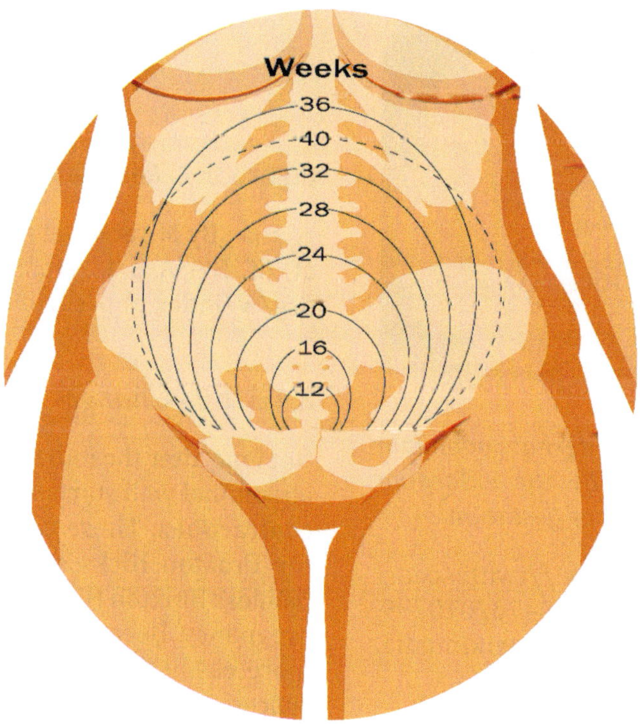

Figure 8.2. *Height of fundus by weeks of normal gestation with a single fetus. Dashed line, height after lightening.*

Source: https://d3i71xaburhd42.cloudfront.net/349bfb309526ddbd7a73395e456b020f8283c469/6-Figure8-2-1.png.

The uterus often rotates to the right as it elevates because of the rectosigmoid colon on the left side, but because of the extensive hypertrophy (enlargement) of the round ligaments, the uterus stays in the midline. As the growing uterus touches the anterior abdominal wall, the intestines eventually move to either side of the abdomen. Because the bulk of a pregnant woman's uterus presses against the anterior abdominal wall when she stands, her center of gravity is altered (Figure 8.3).

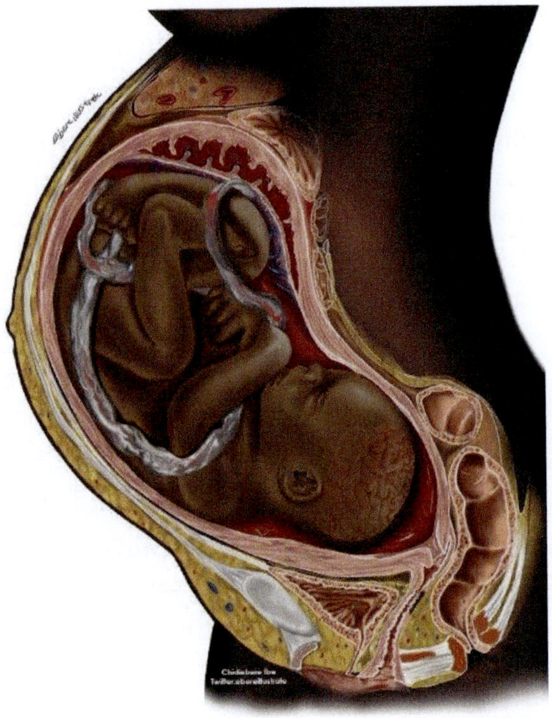

Figure 8.3. *Displacement of internal abdominal structures and diaphragm by the enlarging uterus at 4, 6, and 9 months of gestation.*

Around 6 weeks of gestation, the lower uterine segment, or uterine isthmus, starts to soften and compress (Hegar sign). This leads to an increase in uterine anteflexion during the first trimester of pregnancy. Because the uterine fundus is pressing against the bladder, the woman has frequent urination (Figure 8.4).

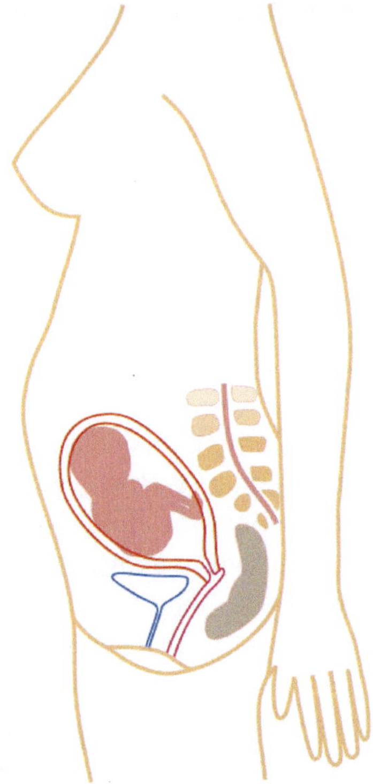

Figure 8.4. *Representation of the fifth month.*

8.1.5.1.2. Changes in Contractility

Not long after the fourth month of pregnancy, the abdominal wall starts to feel the force of uterine contractions. These contractions are known as the Braxton Hicks sign. Periodically, irregular, painless Braxton Hicks contractions occur during pregnancy. Because the uterine blood can pass more easily through the placenta's intervillous spaces as a result of these contractions, the fetus receives more oxygen. Though Braxton Hicks contractions are not painful, some women find them bothersome. After the 28th week, these contractions become much more regular, but they usually stop when you walk or exercise. Braxton Hicks contractions can be confused for labor even though they don't cause cervical dilation or increase in frequency or intensity.

8.1.5.1.3. Uteroplacental Blood Flow

Placental perfusion requires the mother's blood to flow into the uterus. Blood flow rapidly increases as the uterus grows larger. When this happens, the uterine blood flow increases 20-fold, but the fetoplacental unit grows more quickly. Consequently, the uterine blood is used to extract more oxygen during the later phases of pregnancy. In a normal-term pregnancy, the uterine vascular system contains one-sixth of the mother's total blood volume. The gravid uterus requires more oxygen to meet the needs of the developing fetus, and the average blood flow rate through the uterus is 500 ml/min.

Three factors—low maternal arterial pressure, uterine contractions, and the supine position—are known to decrease blood flow in women. Estrogen stimulation may cause an increase in uterine blood flow. Doppler ultrasonography examination is a useful tool for measuring uterine blood flow velocity, especially in pregnancies that are at risk because of factors such as diabetes mellitus, intrauterine growth restriction, hypertension, and multiple gestations, which are associated with reduced placental perfusion. A fetal stethoscope or an ultrasound device can be used by the healthcare provider to detect the uterine souffle, which is the sound made by blood in the uterine arteries that is synchronous with the mother's pulse, or the funic souffle, which is the sound made by blood rushing through the umbilical vessels and synchronous with the fetal heart rate.

8.1.5.1.4. Cervical Changes

A softening of the cervical tip known as the Goodell sign may be observed at the beginning of the sixth week in a normal, unscarred cervix. This sign, which is accompanied by increased vascularity, mild hypertrophy, and hyperplasia (increase in number of cells), is caused by the muscle and its collagen-rich connective tissue, which becomes loose, edematous, highly elastic, and increased in volume. Because the glands near the external so multiply beneath the stratified squamous epithelium during pregnancy, the cervix appears velvety. Mild bleeding during deep penetration coitus or vaginal examination may be caused by increased friability. Pregnancy may also cause the squamocolumnar junction, the site of cell collection for cervical cancer screening, to be farther away from the cervix. Because of all these changes, evaluating abnormal Papanicolaou (Pap) tests during pregnancy can be difficult. All expectant mothers should, however, undergo a thorough examination because about 3% of cervical cancer cases are detected during pregnancy.

The cervix of the nullipara is rounded. Almost always, childbirth results in cervical lacerations. But after giving birth, the external so appears as a transverse slit, and the cervix becomes more oval in the horizontal plane, with or without lacerations.

8.1.5.1.5. Changes Related to the Presence of the Fetus

Between weeks 16 and 18, a fetus that is not engaged will usually begin to move passively, a phenomenon known as bloat. Ballottement is the technique of softly hitting a floating structure and palpating it by feeling its return. When the finger is gently tapped upward, the fetus rises to the surface of the vagina when the examiner uses the palpation technique. The fetus then descends and feels like a light tap on the finger (Figure 8.5).

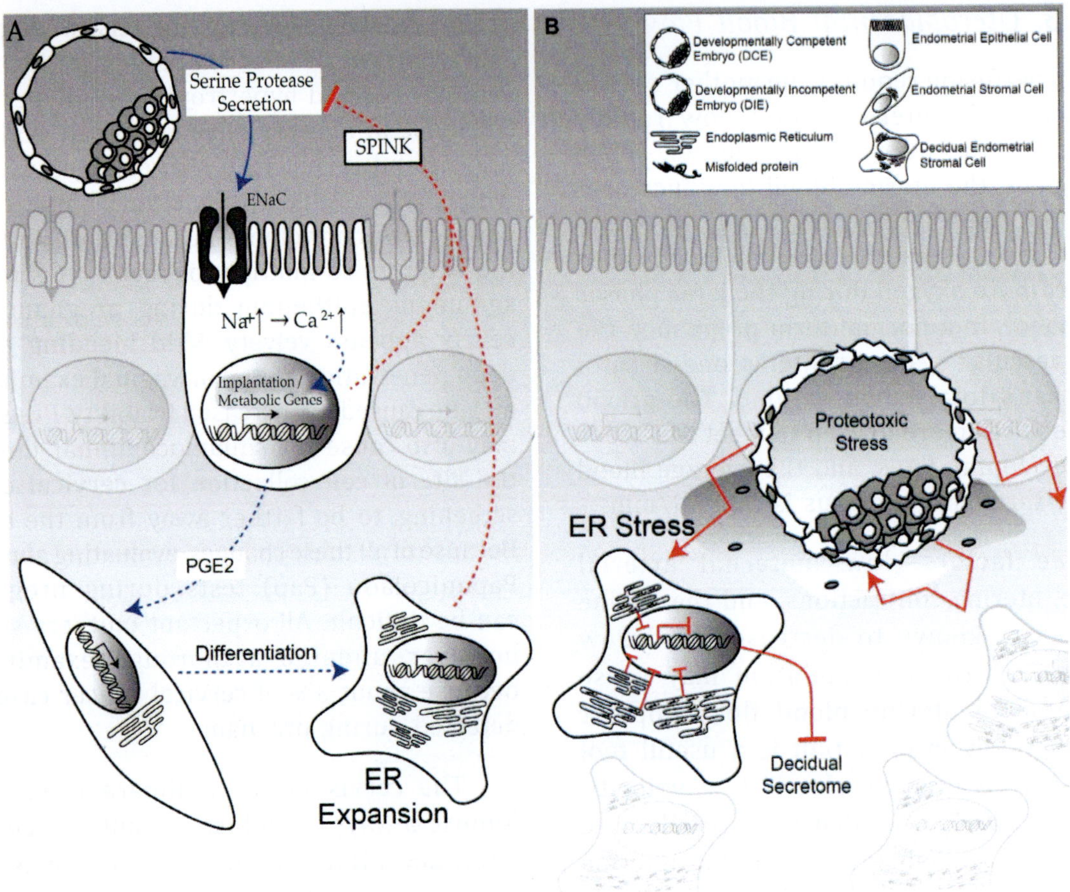

Figure 8.5. *Positive and negative mechanisms contribute actively to the selection of human embryos at implantation. (A) Developmentally competent human embryos secrete serine proteases that activate epithelial Na1 channel (ENaC) that induce genes involved in implantation and post-implantation embryo development. (B) Developmentally compromised embryos, by contrast, induce excessive protease activity, leading to the accumulation of misfolded proteins and ER stress, compromising decidual cell functions, and triggering early maternal rejection.*

Source: Benagiano, G., Mancuso, S., Guo, S. W., & Di Renzo, G. C., (2023). Events leading to the establishment of pregnancy and placental formation: The need to fine-tune the nomenclature of pregnancy and gestation. International Journal of Molecular Sciences, 24(20), 15420. https://doi.org/10.3390/ijms242015420.

It is possible for a multiparous woman to feel life, or the first fetal movements, as early as the 14th or 16th week. The nulliparous woman may not become aware of these feelings until the 18th week or later. Quickening is frequently described as a flutter, and it can be difficult to distinguish it from peristalsis. The frequency and intensity of fetal movements gradually increase. The week that quickening occurs provides a ballpark estimate of the gestational period.

8.1.5.2. Vagina and Vulva

To prepare the vagina for stretching during labor and delivery, pregnancy hormones cause the vaginal mucosa to thicken, the connective tissue to loosen, the smooth muscle to hypertrophy, and the vaginal vault to lengthen. Because of the increased vascularity, the cervix and vaginal mucosa have a violet-bluish tint. The deepened color sometimes referred to as the Chadwick sign, first appears as early as the sixth week of pregnancy, but by the eighth week, it becomes most apparent.

Leukorrhea is a mucoid discharge that is white or slightly gray in color and has a faint musty odor. The cervical cavity is stimulated by progesterone and estrogen, which leads to an abundance of mucus fluid. The fluid is whitish because of the hyperplasia associated with a normal pregnancy, which results in an abundance of exfoliated vaginal epithelial cells. This vaginal discharge never itches or leaves blood stains. In contrast to an amniotic fluid smear, ferning usually does not happen in a dried cervical mucus smear because of the progesterone effect. Instead, the dried mucus crystallizes into a pattern that looks like beads. The mucous plug, or operculum, forms as a result of the mucus filling the endocervical canal. The operculum serves as a barrier against bacterial invasion during pregnancy (Figure 8.6).

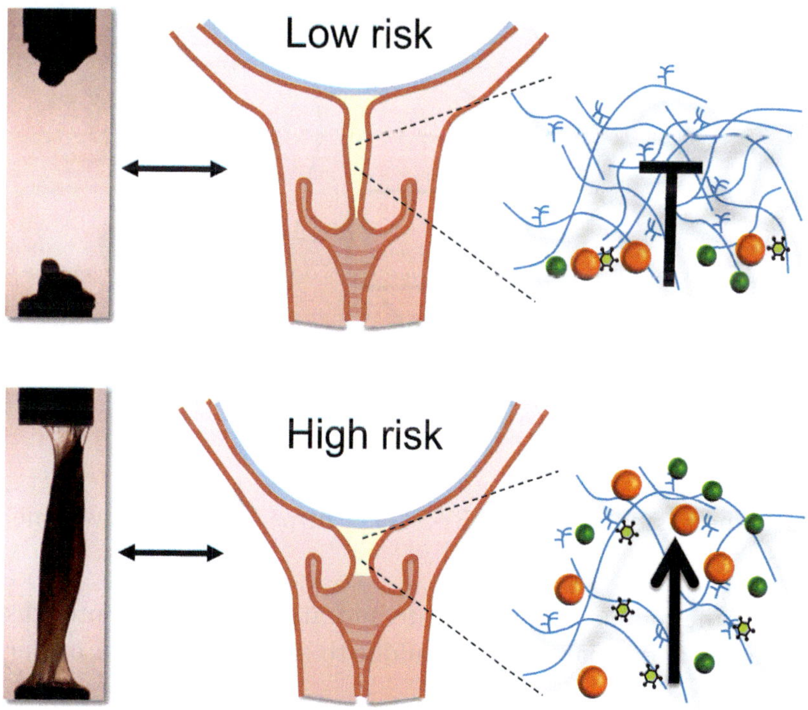

Figure 8.6. *A cervix mucus plugs during pregnancy.*

Source: Critchfield, A. S., Yao, G., Jaishankar, A., Friedlander, R. S., Lieleg, O., Doyle, P. S., Critchfield, A. S., Yao, G., Jaishankar, A., Friedlander, R. S., Lieleg, O., Doyle, P. S., et al., (2013). Cervical mucus properties stratify risk for preterm birth. PLoS ONE, 8(8), e69528, CC BY-SA 4.0, https://commons.wikimedia.org/w/index.php?curid=143483174.

Because Lactobacillus acidophilus acts on glycogen in the vaginal epithelium to produce more lactic acid, the pH of vaginal secretions rises (from roughly 3 to 6 [normal 4 to 7]) during pregnancy. This is probably due to elevated estrogen levels. Because *Candida albicans* thrives in an environment rich in glycogen, the pregnant woman is more susceptible to infections other than yeast infections, even though she is better protected from some organisms by this acidic environment.

The increased vascularity of the vagina and other pelvic viscera causes a significant increase in sensitivity. Particularly in the second trimester of pregnancy, the increased sensitivity may cause a high level of sexual interest and arousal. The heavy uterus, relaxed blood vessel walls, and increased congestion can all lead to edema and vulva varicosities. The edema and varicosities typically disappear during the postpartum period.

External structures of the perineum are enlarged during pregnancy because of an increase in vasculature, hypertrophy of the perineal body, and deposition of fat (Figure 8.7).

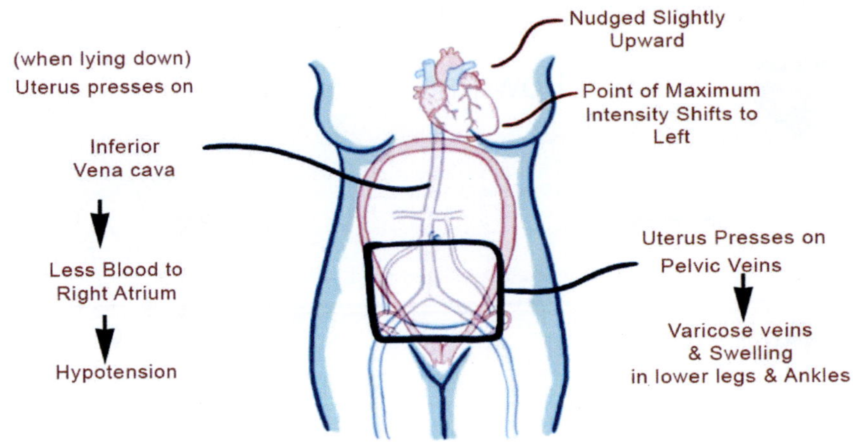

Figure 8.7. *Alterations.*

Source: By Osmosis – open.osmosis.org, CC BY-SA 4.0, https://commons.wikimedia.org/w/index.php?curid=64758143.

The labia majora of the nullipara approximate and hide the vaginal introitus, while the labia of the parous woman gape and separate after childbirth and after vaginal or perineal trauma.

8.1.5.3. Breasts

Elevated progesterone and estrogen levels early in pregnancy result in fuller, more sensitive, tingly, and heavier breasts. Breast sensitivity can cause anything from a mild tingling feeling to excruciating pain. Secondary pinkish areolae form and extend beyond the primary areolae, the nipples become more erectile, and the pigmentation of the nipples and areolae increases. The sebaceous (oil) glands embedded in the primary areolae around the nipples may exhibit hypertrophy; these are referred to as Montgomery tubercles. These sebaceous glands might offer defense by keeping the nipples lubricated while nursing.

The richer blood supply causes the blood vessels under the skin to enlarge. The previously barely noticeable blood vessels now stand out and often form a complex blue network just below the skin's surface. Venous congestion in the breasts is more obvious in primigravidas. Striae gravidarum may manifest on the outside of the breasts. Mammary gland growth causes breast enlargement, which happens gradually in the second and third trimesters. When the breasts are palpated, a broad, coarse nodule is felt due to the stimulation of the lobule-alveolar tissue and lactiferous ducts by the high levels of luteal and placental hormones associated with pregnancy. The glandular tissue pushes the connective tissue aside, causing the tissue to become softer and looser.

Although by midpregnancy the mammary glands have fully developed, lactation is not allowed until after birth. This is brought on by a decrease in estrogen. Precolostrum, a thin, transparent, viscous secretory material, is visible in the acini cells by the third month of pregnancy. The nipples may begin to release colostrum, a creamy, white to yellowish to orange premilk fluid, as early as 16 weeks of gestation (Cunningham et al., 2005).

8.2. Stages of Labor and Childbirth

There are multiple phases to labor and delivery, each with special traits and physiological functions. The latent phase, sometimes referred to as early labor, is when the journey usually starts. Contractions may start mild and erratic and then get progressively stronger and more frequent. In order to facilitate the baby's passage, the cervix begins to dilate and efface. The intensity, duration, and frequency of contractions increase as labor advances into active labor. The cervix keeps dilating and usually reaches a length of 6 to 7 centimeters. The baby's head descends further into the birth canal at this point. Active labor is followed by transition, which is sometimes regarded as the most intense stage of labor. Strong and frequent contractions intensify, and the cervix fully dilates to 10 centimeters, indicating that the baby is about to arrive. Women may experience a range of emotions at this time, including excitement, anxiety, and a sense of urgency.

Once the cervix is fully dilated and the baby's head is engaged in the pelvis, the second stage of labor, pushing, begins. To help the baby pass through the birth canal, women are advised to push during each contraction. Women are working extremely hard and long hours to bring their babies into the world during this stage. Healthcare professionals keep a close eye on both the mother and the child and offer assistance when required. The baby's body emerges in a controlled manner, with the head emerging first. Depending on the baby's position and the mother's strength and endurance, the pushing experience can last anywhere from a few minutes to several hours, with varying intensities among women.

The placenta is delivered during the third stage of labor, which is the last stage. The placenta separates from the uterine wall when the baby is born because the uterus keeps contracting after the birth. When the placenta and remaining membranes are pushed out, women may feel slight contractions. To prevent complications, healthcare providers check the placenta to make sure it is whole and that no pieces have broken off and are still inside the uterus. After the placenta is ejected, the uterus keeps contracting, which aids in uterine involution and helps regulate bleeding. At this point, women start their postpartum recovery journey after completing the labor and delivery process.

The body's normal childbirth process is called labor. For a first birth, it takes between

12 and 24 hours on average. After that, labor usually lasts less time. There are three stages to labor. From the moment you begin having regular contractions until you're prepared to give birth, which is the first stage. It consists of three phases: an active phase, when most of the work is done to prepare your body for delivery, a transitional phase when you start feeling the need to push, and an early or latent phase, when contractions are mild, and the cervix starts to change to allow the baby to pass through.

8.2.1. Childbirth

When one or more babies are delivered via vaginal delivery or cesarean section, the term "childbirth," which is another word for labor and delivery, describes the conclusion of a pregnancy. In 2019, there were approximately 140 million births worldwide. In developing countries, most births occur at home, while in developed countries, most deliveries occur in hospitals.

Worldwide, the most popular delivery method is vaginal delivery. It happens in four stages: the first is when the cervix shortens and opens; the second is when the baby descends and is born; the third stage is when the placenta is delivered; and the fourth stage, which is called postpartum, is when the mother and child recover. During the initial phase, the mother might feel back pain or cramps in her abdomen that last for about 30 seconds every 10 to 30 minutes. As the contractions get stronger and closer together, they will become more frequent. When the baby is fully born, the second stage comes to an end. The placenta is delivered during the third stage. The mother's recuperation, a postponed umbilical cord clamping, and infant observation comprise the fourth stage. Regardless of the delivery method, major health organizations recommend skin-to-skin contact as soon as possible after birth and postpone medical procedures on the newborn for at least one to two hours or until after the first feeding.

A vaginal delivery is recommended over a cesarean section due to the increased risk of complications from the latter and the inherent benefits of the former for both mother and child. Spinal blocks, relaxation methods, and opioids are a few pain management strategies. It is best practice to limit the number of interventions during labor and delivery, such as elective cesarean sections; however, in some circumstances, planning a scheduled cesarean section is necessary to ensure the mother's recovery and successful delivery. An emergency cesarean section may be recommended if unforeseen issues develop or if there is little to no progression through the birthing canal during a vaginal delivery.

An estimated 5,00,000 maternal deaths, 7 million severe long-term problems, and 50 million adverse health outcomes for postpartum women occur each year as a result of pregnancy and childbirth complications; most of these deaths occur in developing countries. Among the mother's complications are obstructed labor, postpartum hemorrhage, eclampsia, and postpartum infection. Among the difficulties the baby faces at birth are prematurity, birth trauma, and low oxygen levels.

8.2.2. Signs and Symptoms

The most obvious indication of labor is a strong, repeated contraction in the uterus. Some people have compared the pain during contractions to extremely intense menstrual cramps. A strong stretching and burning sensation may be felt during crowning. The Lamaze method of childbirth teaches that making noises such as moaning, groaning, grunting, repeating words over and over, and any sound that one's body may wish to naturally make may help to relieve pain and help labor progress. While the media would have you believe that every woman giving birth screams, this is not the case, according to Lamaze. Screaming, it is said, could indicate that the laboring woman is starting to feel panicked, and the medical staff should assist her in returning to normal breathing (Figure 8.8).

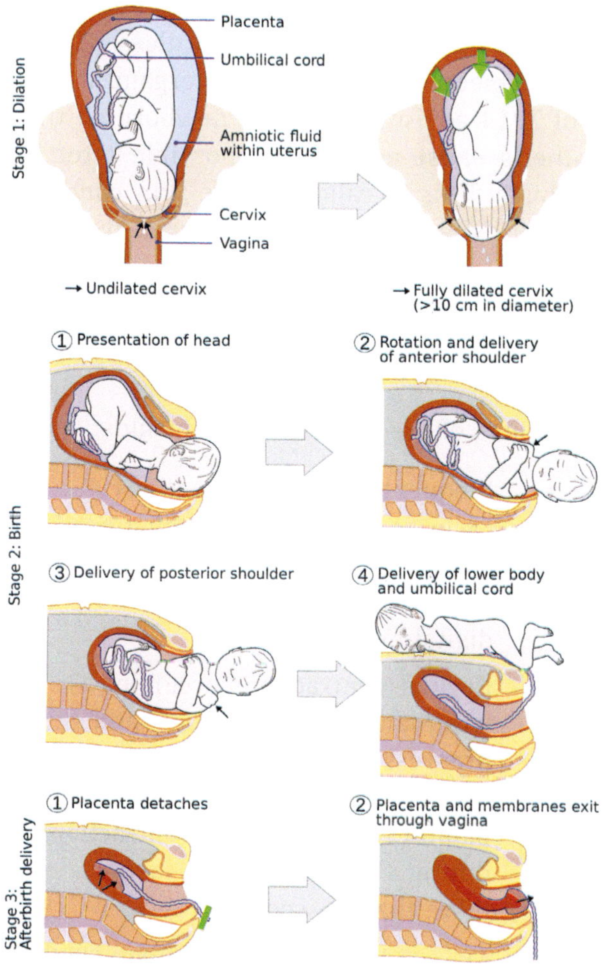

Figure 8.8. *The process of labor.*

Source: By Jmarchn – Own work, CC BY-SA 3.0, https://commons.wikimedia.org/w/index.php?curid=134495995.

Back labor is the name given to a particular kind of pain that women feel during childbirth, specifically in the lower back, right above the tailbone. The breaking of the water, also referred to as membrane rupture, is another obvious indicator of labor.

During pregnancy, a developing baby is surrounded and cushioned by a sac filled with fluid. Usually, the sac bursts at the beginning or during labor. It may cause a woman to experience intermittent or continuous small-scale vaginal leaks. Either clear or pale yellow is the liquid's color. If the amniotic sac hasn't already broken during labor, the medical professional may do an amniotomy. A thin plastic hook breaks the water during an amniotomy by creating a tiny hole in the sac. When the sac ruptures before the onset of labor, it is referred to as a prelabor rupture of the membranes.

Normally, 24 hours after the water breaks, contractions begin. If not, labor induction will usually start in 24 to 48 hours by the healthcare provider. In cases where the baby is born before 37 weeks of pregnancy, the doctor might prescribe medication to postpone the baby's delivery.

8.2.2.1. Psychological

In the later stages of gestation, there is an abundance of oxytocin, a hormone that is known to induce feelings of contentment, decrease anxiety, and feelings of calmness and security around the mate. A mother's behavior and her bonding with her child are thought to be greatly influenced by oxytocin, which is released more frequently during labor when the fetus stimulates the cervix and vagina. According to research, the father of the child also feels his oxytocin levels rise after spending time with the infant.

Furthermore, parents with higher oxytocin levels showed increased synchronization and responsiveness in their interactions with their children. Breastfeeding releases oxytocin, which makes it easier for the baby to access the nipple (Cunningham et al., 2005).

8.2.3. Vaginal Birth

The relationship between the fetal presenting portion and the level of the ischial spines is described by the term "station." The presenting portion is at the ischial spines when the station is zero, which is equivalent to engagement. In cases where a visible segment of the fetus is above the spines, the distance is measured in minus stations, which range in value from –1 to –4 cm. If the presenting portion is below the ischial spines, the distance is indicated using plus stations (+1 to +4 cm). The presenting portion is at the perineum and visible at +3 and +4.

The fetal head may momentarily change shape as it travels through the birth canal, taking on a more elongated or cone-shaped form. This is called molding, and women who are giving birth vaginally for the first time are more likely to experience it. Cervical ripening is the term used to describe the physical and chemical changes in the cervix that take place in anticipation of the fetus eventually stretching as it leaves the uterus and enters the birth canal. A Bishop score scoring system can be used to determine the degree of cervical ripening in women who are at risk of preterm labor, allowing for the prediction of the baby's due date and the onset of labor. Additionally, it is employed to forecast a woman's response to being in labor for an unplanned pregnancy or a medical reason. There are various methods to induce cervical ripening, which allows the cervix to dilate during uterine contractions.

When a baby is delivered vaginally, four stages of labor take place: the contraction and opening of the cervix; the baby's descent and birth; the delivery of the placenta; and the two-hour recovery phase that follows the delivery. The first stage is characterized by 30-minute-long back pain or abdominal cramps. Usually, these cramps happen every 10 to 30 minutes. With time, the contractions and the pain get stronger and closer together. The second stage concludes with the infant's total ejection. The third stage is when the placenta is delivered. The fourth stage of labor includes recovery, the uterus beginning to contract to a pre-pregnancy state, postponing the clamping of the umbilical cord, and keeping an eye on the vital signs and tone of the newborn. Regardless of the delivery method, all major health organizations as of 2014 advise placing the newborn on the mother's chest as soon as possible after a live birth. This is called skin-to-skin contact, and until the baby has experienced its first nursing experience, routine procedures should be delayed for at least one to two hours.

8.2.4. Onset of Labor

Definitions of the onset of labor include:

- Frequent uterine contractions occur at least every six minutes, accompanied by a change in cervical effacement or dilation between digital exams.
- Regular contractions occurring less than 10 minutes apart and progressive cervical dilation or cervical effacement. At least three painful regular uterine contractions during 10 minutes, each lasting more than 45 seconds.

It is well known that many women exhibit the so-called "nesting instinct." Just before going into labor, women report having an energy surge. An obvious sign that labor is about to begin is the "lightning" phenomenon, in which the baby descends from the rib cage while its head is firmly embedded in the pelvis. The pregnant woman may find breathing easier because her lungs have more room to expand, but she may also feel the need to void (urinate) more frequently due to pressure on her bladder. Lightning strikes can occur several weeks in advance, several hours in advance, or even before labor begins. A few days before the onset of labor, some women also experience an increase in vaginal discharge due to the mucus plug, a thick plug of mucus that blocks the uterine opening, pushing out into the vagina. The mucus plug may come loose a few days before labor starts or not at all. The amniotic sac, a fluid-filled membrane, encloses the developing embryo inside the uterus. The sac bursts soon before, at the start of, or during labor. The baby is at risk of infection once the sac ruptures, also known as the "water breaks." If labor has not begun within the amount of time the mother's medical team deems safe for the child, they will determine whether to induce labor.

8.2.5. Stages of Labor

8.2.5.1. First Stage

The latent phase is sometimes included in the definition of labor, and sometimes it is not. The first stage of labor is separated into latent and active phases (Figure 8.9).

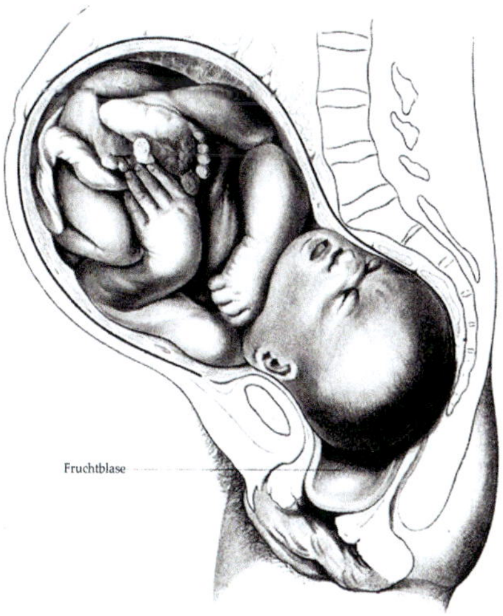

Figure 8.9. *The fetal head.*

Source: By Ernst Bumm and Albrecht Mayer – Grundriss zum Studium der Geburtshülfe 1902, Public Domain, https://commons.wikimedia.org/w/index.php?curid=30131770.

In general, the onset of regular uterine contractions marks the beginning of the latent phase for the woman. However, Braxton Hicks contractions, sometimes referred to as false labor, are uncommon, unpredictable, and only result in mild cramping. They start to occur around week 26 of pregnancy. Braxton Hicks contractions are the contractions of the uterine muscles that occur before the birth of a baby. Cervical dilation and effacement, or the thinning and stretching of the cervix, occur in the last few weeks of pregnancy. Typically, effacement is either fully or nearly fully completed by the time the latent phase ends, and dilation is about 5 cm. Cervical dilation and effacement can be felt during a vaginal exam.

There are regional differences in the definitions of the active phase of labor. The World Health Organization defines the active first stage as the period that includes a high degree of cervical effacement, frequent, painful contractions in the uterus, and a faster rate of cervical dilatation, which begins at 5 cm and continues until full dilatation for the first and subsequent labors. For multiparous moms who had previously given birth, the standard for what constituted active labor was changed from 3 to 4 cm to 5 cm of cervical dilation, and for nulliparous women who had not given birth to 6 cm. The intention behind this was to increase the proportion of vaginal births.

Physicians can use a cervical exam to measure the cervical dilation, effacement, and station to ascertain how far along the mother is in labor. The bishop score is comprised of these elements. The bishop score can also be used to predict how an induction of labor will turn out. During effacement, the cervix merges with the lower portion of the uterus. When uterine muscles contract, the lower segment is drawn upward and the upper segment is shortened, resulting in a gradual expulsive motion. The fetal portion that is currently visible is then permitted to descend. Full dilation occurs when the cervix widens to the point where the baby's head fits through, which for a term baby is approximately 10 cm.

The latent first stage has not been found to have a standard duration and varies widely amongst women. However, the active first stage (from 5 cm to full cervical dilatation) in a first labor (primiparae) usually lasts no longer than 12 hours, and in a second labor (multiparae), it usually lasts no longer than 10 hours. Dystocia of labor is characterized by challenging or unusually slow labor that involves progressive dilation of the cervical canal or non-descent of the fetus. It is also referred to as dysfunctional labor or failure to progress. Friedman's Curve, developed in 1955, was used for many years to diagnose labor dystocia. However, more recent medical research suggests that the Friedman curve may not be relevant at this time [when?] (Figure 8.10).

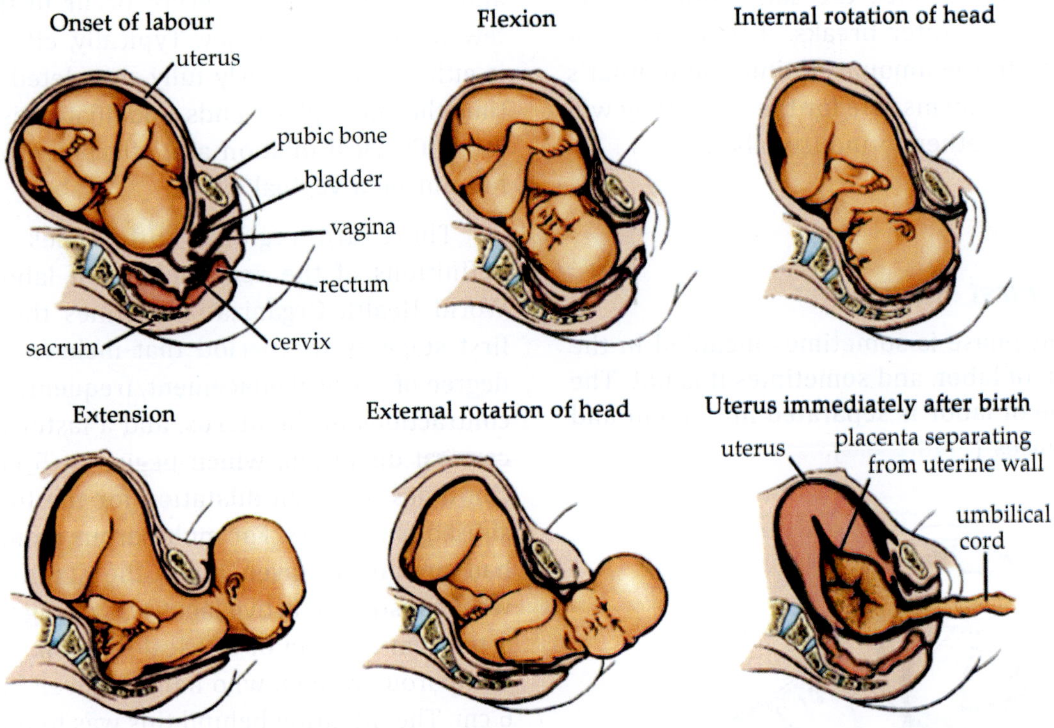

Figure 8.10. *The definitions of the active phase of labor.*

Source: Nsugbe, E., Samuel, O. W., Sanusi, I., Vishwakarma, S., & Adams, D., (2021). Pregnancy labor prediction using magnetomyography sensing and a self-sorting cybernetic model. Engineering Proceedings, 10(1), 60. https://doi.org/10.3390/ecsa-8-11312.

For instance, a woman with a history of mental health problems may be more susceptible to postnatal psychopathology than a woman without such a history, which means that other factors during and after childbirth may not be as important. This is one of the challenges that come with doing research in this area, which produces erratic outcomes. Therefore, it's crucial to consider both the strength of the evidence and the methodological quality of the studies when drawing conclusions.

8.2.5.2. Second Stage: Fetal Expulsion

The expulsion stage ends when the cervix reaches its maximum dilation, and the baby is born. When pressure builds up on the cervix, pelvic pressure rises, causing the urge to push. At the beginning of the normal second stage, the head is fully engaged in the pelvis; its widest diameter has surpassed the level of the pelvic inlet. The fetal head then descends into the pelvis through the vaginal opening and under the pubic arch. This is aided by the extra maternal efforts of bearing down or pushing, which are similar to defecating. The way the fetal head emerges at the vaginal entrance is referred to as crowning. The mother will now feel a sudden, intense burning or stinging sensation.

When the amniotic sac hasn't burst during labor or pushing, an infant can be born if it is intact. This is referred to as delivery in caul. The baby's full expulsion signals the successful end of the second stage of labor. Some babies, especially those born before their due date, have a white substance called vernix on their skin that has a consistency similar to wax or cheese. It is thought to have some protective functions for a few hours after birth and during fetal development. Every woman has a different second phase. First labors usually take three hours to complete, while subsequent labors usually take two hours. Longer than three-hour second-stage labor is associated with lower rates of vaginal births that spontaneously occur, higher rates of infection, perineal tears, obstetric hemorrhage, and a need for critical care for the newborn.

8.2.5.3. Third Stage: Placental Expulsion

The period that immediately follows the fetus's expulsion and the placenta's expulsion is referred to as the third stage of labor or the involution stage. The placenta physiologically separates from the uterine wall at the beginning of the expulsion process. The estimated average time from the baby's delivery to the placenta's full expulsion is 10 to 12 minutes, depending on whether active or expectant management is used. A third stage that lasts longer than half an hour occurs in up to 3% of vaginal deliveries, increasing the risk of placenta retention.

The placenta can be naturally expelled with expectant management, or it can be expelled spontaneously with active management. In addition to administering uterotonic medication within the first minute of fetal delivery, active management entails fundal massage and controlled traction of the umbilical cord following placenta delivery. After that, uterine massage is given for two hours, every 15 minutes. In a joint statement, the World Health Organization, the International Federation of Gynecology and Obstetrics, and the International Confederation of Midwives advocated for active management of the third stage of labor in all vaginal deliveries to help prevent postpartum hemorrhage. Delaying the clamping of the umbilical cord for at least one minute, or until it stops pulsing, could take several minutes, and improve the situation as long as jaundice can be treated. It was long believed that moms who had delayed cord cutting had a higher risk of postpartum hemorrhage, or severe bleeding after giving birth. However, a recent review found that in healthy, full-term infants, delayed cord cutting did not affect the rate of postpartum bleeding and instead led to early hemoglobin concentration, higher birth weight, and increased iron reserves up to six months after birth.

8.2.5.4. Fourth Stage: Postpartum

The period that follows childbirth, lasting roughly six weeks, is referred to as the fourth stage of labor. The terms postpartum and postnatal are often used during this period. The mother's body, including hormone levels and uterus size, returns to a non-pregnant state while the newborn adjusts to life outside the mother's body. The World Health Organization (WHO) considers the postnatal period—when most deaths occur—to be the most critical yet underappreciated period of a mother's and baby's lives.

The mother's perineum is sutured if she has an episiotomy or rips after giving birth. Furthermore, this is the ideal moment for the woman to begin using long-acting reversible contraception (LARC), such as an implanted contraceptive device (IUD) or IUD, which can both be inserted immediately after delivery while the woman is still in the delivery room. The mother is routinely assessed for temperature, heart rate, blood pressure, vaginal bleeding, and fundal height during the first 24 hours after delivery. Some women may experience postpartum chills or an involuntary shivering fit after giving birth. For the first six hours after passing, pee should be noted as soon as it does. The pains last for a few days after they occur and are similar to menstrual cramps, which are brought on by the uterus contracting to stop the blood flow too much. A few weeks are typically all that the term "lochia," or vaginal discharge, lasts. It begins as vivid red and gradually changes to pink, brown, yellow, or white.

Hospital newborns used to be taken from their mothers as soon as they were born and only reunited with them for feeding times. Mothers were told that their children would be safe in the nursery and that being apart would give them more time to relax. Following a period of standard hospital procedures and observation, some hospitals began to offer the option of rooming-in, allowing the baby to share the mother's room as attitudes started to change. By 2020, it has gradually become standard practice in maternity units to stay in a room.

8.2.6. Early Skin-to-Skin Contact

A parent, typically the mother or father, will hold a newborn chest to chest and skin to skin in a technique known as "kangaroo care," or skin-to-skin contact. This means that neither the parent nor the infant should have any shirts or underwear on their chests. Studies have indicated that this technique can lessen baby cries, enhance the length of nursing, improve breathing and heart stability, and control blood sugar levels. Additionally, research has demonstrated that skin-to-skin contact at birth improves the likelihood of a successful nursing bond.

As of 2014, early postpartum SSC is supported by the American Academy of Pediatrics and all other major organizations that oversee infant health. The safe transition of the baby from placental to mammary nutrition signifies the completion of the birthing process, according to the World Health Organization (WHO). It is advised to place the newborn skin-to-skin with the mother following a vaginal birth, or as soon as the mother is conscious and responsive following a Caesarean section. This should delay any routine procedures for at least one to two hours. The father or another support person may also hold the infant SSC until the mother awakens from the anesthesia.

The World Health Organization states that the bonding process can be upset by even a short separation before the baby has had its first feed, so any early observations of the infant should be taken while the child is still near the mother. Furthermore, they advise maximizing skin-to-skin contact during the first few days after giving birth, especially if it is interrupted for any reason.

Women to have a delivery team that includes a support person who will advocate to ensure that:

- The mother and her baby are not separated unnecessarily;
- The baby will receive only her milk;
- The baby will receive no supplementation without a medical reason;
- All testing, bathing, or other procedures are done in the parent's room.

It has long been known that a mother's oxytocin levels rise when she interacts with her child. In 2019, a thorough analysis of the effects of oxytocin found that fathers involved in SSC also have higher oxytocin levels. Two studies show that chest-to-chest contact (i.e., When a baby is placed between a parent's breast and is only wearing a diaper, reduces the parents' post-interaction stress and anxiety (due to increased levels of oxytocin in the father).

8.2.6.1. Discharge

When giving birth in a medical facility, the World Health Organization recommends that women stay in the hospital for at least 24 hours for a simple vaginal delivery and 96 hours for a cesarean section. Based on data collected in 2016, an easy delivery takes an average of less than a day in Egypt and up to six days in (pre-war) Ukraine. The average is 2 + 8 days in Australia and 1 + 5 days in the UK. Two-thirds of women in the UK give birth with the help of a midwife, despite the low percentage; sometimes, the mother chooses a hospital birth to be closer to the extensive emergency care that is offered. However, a woman under a midwife's care may leave the hospital after giving birth, and her midwife will still provide care for her at home. Within the U. S. From 4 1½ days in 1970 to 2 days now, the average length of stay has decreased over time. The CDC attributed the decline in hospital stays to rising healthcare costs and stated that people could no longer afford to stay there. To keep it from dropping any further, Congress passed the Newborns' and Mothers' Health Protection Act in 1996. This act requires insurers to cover basic deliveries for a minimum of 48 hours (Cunningham et al., 2005).

A Closer Look

Placental Perfusion

Placental perfusion is a vital process during pregnancy, ensuring the efficient exchange of nutrients, oxygen, and waste products between the maternal and fetal circulatory systems. This intricate mechanism involves the intricate interplay of maternal and fetal blood vessels within the placenta.

Maternal blood, rich in oxygen and nutrients, flows into the placenta through uterine arteries. Upon reaching the placenta, it enters a network of chorionic villi, finger-like projections containing fetal blood vessels. These villi are bathed in maternal blood, facilitating the exchange of substances between maternal and fetal circulations through a process known as diffusion.

Fetal blood, low in oxygen and nutrients, passes through the fetal vessels within the chorionic villi. As it flows through these vessels, fetal blood picks up oxygen and nutrients from the maternal blood, while simultaneously releasing waste products like carbon dioxide. This exchange is made possible by the proximity of maternal and fetal blood within the villi, separated only by thin layers of tissue. Effective placental perfusion is crucial for the optimal growth and development of the fetus. Any disruption in this process can lead to complications such as intrauterine growth restriction or preeclampsia, highlighting the importance of understanding and monitoring placental perfusion during pregnancy (Cunningham et al., 2005).

Summary

- Pregnancy, the physiological process by which a woman carries and nurtures a developing fetus, culminates in parturition, commonly known as childbirth.
- The pregnant uterus undergoes remarkable changes to accommodate and support the developing fetus, and these changes are closely intertwined with the structure and function of the placenta.
- The hormones associated with pregnancy and the mechanical pressures resulting from the growing uterus and other tissues are thought to be responsible for maternal physiologic adaptations.
- The term "childbirth," which is another name for "labor and delivery," refers to the end of a pregnancy when one or more babies are delivered by vaginal delivery or cesarean section.
- Skin-to-skin contact, also known as kangaroo care, is a method of caring for newborns where they are held chest-to-chest and skin-to-skin with a parent, usually their mother or father.
- Women receiving obstetric care are frequently subjected to institutional routines, which may negatively impact the course of labor. In order to reduce the need for obstetric intervention, supportive care during labor may include information and advocacy, comfort measures, emotional support, and information that may enhance both the physical process of labor and women's feelings of competence and control.

References

1. Aminoff, M. J. (2007). A decade at the helm of muscle & nerve; Editorial: Michael J. Aminoff. *Muscle & Nerve, 36*(6), 731–733. https://doi.org/10.1002/mus.20914.
2. Cole, K., et al. (2004). Accuracy of home pregnancy tests at the time of missed menses. *American Journal of Obstetrics and Gynecology, 190*(1), 100–105. https://doi.org/10.1016/S0002-9378(03)00855-5.
3. Cunningham, F., Leveno, K., Bloom, S., Hauth, J., Gilstrap, L., & Wenstrom, K. (2005). *William's obstetrics* (22nd ed.). McGraw-Hill.
4. Eberling, J. L., Jagust, W. J., Christine, C. W., Starr, P., Larson, P., Bankiewicz, K. S., & Aminoff, M. J. (2009). Results from a phase I safety trial of hAADC gene therapy for Parkinson's disease. *Neurology, 70*(21), 1980–1983. https://doi.org/10.1212/01.wnl.0000345613.82006.a1.
5. Furneaux, E., Langley-Evans, A., & Langley-Evans, S. (2001). Nausea and vomiting of pregnancy: Endocrine basis and contribution to pregnancy outcome. *Obstetrical and Gynecological Survey, 56*(12), 775–782. https://doi.org/10.1097/00006254-200112000-00023.
6. Hermida, R., Ayala, D., Mojon, A., & Fernandez, J. (2001). Time-qualified reference values for ambulatory blood pressure monitoring in pregnancy. *Hypertension, 38*(3 Pt 2), 746–752. https://doi.org/10.1161/hy1001.093959.

7. Padua, L., Aprile, I., Caliandro, P., Carboni, T., Meloni, A., Massi, S., et al. (2001). Symptoms and neurophysical picture of carpal tunnel syndrome in pregnancy. *Clinical Neurophysiology, 112*(10), 1946–1951. https://doi.org/10.1016/S1388-2457(01)00631-4.

8. Valles, F., Fiandaca, M. S., Eberling, J. L., Starr, P. A., Larson, P. S., Christine, C. W., & Bankiewicz, K. S. (2010). Qualitative imaging of adeno-associated virus serotype 2-human aromatic L-amino acid decarboxylase gene therapy in a phase I study for the treatment of Parkinson's disease. *Neurosurgery, 75*(5), 1377–1385. https://doi.org/10.1227/NEU.0b013e3181f361cf.

Chapter

REPRODUCTIVE DISORDERS AND DISEASES

9

Contents

Unit Introduction

The term "reproductive disorders and diseases" refers to a broad category of illnesses that impact the reproductive system, which includes the testes, prostate gland, uterine tubes, uterus, and ovaries. These conditions can have a serious effect on a person's ability to conceive, general health, and quality of life. Diseases affecting the human reproductive system are collectively referred to as reproductive system diseases. These include the testicles, ovaries, and other endocrine glands like the pituitary, thyroid, and adrenals producing hormones abnormally. Infections, tumors, genetic or congenital anomalies, and illnesses with no apparent cause can also result in these diseases.

Polycystic ovarian syndrome is one of the most prevalent reproductive disorders that women experience (PCOS). Hormonal imbalances that can result in ovarian cysts, irregular menstrual cycles, and problems ovulating are the hallmarks of PCOS. It can raise the risk of infertility, obesity, diabetes, and cardiovascular disease, and it affects about one in 10 women who are of reproductive age. Treatment frequently consists of hormone-regulating drugs and symptom-management lifestyle modifications like diet and exercise. Endometriosis is a common reproductive disorder where tissue resembling the uterine lining grows outside the uterus, leading to symptoms like pelvic pain, painful periods, and infertility. Though the exact cause is unclear, treatment options may include medication, surgical removal of the abnormal tissue, or assisted reproductive technologies for those affected by infertility.

Both men and women can experience infertility, which can be brought on by many conditions such as hormonal imbalances, anatomical anomalies, or genetic problems. Infertility in men can result from a variety of conditions, including low sperm counts, erectile dysfunction, and reproductive tract blockages. Fertility in women can be impacted by age, ovulation disorders, uterine or uterine tube problems, and other factors. *In vitro* fertilization (IVF), intrauterine insemination (IUI), and surrogacy are examples of assisted reproductive technologies that can help individuals and couples overcome infertility obstacles.

Reproductive health can also be impacted by sexually transmitted infections (STIs). If left untreated, sexually transmitted infections (STIs) like chlamydia, gonorrhea, and syphilis can inflame, scar, and harm reproductive organs. Untreated STIs in women can result in pelvic inflammatory disease (PID), which raises the possibility of an ectopic pregnancy or can cause infertility. STIs in men can cause prostatitis or epididymitis, which can impair sperm production or result in infertility.

Significant health risks are associated with reproductive cancers, which include testicular, ovarian, uterine, prostate, and cervical cancers. Improving results requires early detection through routine screenings and quick treatment. Depending on the type and stage of cancer, treatment options may include radiation therapy, chemotherapy, surgery, or a combination of these. Reproductive illnesses and disorders can have a significant impact on a person's ability to become pregnant, keep a pregnancy going, and maintain good reproductive health. The prevention, early detection, and efficient management of these conditions depend on education, awareness, and access to healthcare services (Makar & Toth, 2002; Cousineau & Domar, 2007; Parasar et al., 2017).

Orientation and Directional Terms:

Terms	Definition	Illustration
Endometriosis	Endometriosis is a disease in which tissue similar to the lining of the uterus grows outside the uterus.	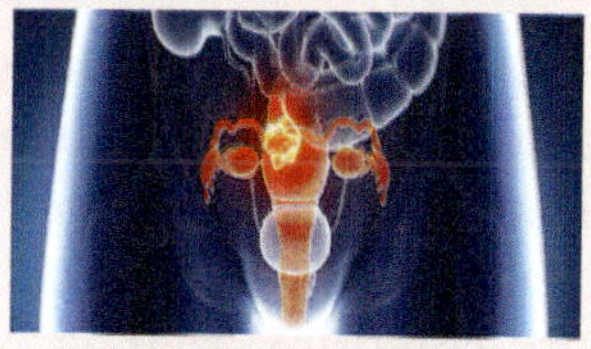
Pelvic inflammatory disease	Pelvic inflammatory disease (PID) is an infection of one or more of the upper reproductive organs, including the uterus, fallopian tubes and ovaries.	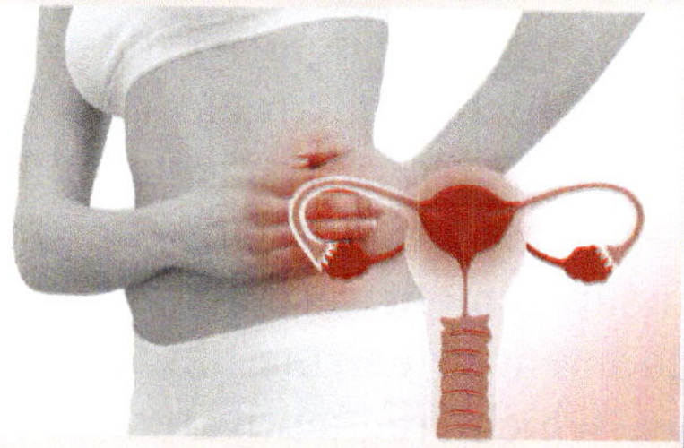
Puberty	Puberty is the process of physical changes through which a child's body matures into an adult body capable of sexual reproduction.	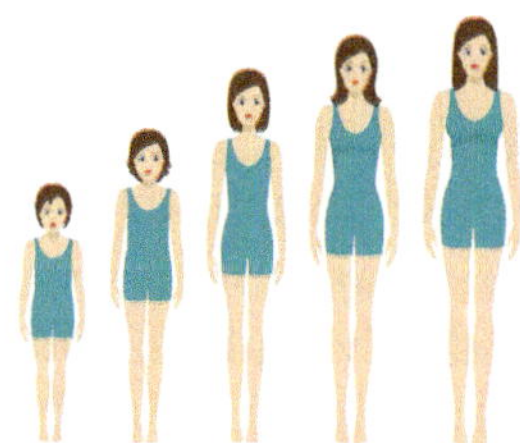
Spermatozoa	A spermatozoon is a motile sperm cell, or moving form of the haploid cell that is the male gamete.	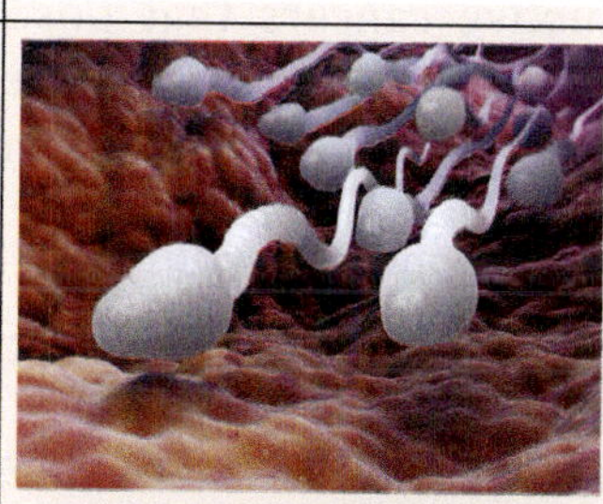
Scrotum	The scrotum is a part of a male's body that is located below the penis. The scrotum is the sac (pouch) that contains the testes, epididymis, and the lower part of the spermatic cord (blood vessels and vas deferens).	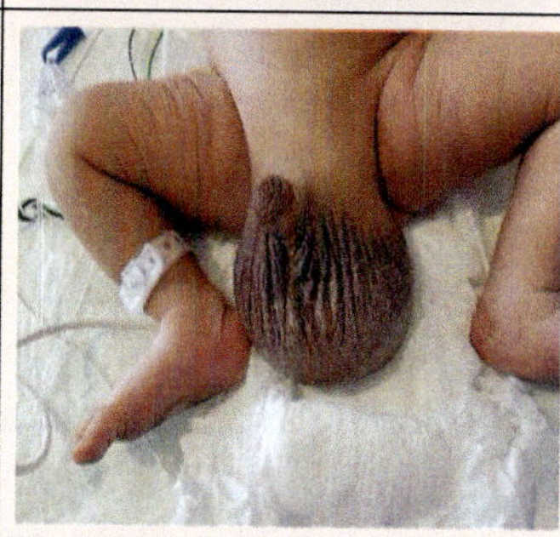

9.1. Common Disorders Affecting the Male and Female Reproductive Systems

The health and fertility of individuals can be greatly impacted by common disorders that affect the male and female reproductive systems, making awareness, diagnosis, and treatment necessary. One condition that is particularly common in women is polycystic ovary syndrome (PCOS), which is characterized by hormonal imbalances that result in irregular menstruation, ovarian cysts, and problems ovulating. Another prevalent ailment called endometriosis is the development of uterine-like tissue outside the uterus, which frequently results in infertility, irregular menstruation, and pelvic pain. Furthermore, untreated sexually transmitted infections (STIs) like gonorrhea, syphilis, and chlamydia pose serious risks to reproductive health, as they can result in ectopic pregnancy, infertility, and pelvic inflammatory disease (PID). Cervical, ovarian, and uterine cancers are among the reproductive cancers that pose a serious risk. Early detection and routine screenings are crucial for the best possible outcomes.

Sexual function and fertility can be affected by disorders such as erectile dysfunction in men, which is characterized by difficulty getting or keeping an erection. Moreover, male infertility poses difficulties for couples trying to conceive because it is frequently linked to low sperm count, poor sperm motility, or structural abnormalities in the reproductive tract. If left untreated, sexually transmitted infections, including those that affect the male reproductive system like gonorrhea and chlamydia, can cause complications like prostatitis or epididymitis, which can reduce fertility. Male reproductive health is also at risk from diseases like testicular cancer, which emphasizes the significance of early detection and treatment.

9.1.1. Functional Genital Disorders: Affecting Both Male and Female Systems

9.1.1.1. Delayed Puberty

The term "delayed puberty" may be misleading because puberty that occurs after the age of 19 is a permanent failure of sexual development caused by hypogonadotropic eunuchoidism, a condition in which the pituitary gland secretes an abnormally low amount of gonadotropic hormone, the hormone that stimulates the growth and activity of the sex glands. Typically, boys who develop more slowly than average but eventually reach full sexual development are referred to as having delayed puberty. Therapy for sexual underdevelopment may include chorionic gonadotropin (CGT), a hormone made by the placenta and extracted from the urine of pregnant women if social and psychological issues are present. If puberty is only postponed, it will typically resume as usual following this course of treatment. If it doesn't advance, the individual has hypogonadotropic eunuchoidism rather than delayed puberty.

9.1.1.2. Precocious Puberty

The earliest indication of puberty, which is the onset of pubic hair and breast growth, has historically been estimated to happen in healthy girls living in temperate climates at a mean age of 10 points 6 years (with a standard deviation of 1 point 2 years). Testicular growth in boys is thought to start at a mean age of 11 points 8, with a one-year standard deviation. A condition known as true precocious puberty occurs when the pituitary-gonadal system activates normally at an unusually young age. Traditionally, "abnormally early" has been defined as younger than 9 years old for boys and younger than 8 years old for girls. However, research conducted since the 1990s suggests that girls in developed nations may be experiencing the normal onset of puberty at a younger age, meaning that the age of precocious puberty for girls could be as low as 6 or 7. Pseudoprecocious puberty is characterized by the emergence of secondary sexual traits in males and females but does not include the production of spermatozoa or eggs.

True precocious puberty can be caused by brain lesions or hypothyroidism (abnormally low thyroid gland secretion); most cases have no known cause. Female ovarian tumors or cysts, tumors of the adrenal cortex (the outer layer of the adrenal gland), or congenital hyperdevelopment of the adrenal gland can all lead to premature pseudopuberty. Males are more likely to develop congenital hyperadrenal hyperplasia, adrenal cortex tumors, tumors involving the interstitial cells in the testes, and teratomas, which are tumors that contain a variety of tissue types, including adrenal-cortical tissue.

9.1.1.3. Genetic and Congenital Abnormalities

9.1.1.3.1. In the Male

Seldom occurring congenital abnormalities of the prostate gland and seminal vesicles include their absence, hypoplasia (underdevelopment), or the presence of cysts, which are sacs filled with fluid or semisolid material. Prostatic utricle cysts, or the male uterine remnant, are frequently discovered in conjunction with advanced stages of pseudohermaphroditism, a disorder in which the presence of sex glands is accompanied by an ambiguous bodily appearance regarding sex, and hypospadias, a defect in the urethra, i.e., the secondary sexual traits are not fully formed. Due to localized pressure on the bladder neck, cysts can also result in symptoms of urinary obstruction.

Rarely, severe penile abnormalities are typically linked to systemic conditions that make life unlivable, such as urinary problems. The penis can exhibit anomalies in the following ways: absence, transposition, torsion (twisting), and duplication. Males who have dwarfism, an overactive pituitary, adrenal tumors, or premature puberty often have an abnormally large penis. A small penis is associated with infantilism, underdevelopment of the genitalia, pituitary, or pineal gland under secretion, and failure of the corpora cavernosa (the dorsal side of the penis, which is where the erection occurs) to develop.

Congenital phimosis is the only abnormality of the foreskin. It is characterized by a contracture of the foreskin, or prepuce, which prevents it from retracting over the glans, the conical structure that forms the head of the penis. Urine flow may be impeded by the preputial opening. Circumcision is used to treat the condition.

The range of urethral anomalies is quite large. The most frequent type is stenosis (contracture) of the external opening (meatus), though congenital stricture of the urethra can also happen at other locations. Males who are born with congenital urethral obstruction may have flaps or valves across the anterior or posterior portion of the urethra. The verumontanum, a tiny protrusion in the back wall of the section of the urethra that surrounds the prostate gland, is typically connected at one end of the deep folds of mucous membrane that make up posterior urethral valves, which are more common than anterior valves. The urethra could become obstructed, and the kidneys could be harmed by overly tight valves.

Incomplete closure of the urethra is linked to a number of defects. One of the most prevalent is hypospadias, a condition in which the urethral canal's outer end is open for a considerable amount of distance on the ventral side. The penis also often curves downward beyond the meatus, and the meatus is often narrowed. Urinary control is maintained since the posterior portion of the urethra is never affected, allowing the muscle responsible for closing it to contract normally. While both sexes can have the condition, men are more likely to have it. Small external and internal genitalia, cryptorchidism (the failure of one or both testes to descend into the scrotum), and partial or complete failure of the testes to develop are all very common. Compared to hypospadias, epispadias, or an opening in the upper (dorsal) side of the penis, is much less common. Urinary incontinence is typically caused by the defect extending past the urinary sphincter, although dorsal curvature may also be present. A urethral diverticulum, which is a pouch in the urethral wall, urethrorectal fistula, which is an opening between the urethra and the rectum, complete absence of the urethra, double urethra, and urethral fistula are among the other, less common urethral anomalies. Surgery is an option for most of the conditions (Makar & Toth, 2002; Cousineau & Domar, 2007; Parasar et al., 2017).

Rarely occurring anorchism, which is the absence of one or both testes, may be linked to the absence of other spermatic tract structures. In most cases, when one testis—also known as a testicle—is missing, the other is discovered inside the abdomen as opposed to the scrotum. Small testes at birth may be the result of a primary disorder or pituitary underactivity. There is some weakness in libido and potency as well as a lack of development of secondary sexual traits in both disorders. Supernumerary testicles are incredibly uncommon; when they do occur, one or more of them typically exhibit some kind of abnormality, such as spermatic cord torsion. The fusion of the two testicles into a single mass, known as a synorchism, can happen in the abdomen or scrotum. The most common spermatic tract anomaly, cryptorchidism, is the inability of one or both testes to descend into the scrotum on their own. Hormonal therapy may help treat the condition, but surgery is typically required to correct it.

9.1.1.3.2. In the Female

Although the female genitalia are less complex than the male genitalia, they do have some anomalies that can occasionally seriously impair the ability of the female urogenital tract to function. In certain situations, the clitoris—an erectile structure that resembles the penis but lacks the urethra—may be absent, but in other situations, it may be enlarged due to a congenital or hormonal condition. A tiny unfused area is typically left just below the clitoris, through which urine and menstrual fluid can flow. Fusion of the labia minora, or the tiny folds of skin covering the clitoris, the urethral opening, and the vaginal opening, is a midline "sealing together." Urine flow obstruction and the resulting urinary tract infection are the main problems associated with this anomaly. The uterus and vagina dilate with fluid other than blood before puberty and with blood following puberty, respectively, due to an imperforate hymen (the membrane that seals off the vaginal opening). These conditions are referred to as hydrometrocolpos and hematocolpometra, respectively. The urethra is sufficiently compressed by the distended vagina to obstruct urination. This condition frequently results in total urine retention in the bladder as well as distension of the upper urinary tract. A stenosed urethral opening and a dense hymenal ring are signs of urethral and hymenal fusion. Persistent urinary infection is frequently the consequence of the ensuing urinary obstruction. Surgery is a common means of treating most conditions.

There are three types of anomalies related to the vagina and uterus: duplication, incomplete development, and total absence. The female urethra can be distended, have an abnormal pouch called a diverticulum in its wall, have a congenitally narrow opening called a meatus, or open abnormally into the vagina. Although it is far less common than in males, hypospadias can occur in females as well. In the female, epispadias is also present. The only available course of treatment is reconstructive surgery. Congenital intercommunication between the rectum and the urethra and vagina, or between the rectum and the urinary bladder and vagina, is one of the rarest and most severe urogenital-tract anomalies, known as urogenital cloaca.

9.1.1.3.3. Intersexuality

Possessing both masculine and feminine traits can be a sign of intersexuality from birth or after puberty. Intersexuality that is evident from birth can be categorized as either true hermaphroditism or female or male pseudohermaphroditism. Female intersex, also known as female pseudohermaphroditism, can be nonadrenal or adrenal in nature. The adrenal type is caused by an inherited error in the metabolism of cortisol, the adrenal hormone, which results in an excess of androgens (male sex hormones) and an increase in corticotropin (ACTH) secretion. The external genitalia of a newborn female with this condition are masculinized due to an excess of male hormone; the clitoris and labia (which are prominent folds of skin that correspond to the scrotum in males) are enlarged and the vagina tends to be connected to the urethra. The newborn female with this condition is a chromosomal female. Adrenaline hormone administration is a viable treatment option (e.g., hydrocortisone), which inhibits the pituitary from reducing its stimulation of the adrenal glands' synthesis of androgenic hormones. Infants whose mothers were administered progestational compounds—substances that stimulate changes in the uterus that further the implantation and growth of the fertilized ovum—or synthetic androgens during pregnancy are susceptible to the nonadrenal type of intersex. On rare occasions, the illness is linked to the mother having an ovarian or adrenal gland tumor. The newborn baby is a female with variable degrees of ambiguous genitalia; puberty is the normal time for normal female development, so no treatment is required.

Males with differing degrees of internal and external virilization are known as male pseudohermaphrodites. Male intersex individuals typically have an enlarged prostatic utricle, a cleft scrotum, an undescended testis, and a markedly hypospadic penis. They may also have a complete uterus and uterine tubes, with the vagina opening into the posterior wall of the urethra. Those who lack ovaries are considered pseudohermaphrodites.

The ovarian and testicular tissue of true hermaphrodites is distinguishable. The internal genitalia differ greatly, often containing both male and female structures, but a uterus is always present. Because of the often-ambiguous external genitalia and the presence of a large phallus, the majority of these children are raised as males. Over 80% of them get enlarged breasts during puberty, and about half of them start menstruating. Most hermaphrodites are chromatin-positive, meaning that they contain chromatin, a material typically found in female cells but absent in male cells, within and close to the periphery of their nuclei. Additionally, more than half of them have a distinctively female set of chromosomes in their peripheral blood cells (Makar & Toth, 2002; Cousineau & Domar, 2007; Parasar et al., 2017).

Based on current physical and psychological findings, surgical and hormonal therapy aims to produce a male or female body configuration. The age at which the diagnosis is made also influences the course of treatment. Intersexuality syndromes that manifest before or after puberty include Klinefelter syndrome, Turner syndrome, and testicular feminization. Males with Kleinfelder syndrome (a genetic disorder) typically have small testes, and enlarged breasts during puberty (gynecomastia), and are infertile due to an extra sex chromosome (XXY). Males who have this syndrome are more likely to develop diabetes mellitus and lupus, two autoimmune diseases.

In the classic form of the condition, females with Turner syndrome carry only one X chromosome (XO). These individuals are typically small, nonmenstruating, and lacking in the female sex hormone estrogen; a characteristic group of congenital anomalies is linked to this syndrome.

Genetic X chromosome mutations that make a man resistant to the effects of androgens (male hormones) are the cause of testicular feminization, also known as androgen insensitivity syndrome. Those who are affected appear to be females with normal development but have a normal male chromosomal sex. The gonads are fully formed testes, and data suggests that testosterone—a male hormone—is produced normally. However, the presence of cellular resistance to this hormone causes the affected individual to change into a female. These gonads are typically removed surgically because they are likely to develop into malignant tumors. The administration of estrogenic hormones then maintains female sexual characteristics.

9.1.2. Infertility

An animal or plant that is infertile is unable to procreate naturally. With a few notable exceptions, it is typically not the normal state of a healthy adult (mostly haplodiploid insects). Because they have not yet reached puberty, the point at which the body begins to prepare for reproduction is the typical state of a human child or other young offspring. The inability to conceive after a year of regular, unprotected sexual activity between a male and female partner is known as infertility in humans. Infertility has a variety of causes, some of which can be addressed with medical intervention. According to estimates from 1997, roughly 5% of heterosexual couples worldwide may be struggling with infertility. However, many more couples—estimates range from 12 to 28%—experience involuntary childlessness for a minimum of one year. Human infertility is primarily caused by aging, and older mothers are more likely to experience spontaneous abortions during their pregnancies.

Around 20% to 30% of cases of infertility are caused by male infertility, 20% to 30% are caused by female infertility, and 20% to 40% are caused by problems in both parts combined. Around 10% to 20% of cases have no known cause. Age is the most common factor contributing to female infertility, which typically shows up as infrequent or nonexistent menstrual cycles. Semen deficiency is the most common cause of male infertility, and semen quality is a proxy for male fecundity. Fertile women go through a window of fertility just before and during ovulation, after which they become infertile for the remainder of the menstrual cycle. The timing of these changes can be determined using fertility awareness techniques, which monitor variations in basal body temperature or cervical mucus.

Around one-third of cases of infertility are caused by deficiencies in the male's sperm production, which affects at least 10% of couples. Male infertility is commonly caused by deficiencies in sperm maturation, orchitis (acute inflammation of the testes, often caused by mumps), which results in testicular destruction; obstruction of sperm passageways; abnormally low thyroid or high adrenal secretion; varicocele (enlargement of the spermatic cord veins); or the production of sperm-specific antibodies by either the male or the female. Semen analysis is the most crucial stage in the assessment of male infertility (Figure 9.1).

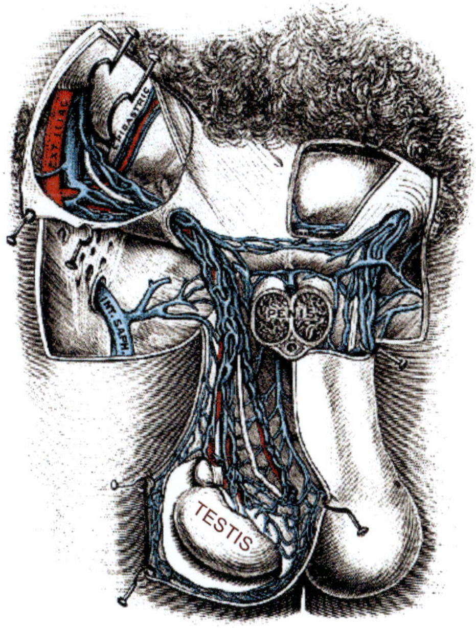

Figure 9.1. *Varicocele, enlargement of the veins of the spermatic cord, is a cause of infertility in men.*

Source: By Henry Vandyke Carter – Henry Gray (1918) Anatomy of the Human Body (See "Book" section below) Bartleby.com: Gray's Anatomy, Plate 1147, Public Domain, https://commons.wikimedia.org/w/index.php?curid=35171305.

A female's inability to conceive is caused by defective ova production or interferences with their ability to unite with spermatozoa. About 25% of female infertility issues are caused by disorders related to ovulation, with oligoovulation (extremely irregular ovulatory cycles) and anovulation (failure to ovulate) being the most common disorders. Infertility can also be caused by blockages and scarring of the uterine tubes, which can be brought on by reproductive tract infections (e.g., endometriosis, uterine fibroids, or pelvic inflammatory disease). Normally, the sperm enter the uterus through the cervical canal and proceed into the uterine tube, where the ovum is fertilized. In the few days preceding ovulation, or the release of an ovum from the ovary, the cervix glands typically secrete a thin, watery mucus that aids in sperm migration and survival. A lack of estrogen or an infection are two examples of variables that can lower mucus quality. Infertility can also be brought on by congenital abnormalities of the reproductive system. Although vaginal causes are rare, obstructions can also be functional, resulting from contraction and enlargement of the levator ani muscles, which form a supporting sheet beneath the pelvic cavity with openings for structures like the vagina and the anus. Alternatively, the obstruction could be the result of an undisturbed hymen. Ovulation may be hampered by thyroid, pituitary, adrenal, or ovarian diseases, as well as by having a high number of ovarian cysts (a condition known as Stein-Leventhal syndrome). Lastly, there's a chance that psychological issues contribute to infertility. The use of different hormones, surgical removal of the tubal blockage, and psychotherapy are the methods of treatment (Makar & Toth, 2002; Cousineau & Domar, 2007; Parasar et al., 2017).

9.1.3. Affecting the Female System

Menstrual abnormalities include dysmenorrhea, which is painful menstruation; menorrhagia, which is excessive blood loss during each menstrual cycle; metrorrhagia, which is irregular bleeding; amenorrhea, which is the absence of menstruation; and dysfunctional uterine bleeding. Premenstrual syndrome is another common condition that many women encounter. It is a collection of emotional and physical symptoms that appear before the start of each cycle. Some women experience mild bleeding from the follicle into the peritoneal cavity during ovulation, which causes brief abdominal pain. This condition can be treated with painkillers like ibuprofen or naproxen, or it can be prevented with oral contraceptives by suppressing ovulation.

9.1.3.1. Dysmenorrhea

During or before menstruation, dysmenorrhea is characterized by excruciating cramps that can occasionally be so bad as to make daily activities difficult. Pain is sufficiently managed with medications that prevent prostaglandin production.

Endometriosis or pelvic diseases involving inflammation of the ovaries and tubes can cause secondary dysmenorrhea. In endometriosis, endometrial deposits are found in the ovaries and other non-normal locations. These deposits form blood-filled cysts, which cause pain and excessive bleeding. The deposits are a cyclic response to ovarian hormones. Premenstrual pain and a feeling of congestion are common in painful menstruation caused by pelvic disease, and excessive menstrual bleeding is frequently experienced during this time. The underlying disorder is the focus of treatment.

9.1.3.2. Menorrhagia

Menorrhagia, or excessive menstrual bleeding, can be brought on by a thyroid or adrenal hormone imbalance, but it can also be brought on by a pelvic organ disease that is localized. This localized illness could be an infection-related inflammation, a benign tumor-like a fibroid, a polyp, protruding mass of endometrium, or cancer, particularly if it manifests after the age of 35. While polyps and some fibroids can be removed without removing the uterus, certain forms of local pelvic disease may necessitate a hysterectomy or treatment with chemotherapy or radiation.

Extremely heavy bleeding can happen as menopause approaches, leading to fatigue, anemia, and poor health. In this case, excess or unbalanced estrogen action leads to the endometrium overdeveloping, which causes menorrhagia. Progestogens can be used to treat younger or childless women; for others, uterine excision may be required.

9.1.3.3. Metrorrhagia

Bleeding during or after menstruation, after sexual activity, and between menstrual periods is often caused by a cervix abnormality; it is important to consider the possibility of cancer. Cervical erosion or a polyp on the cervix may also be the cause of this bleeding. Although cauterization is a simple treatment option, erosions frequently don't require it. Polyps have to be removed. When there is a risk of miscarriage, irregular bleeding can also happen during pregnancy; if any menstrual periods have been missed, this possibility needs to be considered.

9.1.3.4. Amenorrhea

Amenorrhea, or not having a menstrual cycle, is common during pregnancy and for a while after giving birth. Menstruation may not return for up to six months if the mother is breastfeeding her child; this is normal and should be expected if the mother is not making enough milk. The most frequent cause of amenorrhea during the reproductive years is pregnancy.

For a woman who has never had a period before, primary amenorrhea is the lack of menstruation. Primary amenorrhea can occasionally result from gonadal dysgenesis, which is the ovaries' failure to develop normally. Chromosome abnormalities may also play a role in this condition. A patient may have only one X chromosome (Turner syndrome) or even a male pattern of an X and a Y chromosome (Swyer syndrome), as opposed to the typical female complement of 46 chromosomes in each cell, including two X chromosomes. In these individuals, the uterine tubes and uterus are frequently absent, despite the possibility of a female general physique. Absence of the uterus happens occasionally, even in cases with normal ovaries. Vaginal atresia, also known as closure, is a less common abnormality in which the vagina is blocked by a membrane slightly above the hymen; menstruation still takes place, but the discharge is unable to pass through and causes the vagina to dilate. An easy fix for this condition, also known as cryptomenorrhea or false amenorrhea, is to make a cut in the membrane.

Period cessation occurring after the onset of menstruation but before menopause is typically caused by a general illness, mental disorder, or emotional stress. It might also result from an illness of the endocrine system, affecting not just the pituitary gland but also other endocrine glands. Ovarian disease is unlikely to be the cause of secondary amenorrhea because it would take damage to both ovaries for all functions to cease. Instead, it is more likely to result from ovarian removal or radiation therapy. A functional disorder of the ovaries characterized by disrupted estrogen production is called Stein-Leventhal syndrome. This disorder manifests as abnormal facial hair growth due to abnormal androgenic activity, or masculinizing behavior. Arrhenoblastomas, or androgenic hormone-secreting ovarian tumors, are another incredibly rare cause of amenorrhea and abnormal hair growth. It is common for secondary amenorrhea cases to resolve on their own, especially if a general illness or psychological stress is the underlying cause. A thorough pelvic examination and a general medical examination are used to assess the viability of hormone treatment.

9.1.3.5. Dysfunctional Uterine Bleeding

Most often in early adolescence and right before menopause, women experience dysfunctional, or anovulatory, uterine bleeding. It is believed to be brought on by dysfunctional ovarian function. Ovulation does not happen, but endometrial proliferation can be induced by the cycle's production of estrogens. As the estrogens are removed during each cycle, the endometrium degrades and bleeds. These kinds of cycles happen to women who take oral contraceptives. Additionally linked to dysfunctional bleeding are emotional stress, obesity, and excessive exercise (Makar & Toth, 2002; Cousineau & Domar, 2007; Parasar et al., 2017).

9.1.4. Affecting the Male System

9.1.4.1. Impotence

The incapacity of a male to engage in satisfying sexual activity is known as impotence. It can manifest as a variety of symptoms, such as weak erections, early ejaculation, or loss of normal sensation during ejaculation. It could be brought on by abnormal testicular function, diabetes, arteriosclerosis (hardening of the arteries), psychological issues, or a nervous system illness. Sexual function may be negatively impacted by some drugs that are prescribed to treat conditions like psychiatric illness, hypertension, and peptic ulcers. Hormone therapy, psychotherapy, and medication therapy (PDE-5 inhibitors like Viagra) are examples of therapy.

9.1.4.2. Priapism

A painful, prolonged penile erection that isn't brought on by sexual stimulation is called pruritus. Blood solidifies into a sludge-like substance within the corpora cavernosa, where it can stay for several hours or even days. Leukemia, sickle cell anemia, metastatic carcinoma (cancerous development distant from the primary site), and nervous system diseases account for about 25% of the cases; however, in most cases, the cause is unknown. While there are numerous treatment options, medication therapy works best in most situations. Impotence is common following a priapism episode, regardless of treatment, and is more common following multiple priapism episodes.

9.1.5. Sexually Transmitted Infections

Known also as venereal diseases, sexually transmitted diseases (STDs) are typically acquired through sexual contact with an infected partner. The main illnesses that are frequently spread in this way are genital herpes, AIDS, syphilis, gonorrhea, and chlamydia.

9.1.5.1. Syphilis

Treponema pallidum is the bacterial spirochete that causes syphilis. Syphilis has been known in Europe since the 15th century, but it wasn't until about 200 years ago that it was acknowledged as a sexually transmitted illness. Two to four weeks after unprotected sexual contact with an infected partner, it initially manifests as a painless sore on the skin or mucous membranes of the genitals, known as a chancre; however, in rare circumstances, the initial symptoms may also manifest in other areas. Antibodies against *Treponema pallidum* are induced by the infection. Pallidum, which several weeks after the initial infection can be detected in the bloodstream using different tests. If left untreated, secondary syphilis manifests as a genital rash and the disappearance of the chancre. Gumma, or subsurface nodules, first show up in the tertiary stage of the illness. Although the organism attacks the nervous system early on, it frequently takes years for neurologic symptoms, such as behavioral abnormalities, to manifest. The most effective time to treat syphilis is during the primary stage. Antibiotics can also stop a pregnant woman from passing the infection to her fetus, which could lead to a miscarriage or serious congenital abnormalities. The most common antibiotic used to treat syphilis is penicillin.

9.1.5.2. Gonorrhea

Neisseria gonorrhoeae, the bacteria that causes gonorrhea, has a very short incubation period, which makes it challenging to break the chain of transmission. Almost always the result of unprotected sexual contact with an infected partner, infection can be avoided by using a condom. Male gonorrhea is primarily characterized by pain or burning when urinating, though penile discharge is another possible symptom. Approximately 50% of female infections are asymptomatic; in those that are, the symptoms mirror those of the male infection. Localized spread of gonorrhea occurs along mucosal surfaces; in males, it ascends the urethra; in females, it can go through the vagina or the urethra. In addition, the bacteria can spread through the blood to farther locations; systemic symptoms include headaches and, if treatment is not received, arthritis or heart disease.

9.1.5.3. Nongonococcal Urethritis

Although many different microorganisms can cause nongonococcal urethritis (NGU), Chlamydia species are most frequently blamed for the condition, as they are also known to cause lymphogranuloma venereum. An infectious transmission is strongly suspected in about half of the cases. Although they are typically milder than those of gonorrhea, the symptoms are primarily pain and burning when urinating. Antibiotics are used as a treatment.

9.1.5.4. Genital Herpes

Herpes simplex virus type 1 (HSV-1), which causes cold sores on the lips and mouth, and type 2 (HSV-2) are the two viruses that cause genital herpes. In men, the disease initially manifests as clusters of tiny blisters on the penis' surface, while in women's vulva. After two to three weeks, the initial infection resolves on its own, but herpes frequently returns at different intervals, burning or itching at the lesion site. Herpes is typically only contagious when there is an active lesion present; it can be avoided by refraining from sexual activity while the lesion is active. Wearing a condom reduces the chance of transmission. During childbirth, active herpes can be fatal to newborns; in most cases, it results in blindness or brain damage. Cervical cancer in women has also been linked to genital herpes. Early antiviral therapy during the illness may shorten the duration of symptoms. Cytomegalovirus (CMV), another common herpesvirus, is linked to a high death rate in people with compromised immune systems.

9.1.5.5. Chancroid

The bacterium *Haemophilus ducreyi* is the cause of chancroid, also known as a soft sore, which primarily affects underdeveloped nations. After exposure, the bacteria typically produce small red pustules in less than five days. The pustules rupture to form painful ulcers, and the disease can be identified by culturing bacteria from the ulcers. Contrary to syphilis, which it may resemble, chancroid is a genital illness that is only localized. Antibiotics are used as a treatment.

9.1.5.6. Lymphogranuloma Venereum

Chlamydia trachomatis is the cause of lymphogranuloma venereum, a condition that is common in tropical areas but extremely uncommon in temperate ones. It can be contracted in different ways, but sexual contact is usually how it spreads. A brief genital blister is usually followed by localized lymph node inflammation. Genital elephantiasis could develop from this illness if treatment is not received. Antibiotics with a broad spectrum are used as treatment. It might be required to remove diseased tissue surgically.

9.1.5.7. Genital Warts

The virus that causes common warts is related to the human papillomavirus, which causes genital warts, also known as condyloma acuminata. A wart starts as a swelling the size of a pinhead grows larger and eventually becomes pedunculated. A mature wart is frequently made up of numerous smaller swellings and may resemble the genital lesions seen in secondary syphilis.

9.1.5.8. Granuloma Inguinale

Calymmatobacterium granulomatis infection is the primary cause of granuloma inguinale, which is mainly found in tropical and subtropical regions, including the southern United States. Painless papules that develop into ulcers and eventually turn into granulomatous masses that bleed readily are the initial symptoms. These lesions, which can resemble syphilis lesions, appear on the genitalia, thighs, and groin of infected individuals. Granuloma inguinale has been linked to cancer as well. Antibiotics are used as a treatment.

9.1.5.7. Candidiasis

Men almost always get local infections with the yeast *Candida albicans* through sexual encounters, but women, who are far more likely to get candidiasis, can get the infection in many ways. Men who have candidiasis on their glans penis may experience severe burning or itching. Women with candidiasis often experience pain when urinating, a thick white discharge, and vaginal and vulval irritation. Yeast cultures from the affected area are used to make the diagnosis, and local antifungal medications are used for treatment.

9.1.5.8. Trichomoniasis

Sexual contact is not the only way that the flagellate protozoan *Trichomonas vaginalis* infections are transmitted. In men, the illness typically manifests as asymptomatic. Trichomonas can cause a range of symptoms in females, such as vaginal discharge, genital irritation, and pain during urination or sexual activity. Complications like cystitis and arthritis are possible for both sexes; men may also get prostatitis and epididymitis. Standard treatment involves the use of metronidazole, an antibacterial and antiprotozoal agent (Makar & Toth, 2002; Cousineau & Domar, 2007; Parasar et al., 2017).

9.1.6. Endometriosis

Endometriosis, pronounced "en-doe-me-tree-O-sis," is a frequently painful condition in which tissue resembling the uterus's inner lining grows outside of it. It frequently affects the tissue lining the pelvis, uterine tubes, and ovaries. Endometriosis growths can sporadically be discovered outside of the pelvic organ region.

With every menstrual cycle, endometriosis tissue undergoes the same thinning, disintegration, and bleeding as the uterine lining. However, it remains within the body and grows in unwanted areas. Endometriomas, or cysts, can develop in the ovaries because of endometriosis. Damage to the surrounding tissue may result in the formation of scar tissue. Adhesions, which are bands of fibrous tissue, can also develop. These may result in pelvic organs and tissues adhering to one another. Pain can be a symptom of endometriosis, particularly during the menstrual cycle. Issues related to fertility may also arise. However, there are treatments that can help you manage the illness and its aftereffects.

9.1.6.1. Symptoms

Pelvic pain is the primary symptom of endometriosis. It's frequently connected to the menstrual cycle. While many people experience cramps during their periods, endometriosis patients frequently report experiencing much worse menstrual pain than usual. Additionally, the pain might get worse with time.

Common symptoms of endometriosis include:

1. **Painful Periods:** Pelvic pain and cramping may start before a menstrual period and last for days into it. You also may have lower back and stomach pain. Another name for painful periods is dysmenorrhea.
2. **Pain with Sex:** Pain during or after sex is common with endometriosis.
3. **Pain with Bowel Movements or Urination:** You're most likely to have these symptoms before or during a menstrual period.
4. **Excessive Bleeding:** Sometimes, you may have heavy menstrual periods or bleeding between periods.
5. **Infertility:** For some people, endometriosis is first found during tests for infertility treatment.
6. **Other Symptoms:** You may have fatigue, diarrhea, constipation, bloating or nausea. These symptoms are more common before or during menstrual periods.

Your pain level might not be a good indicator of the quantity or size of endometriosis growth in your body. There could be a tiny bit of tissue that hurts a lot. Or you might have little to no pain and a large amount of endometriosis tissue. However, some endometriosis sufferers do not exhibit any symptoms. They frequently learn they have the illness when they are unable to conceive or after undergoing surgery for some other reason.

When a person has symptoms, endometriosis can occasionally appear to be another illness that can cause pelvic pain. These include ovarian cysts and pelvic inflammatory diseases. Alternatively, it might be mistaken for IBS, which is characterized by episodes of diarrhea, constipation, and cramping in the stomach. IBS can also occur in conjunction with endometriosis. This makes determining the precise cause of your symptoms more difficult for your medical team.

9.1.6.2. When to See a Doctor

See a member of your healthcare team if you think you might have symptoms of endometriosis. Endometriosis can be a challenge to manage. You may be better able to take charge of the symptoms if:

- Your care team finds the disease sooner rather than later.
- You learn as much as you can about endometriosis.
- You get treatment from a team of healthcare professionals from different medical fields if needed.

9.1.6.3. Causes

The exact cause of endometriosis isn't clear. But some possible causes include:

1. **Retrograde Menstruation:** This is when menstrual blood flows back through the uterine tubes and into the pelvic cavity instead of out of the body. The blood contains endometrial cells from the inner lining of the uterus. These cells may stick to the pelvic walls and surfaces of pelvic organs. There, they might grow and continue to thicken and bleed throughout each menstrual cycle.
2. **Transformed Peritoneal Cells:** Experts suggest that hormones or immune factors might help transform cells that line the inner side of the abdomen, called peritoneal cells, into cells that are like those that line the inside of the uterus.
3. **Embryonic Cell Changes:** Hormones such as estrogen may transform embryonic cells — cells in the earliest stages of development — into endometrial-like cell growths during puberty.
4. **Surgical Scar Complication:** Endometrial cells may attach to scar tissue from a cut made during surgery to the stomach area, such as a C-section.
5. **Endometrial Cell Transport:** The blood vessels or tissue fluid system may move endometrial cells to other parts of the body.
6. **Immune System Condition:** A problem with the immune system may make the body unable to recognize and destroy endometriosis tissue.

9.1.6.4. Risk Factors

Factors that raise the risk of endometriosis include:

- Never giving birth.
- Starting your period at an early age.
- Going through menopause at an older age.

- Short menstrual cycles — for instance, less than 27 days.
- Heavy menstrual periods that last longer than seven days.
- Having higher levels of estrogen in your body or a greater lifetime exposure to estrogen your body produces.
- Low body mass index.
- One or more relatives with endometriosis, such as a mother, aunt, or sister.

An additional risk factor for endometriosis is any medical condition that stops blood from leaving the body during menstruation. Reproductive tract ailments may also qualify. Symptoms of endometriosis frequently appear years after the onset of menstruation. During pregnancy, the symptoms might temporarily get better. Menopause-related pain may gradually lessen if you don't take estrogen therapy.

9.1.6.5. Complications

The main complication of endometriosis is trouble getting pregnant, also called infertility. Up to half of people with endometriosis have a hard time conceiving.

9.1.6.5.1. Infertility

An ovary must release an egg for pregnancy to occur. After that, the egg must pass through the uterine tube so that a sperm cell can fertilize it. For the fertilized egg to begin developing, it must next adhere to the uterine wall. The tube may become blocked by endometriosis, preventing the union of the egg and sperm. However, the illness also appears to have indirect effects on fertility. For example, it might harm the egg or sperm (Figure 9.2).

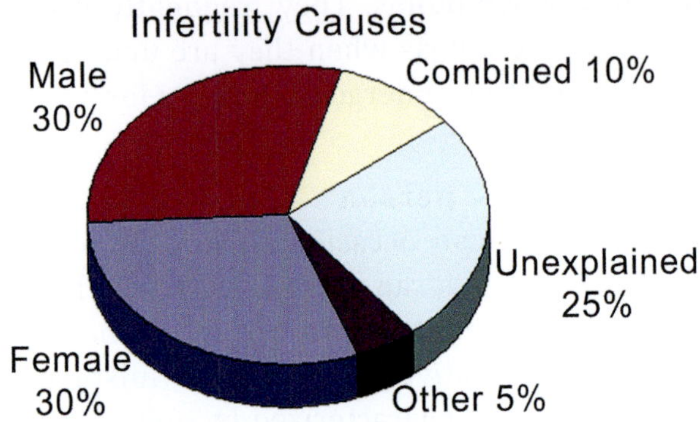

Figure 9.2. *Infertility.*

Source: By Mikael Häggström. When using this image in external works, it may be cited as Häggström, Mikael (2014). "Medical gallery of Mikael Häggström 2014." Wiki Journal of Medicine, 1(2). doi: 10.15347/wjm/2014.008. ISSN 2002-4436. Public Domain or By Mikael Häggström, used with permission. Own work, Public Domain, https://commons.wikimedia.org/w/index.php?curid=11060402.

Many people with mild to moderate endometriosis can still become pregnant and bring their child to term, despite this. Sometimes medical professionals tell people who have endometriosis not to put off having children. This is because the illness could get worse over time.

9.1.6.5.2. Cancer

Endometriosis may increase the risk of ovarian cancer, according to certain studies. However, there is initially a low lifetime risk of ovarian cancer. And in those who have endometriosis, it remains relatively low. Endometriosis-associated adenocarcinoma is an uncommon but potentially fatal cancer that can develop later in life in endometriosis patients (Makar & Toth, 2002; Cousineau & Domar, 2007; Parasar et al., 2017).

9.2. Diagnosis and Treatment Options for Reproductive Disorders

Reproductive disorders have different diagnoses and treatment options based on the condition and underlying causes. You will study general methods for diagnosing and treating a variety of disorders related to reproduction that impact both men and women.

Reproductive disorders require a comprehensive approach that is customized to each patient's unique needs and specific condition. A thorough medical history and physical examination are usually performed to evaluate symptoms and possible risk factors before making a diagnosis. Laboratory tests offer important diagnostic information. Examples of these tests include blood tests to measure hormone levels and semen analysis to determine male fertility. Imaging tests, such as CT, MRI, or ultrasound scans, can be used to see reproductive organs and spot tumors or structural abnormalities. Endoscopic techniques, like hysteroscopy or laparoscopy, can sometimes be used to directly view and biopsy the reproductive organs, which can help diagnose diseases like endometriosis or uterine fibroids. Furthermore, genetic testing might be advised when there is a possibility that a person has genetic abnormalities linked to reproductive disorders, such as chromosomal abnormalities that result in infertility or genetic mutations that make a person more susceptible to developing a particular type of cancer.

Treatment choices are chosen after a diagnosis has been made, considering the patient's preferences and reproductive objectives in addition to the underlying cause of the reproductive disorder. Medication is essential for treating infections linked to reproductive disorders as well as for controlling symptoms and hormone levels. For example, antibiotics are prescribed to treat sexually transmitted infections (STIs), while hormonal contraceptives are frequently used to manage symptoms of conditions like endometriosis or polycystic ovary syndrome (PCOS). Surgical interventions might be required to treat conditions that don't improve with medication, remove tumors or cysts, or fix structural abnormalities. Less invasive alternatives to traditional open surgery are available, such as robotic-assisted fibroids removal or laparoscopic excision of endometriosis, which also reduce postoperative discomfort and recovery time.

More involved treatments like testicular or hysterectomy may be advised in cases of severe or refractory disease. For single people and couples who are having trouble becoming pregnant, assisted reproductive technologies (ART) offer options. When natural conception is impossible, procedures like intrauterine insemination (IUI), intracytoplasmic sperm injection (ICSI), and *in vitro* fertilization (IVF) provide hope for pregnancy. Aside from diet and exercise changes, stress reduction and other lifestyle adjustments may also be important for maximizing fertility and enhancing general reproductive health.

To give individuals and couples the emotional support and direction they need to deal with the difficulties of living with a reproductive disorder, counseling, and support services are crucial parts of treatment. Healthcare professionals can assist individuals and couples in navigating the complexities of reproductive disorders and achieving their reproductive goals by combining medical interventions, surgical techniques, lifestyle modifications, and supportive care (Makar & Toth, 2002; Cousineau & Domar, 2007; Parasar et al., 2017).

9.2.1. Male Infertility: Causes, Diagnosis, and Treatment Options

The reasons behind male infertility, its diagnosis, and available treatments. Many couples who are trying to conceive are affected by the difficult problem of infertility. Though it's common to associate infertility with women, male infertility is also a significant factor to consider. Knowing the reasons behind infertility, getting a correct diagnosis, and considering your options for treatment are essential if you and your partner are having trouble getting pregnant.

9.2.1.1. Causes of Male Infertility

Male infertility can result from various factors that affect sperm production or delivery. Some common causes include:

1. **Low Sperm Count:** A low number of sperm present in the semen.
2. **Abnormal Sperm Shape or Movement:** Sperm with abnormal shape or impaired movement may have difficulty reaching and fertilizing the egg.
3. **Genetic Abnormalities:** Certain genetic conditions or chromosomal abnormalities can impact sperm production or function.
4. **Hormonal Imbalances:** Hormonal imbalances can disrupt the production of sperm.
5. **Testicular Damage:** Injury or damage to the testicles can affect sperm production.
6. **Varicocele:** Enlarged veins within the scrotum can interfere with sperm production.

9.2.1.2. Diagnosis of Male Infertility

If you suspect male infertility, it's essential to consult a urologist who specializes in reproductive medicine. The diagnostic process may involve the following:

1. **Medical History:** The doctor will review your medical history, including any previous reproductive health issues, surgeries, or exposures that may have contributed to infertility.
2. **Semen Analysis:** A semen sample will be analyzed to assess sperm count, motility, and morphology.
3. **Hormonal Testing:** Blood tests may be conducted to evaluate hormone levels that play a role in sperm production.
4. **Genetic Testing:** Genetic tests may be performed to identify any genetic abnormalities that could affect fertility.
5. **Imaging Studies:** Imaging techniques, such as ultrasound or testicular biopsy, may be used to examine the reproductive organs for any structural abnormalities.

9.2.2. Treatment Options for Male Infertility

The treatment for male infertility depends on the underlying cause and may include:

1. **Lifestyle Modifications:** Adopting a healthy lifestyle, including regular exercise, a balanced diet, and avoiding smoking or excessive alcohol consumption, can improve sperm quality.
2. **Medications:** Certain medications can help address hormonal imbalances or other specific issues affecting sperm production.

3. **Surgical Interventions:** Surgical procedures can correct anatomical abnormalities, such as varicoceles or blockages in the reproductive tract.

4. **Assisted Reproductive Techniques:** In cases where other treatments are ineffective, assisted reproductive techniques, such as *in vitro* fertilization (IVF) or intracytoplasmic sperm injection (ICSI), may be recommended (Makar & Toth, 2002; Cousineau & Domar, 2007; Parasar et al., 2017).

A Closer Look

Irritable Bowel Syndrome (IBS)

The large intestine is affected by the common condition known as irritable bowel syndrome (IBS). A range of symptoms, such as cramps, bloating, gas, diarrhea, constipation, and abdominal pain, are indicative of the condition. The intensity and duration of these symptoms can vary, frequently waxing and waning over time.

Although the precise cause of IBS is unknown, many factors are thought to be involved, such as stress, heightened sensitivity to specific foods, aberrant nervous system activity that controls digestive processes, and abnormal muscle contractions in the intestines.

The presence of distinctive symptoms and the lack of underlying anatomical or biochemical abnormalities in the digestive system are used to diagnose irritable bowel syndrome (IBS). Although there isn't a cure for IBS, management techniques aim to enhance quality of life and reduce symptoms. This could involve altering one's diet, practicing stress reduction, taking drugs to treat symptoms like constipation or diarrhea, and changing one's way of living. IBS can be difficult to live with and may need constant care and assistance. However, many IBS sufferers can successfully manage their symptoms and lead normal, active lives with the correct mix of treatments and lifestyle modifications. Maintaining good communication with medical professionals is critical to controlling IBS symptoms and enhancing general health (Makar & Toth, 2002; Cousineau & Domar, 2007; Parasar et al., 2017).

Summary

- Reproductive disorders and diseases encompass a wide range of conditions that affect the reproductive system, which includes organs such as the ovaries, uterus, fallopian tubes, testes, and prostate gland.
- Common disorders affecting the male and female reproductive systems can significantly impact individuals' health and fertility, necessitating awareness, diagnosis, and treatment.
- Infertility is the inability of an animal or plant to reproduce by natural means. It is usually not the natural state of a healthy adult, except notably among certain eusocial species (mostly haplodiploid insects).
- Abnormalities of menstrual function include painful menstruation, or dysmenorrhea; excessive blood loss during each menstrual cycle, known as menorrhagia; irregular bleeding, or metrorrhagia; absence of menstruation, called amenorrhea; and dysfunctional uterine bleeding.
- Diagnosis and treatment options for reproductive disorders vary depending on the specific condition and its underlying causes. You will explore general approaches to diagnosis and treatment across a range of reproductive disorders affecting both men and women.

References

1. Bulletti, C., Coccia, M. E., Battistoni, S., & Borini, A. (2010). Endometriosis and infertility. *Journal of Assisted Reproduction and Genetics, 27*(8), 441–447. https://doi.org/10.1007/s10815-010-9445-1.
2. Cousineau, T. M., & Domar, A. D. (2007). The psychological impact of infertility. *Best Practice & Research. Clinical Obstetrics & Gynecology, 21*(2), 293–308. https://doi.org/10.1016/j.bpobgyn.2006.12.003.
3. Jangir, R. N., & Jain, G. C. (2014). Diabetes mellitus induced impairment of male reproductive functions: A review. *Current Diabetes Reviews, 10*(3), 147–157. https://doi.org/10.2174/1573399810666140421103317.
4. Makar, R. S., & Toth, T. L. (2002). The evaluation of infertility. *American Journal of Clinical Pathology, 117*(Suppl), S95–S103. https://doi.org/10.1309/YX2C-PEX3-MKYM-AYKM.
5. Nnoaham, K. E., Hummelshoj, L., Webster, P., d'Hooghe, T., de Cicco Nardone, F., de Cicco Nardone, C., et al. (2011). Impact of endometriosis on quality of life and work productivity: A multicenter study across ten countries. *Fertility and Sterility, 96*(2), 366–373.e8. https://doi.org/10.1016/j.fertnstert.2011.05.090.
6. Parasar, P., Ozcan, P., & Terry, K. L. (2017). Endometriosis: Epidemiology, Diagnosis and Clinical Management. *Curr Obstet Gynecol Rep, 6*(1), 34–41. https://doi.org/10.1007/s13669-017-0187-1.
7. Showell, M. G., Mackenzie-Proctor, R., Jordan, V., & Hart, R. J. (2020). Antioxidants for female subfertility. *The Cochrane Database of Systematic Reviews, 8*(11), CD007807. https://doi.org/10.1002/14651858.CD007807.pub4.

1. [illegible] (2019). [illegible] 22(1), 141–145. https://doi.org/10.1007/[illegible]
2. [illegible] (2016). [illegible] of infertility. [illegible]

6. [illegible]

Chapter

REPRODUCTIVE HEALTH AND ETHICS

10

Contents

Unit Introduction

The term "reproductive health" refers to a broad spectrum of conditions in the reproductive system, such as STIs, pregnancy, delivery, fertility, and contraception. To make educated decisions about their reproductive lives, people must have access to comprehensive reproductive healthcare services. These services ought to cover STI treatment, safe and legal abortion, prenatal care, and access to contraception. Education about reproductive health is also essential because it gives people the power to make decisions that are consistent with their preferences and values.

Reproductive health is heavily influenced by ethical issues because choices about pregnancy, abortion, and contraception frequently involve difficult moral and philosophical conundrums. Autonomy, which emphasizes people's right to make decisions about their own bodies and reproductive lives, is one of the fundamental ethical concepts in reproductive health. To respect autonomy, people must have access to reliable information, tools, and assistance so they can make educated decisions regarding contraception, getting pregnant, and giving birth.

Beneficence is a key ethical concept in reproductive health that highlights the duty to advance the welfare of both individuals and communities. This idea emphasizes how crucial it is to give people access to safe, efficient, and culturally appropriate reproductive healthcare services. Healthcare professionals must put their patient's health and well-being first and make sure they receive excellent treatment that respects their autonomy and dignity.

Justice and fairness are two more considerations in reproductive health ethics, in addition to autonomy and beneficence. Equitable access to reproductive healthcare services is necessary to guarantee that people of all socioeconomic backgrounds and backgrounds have equal opportunities to receive care. This entails tackling obstacles that disproportionately impact marginalized communities, such as expense, location, and discrimination.

One of the most morally divisive topics in reproductive health is abortion. Abortion rights advocates contend that people should have the autonomy to make decisions regarding their bodies, including whether to end a pregnancy. They stress that to safeguard women's autonomy and health, access to safe and legal abortion services must be guaranteed. On the other hand, opponents of abortion rights frequently claim that human life begins at conception and should be preserved from the time of fertilization. They base their arguments on moral or religious grounds.

In the end, negotiating the complex ethical issues surrounding reproductive health necessitates carefully weighing opposing beliefs and viewpoints. To advance reproductive health outcomes based on the values of autonomy, beneficence, justice, and respect for human dignity, healthcare professionals, legislators, and individuals must have courteous and open discussions. We can work toward a society where everyone has access to reproductive healthcare services, they need to make educated decisions about their reproductive lives by placing a high priority on the autonomy and well-being of individuals (Benyamini & Todorova, 2017; Değer, 2023).

Orientation and Directional Terms:

Terms	Definition	Illustration
Progesterone	Progesterone is a hormone that plays an important role in your reproductive system.	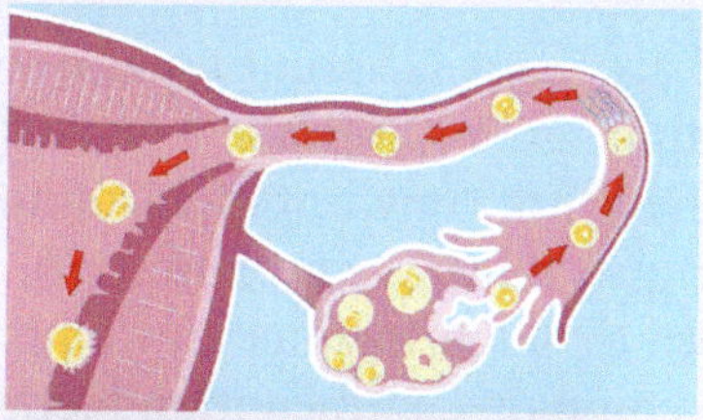
Ejaculation	Ejaculation is the discharge of semen through the urethra in men. It is normally linked with orgasm, which involves involuntary contractions of the pelvic floor.	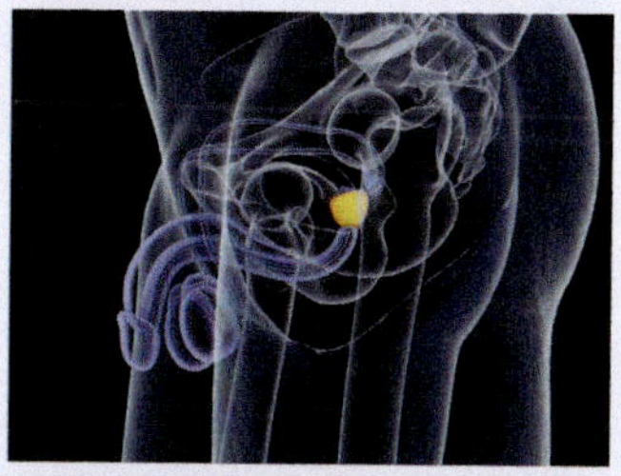
Reproductive health	Reproductive health refers to the condition of male and female reproductive systems during all life stages.	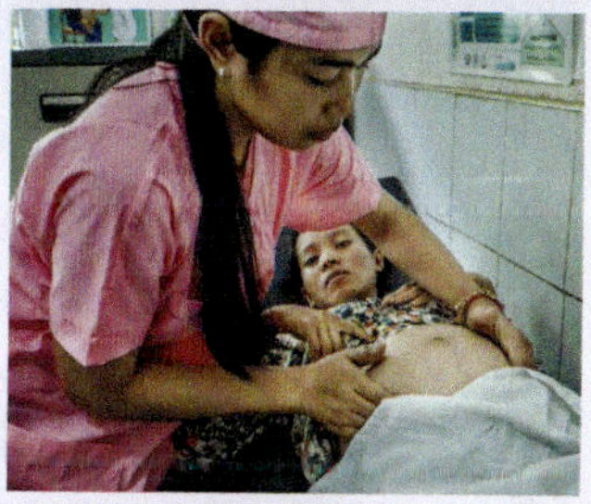
sexual orientation	Sexual orientation is usually divided into these categories: Heterosexual: Attracted to people of the opposite gender	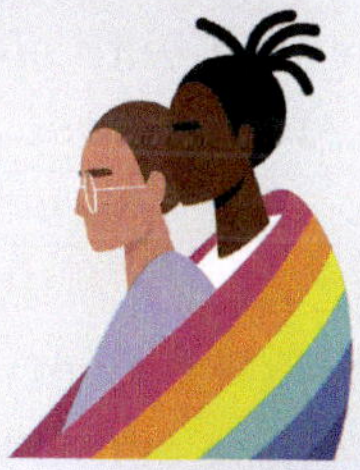
Surrogacy	Surrogacy is an arrangement in which a woman (the surrogate) agrees to carry and give birth to a child on behalf of another person or couple (the intended parent/s).	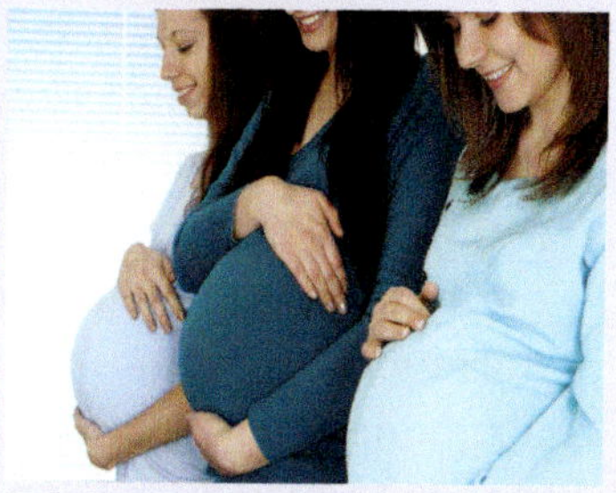

10.1. Contraception Methods and Their Mechanisms of Action

There are many different types of contraception available, giving people a variety of choices for avoiding unwanted pregnancies. Each technique inhibits implantation, fertilization, or both through various mechanisms of action. Some common contraception methods and their mechanisms are discussed in subsections.

10.1.1. Barrier Methods

1. **Condoms:** Both male and female condoms act as physical barriers, preventing sperm from reaching the egg. Male condoms also protect against sexually transmitted infections (STIs) by blocking the transmission of infectious agents.
2. **Diaphragm/Cervical Cap:** These devices are inserted into the vagina to cover the cervix, blocking sperm from entering the uterus. They are often used with spermicide to enhance effectiveness.

10.1.2. Hormonal Methods

1. **Combined Oral Contraceptives (COCs):** These contain synthetic versions of estrogen and progesterone, which prevent ovulation (the release of an egg from the ovary) by suppressing the release of follicle-stimulating hormone (FSH) and luteinizing hormone (LH) from the pituitary gland. They also thicken cervical mucus, making it difficult for sperm to reach the egg, and thin the uterine lining, reducing the likelihood of implantation.
2. **Progestin-Only Pills (Mini Pills):** These pills primarily work by thickening cervical mucus, making it more difficult for sperm to enter the uterus. They may also suppress ovulation in some women.
3. **Contraceptive Patch:** The patch contains estrogen and progestin hormones, which are absorbed through the skin and work similarly to COCs to prevent ovulation, thicken cervical mucus, and thin the uterine lining.
4. **Contraceptive Implant:** A small, flexible rod containing progestin is inserted under the skin of the upper arm. It works primarily by inhibiting ovulation and thickening cervical mucus.
5. **Contraceptive Injection (Depo-Provera):** This injection contains a progestin hormone that prevents ovulation, thickens cervical mucus, and thins the uterine lining. It provides contraception for up to three months per injection.
6. **Intrauterine Devices (IUDs):** Hormonal IUDs release progestin locally in the uterus, where they thicken cervical mucus, inhibit sperm motility, and thin the uterine lining. Some hormonal IUDs may also suppress ovulation to varying degrees.

10.1.3. Non-Hormonal Methods

1. **Copper Intrauterine Device (Cu-IUD):** The copper in the IUD creates an inhospitable environment for sperm, inhibiting their motility and viability. It may also prevent fertilization by altering the uterine

lining, making it less receptive to implantation.

2. **Fertility Awareness Methods:** These methods involve tracking changes in a woman's menstrual cycle to identify fertile days and abstain from intercourse during ovulation.

3. **Withdrawal Method:** Also known as "pulling out," this method involves the man withdrawing his penis from the vagina before ejaculation to prevent sperm from entering the woman's reproductive tract.

Every form of contraception has advantages and disadvantages of its own, and people should speak with medical professionals to choose the best one for them based on their lifestyle, preferences, and medical history.

10.1.4. Practice Essentials

A patient's choice of contraceptive method involves factors such as efficacy, safety, noncontraceptive benefits, cost, and personal considerations.

1. **Periodic Abstinence:** Contraceptive techniques based on periodic abstinence include the following:
   - Coitus interruptus;
   - Lactational amenorrhea;
   - Natural family planning.

2. **Mechanical Barriers:** These contraceptives include the following:
   - i. **Male Condom:** One of the most popular mechanical barriers and, among all the barrier methods, the one that provides the most effective protection of the genital tract from sexually transmitted diseases (STDs).
   - ii. **Female Condom:** Prevents pregnancy by acting as a barrier to the passage of semen into the vagina.
   - iii. **Diaphragm:** Prevents pregnancy by acting as a barrier to the passage of semen into the cervix.
   - iv. **Cervical Cap:** Acts as a mechanical barrier to sperm migration into the cervical canal.
   - v. **Spermicidal Agent:** Prevents sperm from entering the cervical OS by attacking the sperm's flagella and body, reducing their mobility, and disrupting their fructolytic activity, thereby inhibiting their nourishment.

3. **Hormonal Contraceptives:** Hormonal means of contraception include the following:
   - i. **Implants:** The mechanism of action is a combination of suppression of the luteinizing hormone (LH) surge, suppression of ovulation, development of viscous and scant cervical mucus to deter sperm penetration, and prevention of endometrial growth and development.
   - ii. **Injectable Depomedroxyprogesterone Acetate:** Acts by inhibiting ovulation with the suppression of follicle-stimulating hormone (FSH) and LH levels and by eliminating the LH surge.
   - iii. **Progestin-Only Oral Contraceptives:** Mechanisms of action include – (a) suppression of ovulation; (b)

a variable dampening effect on the midcycle peaks of LH and FSH; (c) an increase in cervical mucus viscosity; (d) a reduction in the number and size of endometrial glands; and (e) a reduction in cilia motility in the uterine tube.

iv. **Combination Oral Contraceptives:** Prevention of ovulation is considered the dominant mechanism of action, with the combination of the 2 steroids creating a synergistic effect that greatly increases their antigonadotropic and ovulation-inhibitory effects; these contraceptives also alter the consistency of cervical mucus, affect the endometrial lining, and alter tubal transport.

v. **91-Day Combination Oral Contraceptives:** Reduce the number of menstrual cycles per year.

vi. **Combination Patch Contraceptive:** Releases estrogen and progesterone directly into the skin.

vii. **Contraceptive Vaginal Ring:** Hormones are absorbed directly by the reproductive organs.

4. **Intrauterine Devices (IUDs):** These include the following:

   i. **Copper T380:** T-shaped, polyethylene IUD with fine copper wire wrapped around the vertical stem.

   ii. **Liletta, Mirena:** T-shaped, polyethylene IUD with a reservoir that contains 52 mg of levonorgestrel, a progesterone.

   iii. **Kyleena:** T-shaped, polyethylene IUD with a reservoir that contains 19.5 mg levonorgestrel.

5. Permanent Contraception:

i. **Female Permanent Contraception:** The mechanism of female permanent contraception involves blocking the uterine tubes to prevent conception. It can be surgically done during the interval period or in the postpartum phase using a tiny transverse infraumbilical incision. During the interim, laparoscopy, laparotomy, or colpotomy can be used for sterilization. Uterine tube sterilization techniques include suture ligation with partial or complete salpingectomy, segmental destruction with electrocoagulation, and occlusion with Falope rings, clips, or bands.

The Essure system can be used while the patient is under local anesthesia and does not require any surgical incisions. A microinsert is inserted straight into the uterine tubes using a hysteroscopy. For more details, refer to the description provided below by the US Food and Drug Administration (FDA). On December 31, 2018, Bayer ceased to sell this device in the United States.

ii. **Vasectomy:** Vasectomy involves incision of the scrotal sac, transection of the vas deferens, and occlusion of both severed ends by suture ligation and fulguration.

6. **Emergency Postcoital Contraception:** A variety of emergency contraception methods have been described, including the following:
   - Emergency contraceptive pills (ECP) (e.g., Plan B One-Step OTC, an enteric-coated levonorgestrel ECP that dissolves and is absorbed in the intestine), ovulation inhibition effective until the LH surge.
   - Ulipristal acetate (e.g., Ella), available by prescription, progesterone-receptor modulator effective in ovulation inhibition through the LH surge.
   - Copper T380 IUD, foreign body effect creates toxic milieu preventing implantation, not effective for emergency contraception after implantation has occurred.
   - Progesterone agonist/ antagonist (Benyamini & Todorova, 2017; Değer, 2023).

10.2. Ethical Considerations in Reproductive Medicine

Reproductive medicine involves complex decisions that affect individuals, families, and society at large, making ethical considerations crucial. These factors cover a wide range of topics, such as justice, autonomy, beneficence, and respect for human dignity.

Here are some key ethical considerations in reproductive medicine:

1. **Autonomy:** Respect for autonomy is a foundational principle in reproductive medicine, emphasizing individuals' right to make decisions about their own bodies and reproductive lives. Healthcare providers must ensure that patients have access to accurate information, resources, and support to make informed choices about contraception, fertility treatment, pregnancy, and childbirth.
2. **Informed Consent:** Informed consent is essential in reproductive medicine, requiring healthcare providers to fully disclose relevant information about the risks, benefits, and alternatives of medical interventions. Patients must be able to understand this information and voluntarily consent to or refuse treatment without coercion or undue influence.
3. **Reproductive Rights:** Reproductive rights encompass the right to access comprehensive reproductive healthcare services, including contraception, fertility treatment, prenatal care, safe and legal abortion, and maternal healthcare. These rights are essential for ensuring individuals' ability to control their reproductive lives and make choices that align with their values and preferences.
4. **Beneficence:** The principle of beneficence emphasizes the obligation to promote the well-being of individuals and communities. Healthcare providers must prioritize patients' health and safety, providing high-quality care that respects their dignity and autonomy. This includes addressing the physical, emotional, and social aspects of reproductive health.

5. **Justice:** This involves the fair and equitable distribution of resources and opportunities. In reproductive medicine, justice requires addressing disparities in access to healthcare services, such as disparities based on socioeconomic status, geographic location, race, ethnicity, gender identity, or sexual orientation. Efforts to promote reproductive justice seek to ensure that all individuals have equal opportunities to access reproductive healthcare and make decisions about their reproductive lives.
6. **Respect for Human Dignity:** Respect for human dignity underscores the inherent value and worth of every individual. Healthcare providers must treat patients with respect, compassion, and empathy, acknowledging their unique experiences, values, and cultural backgrounds. This includes respecting patients' privacy, confidentiality, and confidentiality, and ensuring that their autonomy and rights are upheld throughout the reproductive healthcare journey.
7. **Ethical Challenges:** Reproductive medicine presents numerous ethical challenges, including those related to assisted reproductive technologies (ART), such as *in vitro* fertilization (IVF), surrogacy, and preimplantation genetic diagnosis (PGD). These technologies raise complex questions about the creation, selection, and disposition of embryos, as well as concerns about the commodification of reproductive tissues and the welfare of egg donors, sperm donors, and surrogates.

It takes careful thought, honest communication, and cooperation between stakeholders, legislators, ethicists, and healthcare professionals to navigate these ethical issues. We can endeavor to promote reproductive health outcomes that prioritize the rights and well-being of individuals and families by respecting the principles of autonomy, beneficence, justice, and respect for human dignity.

10.2.1. Assisted Reproductive Technologies

When conventional methods fail to produce a child, Assisted Reproductive Technologies (ART) refer to a range of medical procedures intended to help with conception. For individuals and couples struggling with infertility or other reproductive issues, these technologies provide hope.

Here are some common types of ART and their basic principles:

1. ***In Vitro* Fertilization (IVF):**
   - IVF involves fertilizing an egg with sperm outside the body, typically in a laboratory dish, to create an embryo.
   - The process begins with ovarian stimulation to produce multiple eggs, which are then retrieved through a minor surgical procedure called follicle aspiration.
   - The retrieved eggs are fertilized with sperm in the laboratory, and the resulting embryos are cultured for several days.
   - Finally, one or more embryos are transferred into the uterus to establish a pregnancy, while

any remaining embryos may be cryopreserved (frozen) for future use.

2. Intracytoplasmic Sperm Injection (ICSI):
   - ICSI is a specialized form of IVF used in cases of male infertility or low sperm count.
   - In this procedure, a single sperm is directly injected into an egg using a fine needle, bypassing natural fertilization.
   - ICSI can help overcome barriers to fertilization by ensuring that sperm successfully penetrates the egg.
3. Frozen Embryo Transfer (FET):
   - FET involves transferring cryopreserved embryos into the uterus during a natural or medicated cycle.
   - This allows couples to use embryos created during a previous IVF cycle, offering an additional chance at pregnancy without the need for ovarian stimulation or egg retrieval.
4. Donor Gametes (Egg or Sperm Donation):
   - Egg or sperm donation may be used when one or both partners are unable to produce viable gametes.
   - Donor eggs or sperm are fertilized with the recipient's partner's gametes through IVF or ICSI, and resulting embryos are transferred into the recipient's uterus.
   - This allows individuals or couples to achieve pregnancy using donor gametes while experiencing the pregnancy and childbirth process themselves.

• 5. Surrogacy:
   - Surrogacy involves a third-party woman (the surrogate) carrying and delivering a baby for the intended parents.
   - In gestational surrogacy, embryos created through IVF using the intended parents' or donor's gametes are transferred into the surrogate's uterus.
   - Traditional surrogacy involves the surrogate using her eggs, which are fertilized with the intended father's sperm or donor sperm through artificial insemination.

• 6. Preimplantation Genetic Testing (PGT):
   - PGT involves screening embryos for genetic abnormalities or chromosomal disorders before transfer.
   - This can help identify embryos with the highest likelihood of implantation and reduce the risk of miscarriage or genetic conditions in offspring.

Couples and individuals battling infertility can now start or grow their families with the help of assisted reproductive technologies (ART). However, it also brings up moral, legal, and societal issues, such as worries about the well-being and health of surrogates, donors, and their children, as well as problems with accessibility, cost, and fair resource distribution (Benyamini & Todorova, 2017; Değer, 2023).

10.2.2. Surrogacy

Surrogacy is a type of adoption arrangement in which a woman consents to give birth on behalf of another person or people who will raise the child after it is born. This arrangement is frequently backed by a legal contract. For many reasons, including infertility, pregnancy risks or unfavorable aspects, or medical impossibilities, people seek surrogacy.

The gestational carriers are typically referred to as surrogate mothers, even though a surrogacy relationship or legal agreement includes the gestational carrier and the child's parent(s) after birth. In a surrogacy procedure, a woman serves as a surrogate mother by carrying and giving birth to a child on behalf of another person. Usually, matchmakers or other third-party agencies introduce surrogate moms to parent(s) in need of surrogacy. Whether through traditional or IVF methods, they are typically obliged to take part in the processes of insemination, pregnancy, delivery, and early newborn feeding.

Surrogacy arrangements can involve monetary compensation, known as commercial surrogacy, or may not involve payments. The legality and costs of surrogacy vary widely between jurisdictions, leading to fertility tourism and potential issues with international or interstate surrogacy agreements. *For example*, individuals in countries where surrogacy is prohibited may travel to places where it is permitted. In some countries, surrogacy is legal only if there is no financial gain involved. In jurisdictions where commercial surrogacy is allowed, third-party agencies can assist in finding a surrogate and drafting a surrogacy contract. These agencies often coordinate medical tests to ensure a healthy pregnancy and delivery, as well as help with legal matters related to the intended parents and the surrogate.

10.2.2.1. Methods

The two types of surrogacies—gestational and traditional—are determined by the genetic heritage of the egg. Compared to traditional surrogacy, gestational surrogacy is more common and is thought to be less complicated legally.

10.2.2.1.1. Traditional Surrogacy

Classic surrogacy, also called partial, natural, or straight surrogacy, involves the surrogate's egg being fertilized by either the intended father's or a donor's sperm. The surrogate can be inseminated through sexual intercourse (natural insemination) or artificial insemination. If a donor's sperm is used, the resulting child is not genetically related to the intended parent(s). However, if the intended father's sperm is used, the child is genetically related to both him and the surrogate.

Some decide to spread in secret without a doctor's or physician's help. In certain legal systems, intended parents who use donor sperm must go through an adoption procedure to be granted legal parental rights over the offspring. Numerous fertility clinics that offer surrogacy also help the parties with the legal procedure.

10.2.2.1.2. Gestational Surrogacy

Gestational surrogacy, also known as host or full surrogacy, was successfully accomplished in April 1986. This process involves implanting an embryo created using *in vitro* fertilization (IVF) technology into a surrogate, commonly referred to as a gestational carrier.

Gestational surrogacy has several forms, and in each form, the resulting child is genetically unrelated to the surrogate:

- The embryo is created using the intended father's sperm and the intended mother's eggs.

- The embryo is created using the intended father's sperm and a donor egg.
- The embryo is created using the intended mother's egg and donor sperm.
- A donor embryo is transferred to a surrogate. Such an embryo may be available when others undergoing IVF have embryos left over, which they donate to others. The resulting child is genetically unrelated to the intended parent(s) (Benyamini & Todorova, 2017; Değer, 2023).

10.2.3. Abortion

With implications for medicine, law, ethics, and society, abortion is a complicated and divisive subject. When a pregnancy is purposefully ended before the fetus can survive outside the womb, it is referred to as a miscarriage or intentionally terminated through induced procedures.

Here are some key points to consider when discussing abortion:

1. **Legal Status:** The legality of abortion varies widely around the world, with some countries permitting abortion on request under certain circumstances, while others have strict restrictions or outright bans. In countries where abortion is legal, laws often regulate factors such as gestational age limits, reasons for seeking abortion, and the availability of abortion services.
2. **Medical Procedures:** Induced abortions can be performed using different methods depending on gestational age, medical considerations, and individual preferences. Common procedures include medication abortion (using medication to induce abortion in early pregnancy) and surgical abortion (such as vacuum aspiration or dilation and evacuation).
3. **Reasons for Seeking Abortion:** Women may seek abortion for various reasons, including unintended pregnancy, fetal abnormalities or health concerns, socioeconomic factors, relationship issues, or personal beliefs and values. It is essential to acknowledge and respect the complexity of individual circumstances and decision-making processes involved in abortion.
4. **Health and Safety:** Access to safe and legal abortion services is crucial for protecting women's health and well-being. Restrictive abortion laws can lead to unsafe abortion practices, increasing the risk of maternal morbidity and mortality. Ensuring access to comprehensive reproductive healthcare services, including contraception and abortion, is essential for promoting women's reproductive rights and health.
5. **Ethical Considerations:** Abortion raises complex ethical questions related to personhood, autonomy, bodily integrity, and the moral status of the fetus. Debates often center on conflicting rights and interests, including the right to life, the right to reproductive autonomy, and the societal interest in protecting vulnerable populations. Ethical frameworks may vary depending on

cultural, religious, philosophical, and personal perspectives.

6. **Public Discourse and Policy Debates:** Abortion is a deeply polarizing issue that sparks passionate debates and activism on all sides. Discussions often involve moral, religious, scientific, and political arguments, with stakeholders advocating for diverse policy approaches, including legalizing, restricting, or prohibiting abortion. Public discourse plays a crucial role in shaping laws, policies, and societal attitudes towards abortion.

It is crucial to approach conversations regarding abortion with understanding, kindness, and respect for differing viewpoints because of the complexity of the subject and the real-life experiences of those who are impacted by it. Irrespective of individual convictions, promoting policies that advance reproductive rights and health, encouraging candid communication, and endorsing all three can help tackle the complex issues related to abortion (Benyamini & Todorova, 2017; Değer, 2023).

10.3. Gender and Health Perspective

The term "gender" describes the socially constructed roles, behaviors, characteristics, and activities that are deemed appropriate for men, women, boys, and girls, as well as the relationships between them, in each society at a given time and place. In all societies, gender is a social construct that affects men and women, boys and girls, and their attitudes, roles, and responsibilities. Social relations differ amongst societies. It is a people's issue that is influenced by power dynamics in multicultural societies and pertains to women. It addresses issues of humanity that encompass variety and uniqueness. In both developed and developing countries, it has been the most pervasive kind of discrimination that operates across cultural boundaries. The focus of the analysis of the current gender discourse context is how gender influences the politics of knowledge production. Education possesses the inherent capacity to spark societal transformation concerning gender dynamics.

Apex National Organization curriculum frameworks have taken gender issues in education into consideration. Women are subjected to sex discrimination in education in several ways. First, a lot of education sociologists see the school system as a means of social and cultural reproduction. Through both formal and informal processes, the current patterns of inequality—particularly that related to gender inequality—are perpetuated within schools. Given that children pick up gender cues from their surroundings, it makes sense that a child's early school years are crucial for the formation of ideas about gender identity and may even reinforce negative beliefs about the differences between the roles played by men and women.

The process of empowering women involves developing their potential and enabling them to think and act freely, make their own decisions, and take charge of their lives. This helps to lessen discrimination and exploitation against women. It is the process of advancing women in political, social, and economic spheres to enable them to assume roles in society that are comparable to those of men. However, women have frequently suffered for centuries from having fewer rights and a lower social status than men. In many countries, women make up half or more of the total population. Empowering women is the only way to stop the pervasive discrimination against and exploitation of them.

10.3.1. Sex and Health: The Biology of Risk

When providing healthcare, the distinctions between the reproductive systems of men and women have always been crucial. This illustrates how important it is for women to have access to excellent obstetric and family planning services to reach their full health potential. Despite recent advancements, pregnancy, and childbirth still directly cause the deaths of about 5,00,000 women annually, and they also cause serious disabilities of over 10 times as many. Due to the importance of these issues in women's lives, many have made sexual and reproductive rights a focal point of their campaigns.

In response to the "platform of action" formulated at the 1994 International Population and Development Conference in Cairo, several nations have created new services. Given that women are more susceptible to risks related to reproductive health, it is not surprising that most of these programs have focused on meeting their needs. However, since the HIV/AIDS epidemic has brought attention to the risks of STDs for both partners, men are receiving more attention these days. This has created opportunities for men to be educated to take greater responsibility for their partners' health in addition to helping them to improve their health.

The idea that the biological distinctions between the sexes go beyond reproduction has also gained traction. Differential patterns of morbidity and mortality in males and females are shaped by a multitude of genetic, hormonal, and metabolic factors. Cervical and prostate cancers are two of the most prominent examples of diseases specific to a particular sex. Nonetheless, an increasing body of research indicates that there are gender disparities in the occurrence, manifestations, and outcomes of numerous other medical conditions such as HIV/AIDS, tropical infectious diseases, tuberculosis, autoimmune disorders, and coronary heart disease. Men are more biologically predisposed to heart disease than women, which is one of the most significant of these sex differences.

All these gender differences must be taken into consideration when planning and delivering healthcare if health services are to meet the needs of both men and women. However, many other factors also play a role in determining a person's health, not just biological ones. When assessing whether people can reach their full potential for a long and healthy life, socially constructed gender differences also play a significant role (Benyamini & Todorova, 2017; Değer, 2023).

10.3.2. Hazards of Female Gender

Numerous studies have examined the connection between gender divisions and the health of women, exploring various social, economic, and cultural influences on their physical and mental well-being. The research has primarily concentrated on the persistent gender disparities in relationships between men and women. A recent study revealed that no societies exist where women are treated equally to men, ultimately impacting women's health outcomes.

Women are particularly susceptible to poverty due to differences in wealth and income between genders. This makes it challenging for people in some parts of the world to obtain the essentials for health, particularly during the reproductive years when family needs are at their highest. Due to social norms regarding the allocation of responsibilities, many women—particularly those who combine employment with domestic responsibilities, pregnancy, and childrearing—bear exceptionally heavy workloads. Too many women are abused by other family members, and they frequently receive little support from other women in the home. According to a recent study, rape and domestic abuse account for 19% of the overall disease burden that women in developed nations between the ages of 15 and 44 bear. In most parts of the world, women report anxiety and depression at higher rates than men, but there is no proof that women are inherently more prone to these issues.

Gender inequality may not only have an impact on women's health but also restrict their access to services. Because of prejudice and poverty, millions of women worldwide still lack access to basic medical care. One of the primary accomplishments of the NHS in Britain was the removal of these financial barriers. There is evidence, nevertheless, that certain doctors still view women as less valuable than men. This may result in disparate distribution of clinical resources and demeaning attitudes. In the context of medical research, studies have demonstrated that women have far too frequently been excluded from studies for inappropriate reasons. This gender bias is particularly noticeable in this context.

10.3.3. Male Gender: A Mixed Blessing

In the past, there was minimal focus on how gender influences men's health, but that is starting to change as the connection between masculinity and wellness becomes more apparent. While being male may initially appear to have health benefits due to access to resources, further analysis shows a more intricate situation. Despite variations in masculine norms across different groups, the construction and upkeep of a heterosexual male identity often involve engaging in risky behaviors that can be detrimental to one's health.

The realm of paid work presents the most evident instances of these risks. In most societies, men are more likely to die young from work-related accidents because of their traditional role as providers. Even though the labor force's gender composition is shifting, the riskiest jobs are still performed by men from the poorest communities. In addition to these possible hazards at work, a lot of men also feel pressured to take chances to "prove" their masculinity. Because of this, men are more likely than women to be killed in car accidents, violent sports, or murder. They also tend to smoke and drink more than women do in most societies, which raises their biological susceptibility to early heart disease and related issues. They also appear to want unsafe sex more than women do. Once more, men in the poorest communities are probably more likely to experience many of these risks.

There is also growing interest in the effects of masculinity on mental health. There has been a claim made that many men are unable to reach their full emotional potential because they "grew up male." For example, their desire to be viewed as "hard" could keep them from discovering their compassionate side. Many men may not take health promotion messages seriously or see a doctor when problems arise because they are reluctant to acknowledge weakness. Indeed, because a disease has the potential to reduce men to what one recent study has termed "marginalized masculinity," it may be especially feared in and of itself. Therefore, to get the most out of the health services that are available to them, many men must contend with internal limitations (Benyamini & Todorova, 2017; Değer, 2023).

10.3.4. Putting Sex and Gender on the Healthcare Agenda

The intricate connections between biological sex, social gender, and health have been brought to light by this succinct analysis. It is oversimplified in some ways, as there are significant differences between various groups of men and women and noticeable similarities in the healthcare needs of men and women. This does not negate the significance of issues related to male and female identity, though. More awareness of issues related to sex and gender will be required if health services are to be effective and equitable. It will be necessary for research, service delivery patterns, and broader social and economic policies to take this into account.

When it comes to study designs, sex and gender must always be considered important variables if gender bias in medical research is to be eradicated. In the near run, this would advance equity by bridging the knowledge gaps regarding women's health that currently exist. In the long term, it would benefit men as well by raising the standard of medical science.

Improved childcare and transportation options may be necessary for women to have better access to services. There might be a need to offer more services in the community or at work for men (and many women). It is crucial that men and women are treated with respect in all healthcare settings. For example, discriminatory practices or sexist behavior shouldn't degrade or harm women. On the other hand, men shouldn't be held to traditional ideas of what it means to be a heterosexual man. Clinicians must acknowledge the psychological obstacles that male patients may bring to their medical visits, as well as the potential challenges that illness may pose to their sense of self.

Policies that promote health must consider gender equality if they are to have any impact. Too many campaigns target women in their capacity as caregivers for others, neglecting to prioritize their own needs. Too frequently, men believe that messages about health promotion are only intended for women and that their health is their concern. HIV/AIDS campaigns have simultaneously advised men and women to "use a condom," ignoring the very real power and status disparities that govern most sexual interactions. Campaigns that encourage men and women to take care of each other and themselves must be created if this is to change.

Lastly, since the issues are particularly complicated here, we must consider how broader social and economic policies might advance gender equity in health. On the one hand, developing anti-discriminatory laws will help address the social and economic disparities that still have an impact on women's health. Conversely, modifications to the way social security is provided or the nature of work would facilitate men's development of their "female" selves. Men may find it simpler to balance work and home life if, for example, working hours were more flexible and parental leave was more generously offered. The gender relations of the next generation could also be shaped by carefully planned educational initiatives.

These alterations to public policy may contribute to the advancement of gender parity in healthcare. They would, however, still ignore some of the most important issues. Too many men will continue to suffer from avoidable illnesses and even pass away as long as masculinity is defined in ways that are harmful to their health. Simultaneously, a great deal of women will endure harm due to the behaviors of their masculinity-obsessed male partners. Such changes will not be simple to implement because they will require redefining some of the most private aspects of human existence. Gender inequality, however, will remain one of the things preventing both men and women from reaching their full health potential unless it is addressed (Benyamini & Todorova, 2017; Değer, 2023).

10.3.5. Gender Inequalities in Health, Sexism in Medicine

There is a hierarchy of diseases that favors men over women, with women's diseases often seen as less important due to diffuse symptoms and unclear causes compared to men's diseases which have more visible symptoms and affect vital organs. This can result in women receiving less recognition, compensation, and quality service in countries like Norway despite having national medical insurance systems in place. Disease patterns also differ between men and women, with some diseases affecting one gender at different ages or being more prevalent in women, while others are more serious or unique to women only.

Despite this, women's health requirements are frequently thought to be limited to reproductive needs. The gender bias is evident in the way that women's health is restricted to obstetrics and gynecology in medicine and that maternal and child health programs are expected to address all of the health needs of women in public health. This is because women are not viewed as human beings with health needs, but rather as mothers and wives. Women's non-reproductive health is therefore either ignored or invisible. For example, women's occupational health has frequently been disregarded despite their long history of employment. In addition to being determined by a woman's reproductive role, women's health is frequently misinterpreted due to the persistent belief that women are a homogeneous group. In actuality, social class, race/ethnicity, and other factors all influence how differently women experience health issues, whether or not they are related to reproduction. For example, cervical cancer tends to afflict more poor women than wealthy ones, but breast cancer is more common among older women. According to research, black women are more likely than white women to have hypertension at all income levels. Such a social patterning of disease indicates that biology and/or sex are not sufficient explanations for women's health problems.

What she refers to as socialist feminist epidemiology is the understanding of women's health and illness concerning the patriarchal and capitalist aspects of society. She emphasized the impact of female roles and socialization on women's health when examining the main occupational diseases that affect women. Housewives are found to suffer from depression as a major occupational illness because women are socialized to express their problems through depression. Because husbands assume sexual access and control, women lack the decision-making power to negotiate about sex, childbearing, and contraception when it comes to reproductive health, such as the use of contraceptives and family planning. While a husband may, and frequently does, refuse to use contraceptives despite his persistent demands for sexual relations, women are caught between having sole responsibility for family planning and being expected to be sexual partners. In certain developing nations, sick women still require their husbands' consent to leave the house and seek medical attention. Or, when they do get to the hospital, their husbands' signatures are needed for many medical procedures. Therefore, it is evident that women's health and well-being are supported by gender roles and male-female power dynamics rather than biology (Benyamini & Todorova, 2017; Değer, 2023).

10.3.6. Medical Education and Research: Gaps and Gender Bias

10.3.6.1. Medical Education

The previous narrative demonstrated how medical practice and health services have a pervasive disregard for women and have reduced women's health and illness to biological issues. According to reports, during the first few decades of the 20th century, these ideas were institutionalized in scientific medicine and the emerging field of public health in the United States. Thus, in medical and public health practices, biologically deterministic perspectives on sex and gender differences have since been accepted as normal and essential components of curricula and research agendas. Even though the Hippocratic Oath, with its explicit prohibition against providing women with the means to have an abortion, is arguably out of date and not quite the model to follow, the 35th World Medical Assembly's 1983 amended Declaration of Geneva still addresses colleagues as my brothers.

While the percentage of female applicants to medical schools has increased in the United States from approximately 5% in the mid-1970s to 40% in the 1990s, women's health issues are not addressed in the medical curriculum. Furthermore, it is common for white men to teach lectures and clinical skills about and to white men. Even in the teaching of biological and basic science courses, such as the typical human body and its functions, gender bias is evident. For instance, since women's and men's sexual organs are essentially the same, lectures on male genitalia could take place over the course of three days, but none on women's. Medical textbooks still view men as the standard or point of reference for every subject and view women as the exception to this rule.

The medical curriculum's disdain for women's health is most evident in the way fundamental clinical skills like physical examinations are taught. The head, neck, abdominal regions, and cardiovascular and neuromuscular systems, except for the breast and pelvis, are all examined by medical students. Rather, students are forced to practice on underprivileged patients who are already in pain to acquire these fundamental skills that are essential to women's health care. On the other hand, it has been claimed that students were instructed to perform pelvic exams on surgical patients who were sedated. There are at least two major consequences of these medical education methods that are detrimental to women's health care. Such clinical examination teaching methods for women's breasts and pelvises would undoubtedly not help treat or prevent breast and cervical cancers, which are among the leading causes of death for women according to statistics. The second, more pernicious long-term impact is that medical students' understanding of women's health is now based on the practice of examining a woman who is in pain. Thus, teaching medical students how to perform competent, sensitive, and painless breast and internal examinations for women has not been an essential component of medical teaching practice until very recently, when and where the use of teaching associates is practiced. This explains why, among many other instances of needless suffering that women go through when receiving medical examinations or treatment, women anticipate and feel pain during what should be routine internal examinations.

Women's health electives, which are optional courses that address health issues that specifically affect women, such as osteoporosis, incontinence, heart disease, breast cancer, and menopause, are offered by about 25% of medical schools, according to a survey. It's unclear if these electives on women's health address gender perspectives and gender analysis of health.

Examining the medical curricula of two reputable medical schools taught in Malaysian public universities revealed that efforts have recently been made to counteract the biomedical bias in favor of the patient's integration into the family, community, and society. For example, this is mirrored in the goals of medical school, which are to create qualified physicians who practice medicine holistically and who will be essential members of the medical community. Medical curricula continue to be heavily biomedical despite such integrative innovations, with psycho-social and cultural courses being viewed as soft subjects. Regarding clinical examinations that are essential to women's health, general surgeons teach breast examinations using female patients who have diseases like tumors or abscesses. Previously, groups of 10 students studied each breast examination; currently, only one student studies at a time. During the Obstetrics posting, when students watch and assist with birth deliveries, and during the Gynecology posting, when women patients are put to sleep for surgical procedures, they learn about vaginal examinations. It is said that because of their relative lack of experience with female anatomy, preconceived notions about female sex and sexuality, and patients' reluctance to be examined by trainee students, male medical students find breast and pelvic exams to be particularly challenging. Neither elective nor integrated courses on women's health are offered in the medical curriculum. In courses like Family Health, women are studied as members of the family, particularly as mothers, which perpetuates the stereotype that women's health is only relevant to reproduction. Furthermore, women's reproductive health is still primarily addressed from a biomedical perspective. For example, medical students are emphasized on the biological aspects of the side effects of different forms of contraception. Given the multi-ethnic background of our patients, the latter are exposed to cultural and religious barriers to family planning; however, the underlying issues of male-female power relations affecting sex, sexuality, and contraception are rarely discussed, if at all, in the classroom.

Nonetheless, it is encouraging to see that in some of the other Asia Pacific nations, creative strides have been taken to change the biomedical bias of medical education. For example, through its Department of Community Health Sciences (CHS), Aga Khan University, a private medical college in Pakistan, has introduced gender into the context of primary health care. Medical students learn about topics like "Women and the Environment" and "The Role of Women in Health" during their non-clinical years, while nursing students learn about social issues related to women's health through the Culture, Health, and Society course. To advance reproductive health in the nation and capitalize on various approaches—possibly including non-biomedical and more gender-sensitive ones—to women's health, the CHS recently launched the Pakistan Reproductive Health Network (PRHN), a network of medical and non-medical professionals. The University of the Philippines, Manila (UPM), a public institution in the country, provides creative programs that address the health and social needs of the Filipino populace. To instill social awareness in medical students, its College of Medicine offers the Integrated Liberal Arts-Medicine program, which attempts to give medical students as much exposure to social sciences and humanities as possible. The UPM medical curriculum appears to be less biomedical than some of the more traditional medical education offered in the area, even though it's unclear if social awareness entails gender awareness.

It can generally be stated that the curricula for the education of other health professionals, especially nurses, contain comparatively more courses in social science related to patient care and health behavior. To what extent they are aware of the gender perspective, however, will largely depend on the individual educational institutions and their faculty members.

10.3.6.2. Medical Research

Even though men and women are affected by diseases like heart disease, depression, and AIDS differently, many medical studies on illnesses, treatments, and outcomes—whether expensive or not, short- or long-term—have only used male subjects. It has been suggested that women have been routinely left out of medical research, in addition to gender bias existing within the field. This is evidenced by the following observations: women were not included in studies of heart disease; lack of funding for diseases that disproportionately affect women, viz. breast cancer; and the effectiveness and safety of medications that are only tested on men but are prescribed to women. According to reports from the National Institute of Health, just 13% of the money allocated by the U.S. government, which is the main source of funding for medical research, has been used to address issues related to women's health. Around 22,071 men and no women were studied in a five-year Physician's Health Study, funded by the NIH, on aspirin consumption and heart attack prevention. During the first 20 years of a prospective study on health and aging, only men were included, even though women make up the majority of those over 65. As unbelievable as it may seem, only men were used as study subjects in one Rockefeller University study on the relationship between obesity and women's propensity to develop endometrial or breast cancer.

In general, developed nations have produced and published a relatively greater number of critical or feminist analyses of medical research than developing nations. However, it's crucial to remember that gender relations are frequently overlooked for research, especially in the field of family planning health studies conducted in developing nations. The research methodology known as the Knowledge, Attitudes, and Practice (KAP) survey, which was widely employed to ascertain the infamous unfulfilled need for family planning in developing nations in the 1960s, has faced significant criticism for being culturally biased and Eurocentric. The traditional definition of unmet need is the desire to delay or abstain from having children while utilizing contemporary methods of contraception like sterilization, intrauterine devices, oral contraceptives, and condoms. In the 1960s and 1970s, the unmet need estimate derived from KAP and the Demographic and Health survey data, funded by USAID, became a crucial tool for policymakers as they conceptualized and created family planning programs and population policies throughout the developing world. My disagreement with the traditional definition of unmet need is that it ignores the widespread use of traditional and non-program methods like breastfeeding and withdrawal in favor of using contemporary contraceptives as the only effective criterion for spacing or limiting births. Apart from its cultural prejudice, this universal metric ignores fertility control strategies that are presently employed in developing nations by men and women alike, such as withdrawal and breastfeeding. These indigenous techniques involve men, have no negative effects, and are user-controlled. However, the foundation of their success and long-term viability has been some pre-arranged agreements and understandings between the partners regarding their sexual interactions. Family planning programs that promote modern contraceptives tend to overlook the intimate and power relations between men and women. This could be the reason behind the greater number of failures rather than successes associated with these methods. Both men's and women's sexual and reproductive rights have been flagrantly abandoned in these gender-insensitive family planning programs to meet the demographic and economic objectives of state population policies.

The gaps and gender biases within medical education and research have led to a situation where doctors have been providing men's healthcare to women. This not only puts women's health and healthcare at risk, but it can also endanger their lives. Some scientists and medical researchers justify excluding women from their studies by claiming it is to protect a woman's potential pregnancy, leading to the belief that it is for women's benefit. They also argue that women's menstrual cycles could complicate research, increase costs, and introduce confounders and outliers into the data. These justifications demonstrate a skewed perspective that views normal bodily functions unique to women as diseases or medical conditions. This reinforces the misconception that women's health issues are caused by their biology and cannot be improved or changed, leading to the exclusion of women from medical research efforts.

The fundamental justification for exclusively male participation in medical research and studies is that society values men, not women, for medical purposes. This is a segment of the spectrum of unequal gender relations, wherein men's lives, and labor are valued more highly than women's. Since we are taught to study the lives of men in history, politics, and the arts, why should this be any different in the medical field? In fact, there have been accusations that the scientific medical establishment not only perpetuates gender inequality in society at large but also actively contributes to it through medical knowledge and practice (Benyamini & Todorova, 2017; Değer, 2023).

10.3.7. Gender-Sensitive Medical Education and Research

To ensure the successful implementation of the Beijing Platform's recommendations on women and health and the mainstreaming of gender into the health sector, what new philosophy, values, objectives, contents, teaching, and learning strategies will these changes to medical education and research take? The discussion that came before it on gender bias in medical education and gender inequalities in health compels us to adopt a gender approach to medical education that would fully account for existing gender differences in healthcare provision at all levels. Additionally, it would highlight how women participate in the healthcare system. Training medical professionals to treat women holistically—not just from the waist down—is the ultimate goal.

Over the past 25 years, the women's health movement has achieved great success and made significant contributions. By establishing social-action groups and women's health centers focused on providing healthcare by and for women, this movement has worked to make medical knowledge more accessible and less intimidating. Women have been encouraged to trust their own experiences and observations of their bodies, challenging traditional clinical knowledge, and emphasizing the importance of subjective understanding in addressing women's health issues. This feminist health education practice has emerged as a result, promoting the development of new skills and areas of knowledge within the women's health movement.

A study, that examined 73 women's health organizations across nine Western nations, proposed that the women's health movement has given rise to a unique specialty in women's healthcare (WHS). Women-only services; the establishment of a woman-space; self-help and holism; feminist counseling and woman-to-woman support; feminist teamwork; diverse health care; information sharing and social action; and, finally, accessibility are the eight key features she has identified for the specialty. Hunt elucidated that diversified healthcare pertains to the various variances among female patients or healthcare consumers, such as differences in social class, sexual orientation, culture, ethnic groupings, and so on. On the other hand, women are treated uniformly in the medical care model. The Women's Health Specialty believes that creating woman space in social, physical, and temporal dimensions is crucial. In addition to making women feel secure and appreciated, this cozy, homey ambiance helps them relax and avoid the cold, clinical atmosphere of a medical facility. The three tenets of the WHS and the cornerstones of the women's health movement, according to Hunt, are feminism, empowerment, and the social model of health. However, how these ideas are applied differs depending on the particulars of each local circumstance. The WHS has expanded the definition of health beyond its biological foundation to include the social environment in which women live. Hunt insists that the social model of health be used as the framework for teaching both feminist principles and empowering practices when advocating for the inclusion of the WHS in postsecondary curricula. There will be many challenges, particularly in relation to the monopolization and appropriation of these ideas, which increases the likelihood that they will be appropriated and made into songs. There are several women's health groups and organizations that focus on reproductive health, especially in Indonesia and the Philippines, even though the concept of a women's health center as it is known in Australia, Canada, or the USA is not as common in the South-east Asian region (personal communication with Lynne Hunt). Relatively few women's organizations in Malaysia, aside from the voluntary family planning associations, can be said to offer women's health services and health education. Since published studies and research are not readily available, there is also comparatively little information about how much the experiences of these women's health groups could be incorporated into medical education in the area.

In fact, a good place to start would be integrating the gender perspective into the medical curriculum through the application of the women's health specialty's guiding principles and practices. However, the question remains: How can we operationalize and translate Hunt's WHS model in a medical setting? To begin with, this kind of transformation will require significant ideological shifts rather than merely curriculum reforms. These days, medical students are more likely to focus only on developing their clinical skills rather than challenging the philosophy and underlying values of medicine. Concepts of social justice, feminism, empowerment, and social action are new and meaningless to many medical students who have been accepted into medical programs that do not require any basic or general education in the liberal arts. Instead, these students have been streamed into the "hard" sciences. Medical students are typically not taught to conceptualize what they are learning, so they either cannot or do not do so. How can the right pedagogy be used to close this ideological gap?

Secondly, what specific instructional strategies and courses are required in the lecture halls so that, upon graduation, the physician not only possesses the necessary skills in reproductive medicine and technology but also can enable a woman patient to exercise her right to an abortion? How could a medical student, intern, nurse, or qualified physician in the hospital save the mother who is lying at home, dying from a postpartum hemorrhage, but is unable to visit the hospital without her husband's consent because he is out of town? Will they be able to acknowledge her right to control her own body and, in a culturally acceptable manner, stand up against her husband and her husband's family? Thirdly, evaluation is intimately tied to instructional strategies. What cutting-edge test will be appropriate to gauge the aforementioned beliefs, commitment, and values of aspiring gender-sensitive physicians?

When it comes to strategy, should we establish a women's health specialty separate from medicine or integrate the gender perspective throughout medicine? While there is a need for specialized health services for women, is creating a separate specialty just preaching to the converted, or will it simply become another branch of specialized medicine? How can we incorporate gender into the health sector when gender inequalities persist in society? Will this require broader political change? These are important questions regarding the integration of the gender perspective in medical education and the implementation of women's health specialty models in medical practice (Benyamini & Todorova, 2017; Değer, 2023).

10.4. Reproductive Health and Ethical Problems in Women's Health

The term "reproductive health" refers to a broad range of topics that are essential to women's health, including family planning, access to contraception, treatment, and prevention of sexually transmitted infections (STIs), infertility, and maternal health. But even with major progress in healthcare, there are still a lot of ethical issues that women must deal with. Regarding women's reproductive health, one of the most important ethical conundrums concerns the right to autonomy and well-informed decision-making. Without interference or criticism, women ought to be allowed to make decisions about their bodies and reproductive lives. However, these choices can be influenced by cultural norms, societal expectations, and even the prejudices of medical professionals. For example, due to the personal beliefs of healthcare providers or prevailing societal attitudes, women may be denied access to contraceptives or face pressure to undergo certain reproductive procedures.

Furthermore, there are connections between the reproductive justice movement and more general social injustices related to socioeconomic status, race, and class. Systemic obstacles frequently prevent women from marginalized communities from accessing reproductive healthcare services. This inequality feeds cycles of injustice and poverty while also undermining their ability to make reproductive decisions for themselves.

Concerns about ethics also surface when discussing assisted reproductive technologies (ART), like surrogacy and *in vitro* fertilization (IVF). Although these technologies give hope to those who are experiencing infertility, they also bring up difficult moral issues related to the exploitation of women's bodies, the commoditization of reproductive labor, and the possibility of social and economic coercion. The commercialization of fertility treatments has the potential to worsen already-existing inequalities by further marginalizing underprivileged groups by making access dependent on financial resources.

Moreover, the discussion of reproductive rights touches on more general issues related to abortion and bodily autonomy. There is intense debate over the moral and legal implications of abortion, with the main points of contention being the rights of the unborn child vs those of the pregnant person. Legislative restrictions or social stigma pertaining to abortion impede women's autonomy in making decisions regarding their own bodies and reproductive futures. Women are frequently pushed toward risky and covert procedures by the criminalization of abortion, endangering their health and well-being.

Furthermore, there is a close relationship between women's reproductive health and their overall health and well-being, which includes their mental health. Women's health outcomes are severely hampered by problems like postpartum depression, pregnancy-related complications, and reproductive cancers. However, stigma and weak support networks might keep women from getting the care they need on time or from accessing the resources they need, which would exacerbate these health inequalities.

Gender equity, autonomy, and social justice must be given priority in a multifaceted approach to addressing the ethical issues surrounding women's reproductive health. This means making sure that all women, regardless of their identity or socioeconomic status, have access to comprehensive and inclusive healthcare services. Policies should be developed to remove structural obstacles and support reproductive rights, and healthcare professionals must be taught to respect the values of patient autonomy and cultural competence. Furthermore, the development of a more just and moral environment for women's reproductive health depends on encouraging candid communication and questioning cultural norms surrounding gender, sexuality, and reproduction. In the end, we can work toward a future where everyone has the chance to lead healthy and fulfilling reproductive lives by emphasizing women's agency and dignity.

Certain cultural connotations and representations of femininity exist, but they are frequently linked to motherhood, which is frequently connected to women's innate capacity for nurturing. Although being a mother is an esteemed and affirmative identity, the prevalent role of motherhood in numerous cultures serves to minimize the diversity among women. Among the most prevalent stereotypes in society about women are those of being "good mothers," "bad mothers," "permissive mothers," "childless mothers," etc. These discourses expose women to stigmatization. For instance, stigmatization occurs in many societies when a woman chooses not to become a mother or experiences infertility, despite failing to fulfill her socially and personally expected roles. Such accusations and stigmatization could have detrimental effects by forcing them to undergo interminable fertility treatments that could jeopardize their health and make people insensitive to women's health issues. Additionally, patriarchal discourses that view women as weak, illiterate, and in need of protection or guidance are frequently combined with the stigmatization of reproductive decisions or circumstances. As a result, women's reproductive health has many facets, and different people around the world experience different aspects of women's health.

The 1948 World Health Organization health definition had a significant impact on efforts to define sexual health. An agreement on an expanded definition of reproductive health, including sexual health, was reached at a conference named the International Population and Development Conference on International Conference and Development/ICPD, which was held in Cairo in 1994. Public access to these services was also stressed. The International Conference on Population and Development (ICPD) defined sexual health as a component of reproductive health; this definition has been the subject of debate in recent years. It is commonly acknowledged that sexual health is distinct from reproductive health and should be viewed as such. The report's first section explains that rather than being a component of or a prerequisite for reproductive health, sexual health is the foundation for access to it.

While most sexual activity is not directly related to reproduction and has an impact on an individual's entire life, sexuality, and sexual relations are central to both reproductive and sexual health. As such, it is possible to view sexual health as a more expansive concept. Human rights and sexual health issues are still being discussed, and papers on international human rights are being used more frequently to promote and support private and public efforts to guarantee and fulfill governments' respect for sexual and reproductive rights as well as to guarantee the security and fulfillment of governments. Sexual and reproductive health are conceptually integrated. The WHO defines sexual health as a condition of social, mental, and physical well-being associated with sexuality. It necessitates not only a positive and courteous perspective on sexuality and relationships, but also the possibility of enjoyable and safe sexual experiences free from all forms of coercion, discrimination, and violence. The entirety of the reproductive system's components, operations, and procedures are the focus of reproductive health.

There is growing agreement that certain human rights must be respected and protected to achieve and maintain sexual health. It is important to discuss sexual rights in this context. The sexual right adds to the continuing conversation about human rights related to sexual health. Sexual rights are the existing human rights that are applied to sexuality and sexual health. Sexual rights uphold everyone's ability to experience, express, and benefit from their sexual health while also protecting their rights within the parameters of anti-discrimination laws. Sexual health and the degree to which human rights are upheld, safeguarded, and realized are correlated. Certain human rights are covered by sexual rights; these rights are already acknowledged in national laws, relevant agreements, and international and regional human rights documents.

Critical rights for the maintenance of sexual health include:

- Rights for maintaining equality and avoiding discrimination.
- Right not to be tortured or exposed to cruelty, inhuman or humiliating treatment or punishment.
- The right to have privacy.
- The highest accessible health standard (including sexual health) and social security rights.
- The right to get married and have a family involves the free and full consent of future spouses for marriage contracts and the right to equality in divorce.
- The right to decide on the number and the interval of birth of children by the parents.
- The right to obtain information and receive education.
- The rights of freedom of thought and expression.
- The right to apply for an effective legal path for violations of fundamental rights.

Everyone must respect others' rights to use human rights responsibly. Different health issues are brought on by the biological differences between men and women. One of the aspects of this difference that is immediately apparent is the onset of a new life period called menopause, which coincides with the end of fertility. Other aspects include the pregnancy and birth processes that are specific to women's physiology and the unique illnesses that are more common among women. Furthermore, because some diseases and conditions in women form a different risk group that varies according to age, diseases seen in the reproductive organs in cases caused by female physiology are very severe. Thus, it can be concluded that unique solutions should be created in this area and that health issues unique to women should be addressed separately (Benyamini & Todorova, 2017; Değer, 2023).

10.4.1. Sexual Health (SH) and Reproductive Health (RH) Problems of Women

The women live a large portion of their lives during what is referred to as "the age of fertility." Most women's experiences with pregnancy-related complications occur during this time, which spans the ages of 15 to 49. In many developing nations around the world, unfavorable pregnancy and delivery outcomes are regarded as the leading cause of disease and mortality for fertile women (Table 10.1).

Table 10.1. *Sexual Health (SH) and Reproductive Health (RH) Problems of Women Over Age Periods*

Fetal and Childhood Period (0–9 Ages)
· Gender choice, female circumcision, early menarche because of hormonal imbalances.
· Neglecting the health status of girls and restricting them from health services because boys are favored or pampered by the family.
· Malnutrition in girls because of less breastfeeding and insufficient nutrition.
· Inadequacy in immunization.
· Infections (such as pneumonia, diarrhea).
· The rate of morbidity and mortality is higher in girls aged between 2 and 5 years than in boys.
· Sexual abuse, harassment (incest relationship, child pornography, etc.).
Adolescent Period (10–19 Ages)
· Physiological change in the reproductive system (development in Menarch, Telarch, and secondary sexual characters).
· Failure to benefit from sexual and reproductive health services.
· Social gender discrimination and pressure.
· Sexual harassment and abuse (such as prostitution, incest relationships, pornography, etc.).
· Early marriage.
· Adolescent pregnancy.
· Unhealthy abortion.
· Sexually transmitted diseases (STD such as HIV).
· Harmful habits (such as alcohol, smoking, and drugs).
· Depression, suicide.
· Violence.
· Anemia is malnutrition because of insufficient and unbalanced nutrition.
· Eating disorders (such as anorexia neurosis and bulimia neurosis).
· Female genital mutilation.
Adulthood/Fertile Period (15–49 Ages)

• Problems with pregnancy, birth, and postpartum period.
• Unwanted pregnancy.
• Deliberate abortion.
• Deaths due to pregnancy and mother deaths.
• Infertility.
• Traditional applications are harmful to health.
• Sexual health problems (vaginismus, abortion sexual desire and disgust, orgasmic disorders, dyspareunia, etc.)
• Sexual health problems (vaginismus, sexual desire and disgust, orgasmic disorders, dyspareunia).
• Anemia and malnutrition.
• Violence.
• Sexual harassment and abuse.
• Harmful habits (alcohol, smoking).
• Sexually transmitted diseases (such as HIV).
Menopause and Post-Menopause Period (50 Age and Over)
• Menopausal complaints (such as fever, night sweats, insomnia, and dyspareunia).
• Pelvic organ prolapsed.
• Incontinence.
• Vaginal infection and irritation.
• Decrease in sexual desire.
• Violence.
• Increased incidence of especially breast, lung, and colon cancer.
• Postmenopausal bleeding.
• Chronic diseases (such as cardiovascular problems and diabetes).
• Postmenopausal problems (genital atrophy, osteoporosis, and increased risk of vulva cancer).
• Mental and psychological problems (such as loneliness, decreased self-esteem, depression, and dementia.

Source: Bayram, D. V., (2023). Reproductive health and ethical problems in women's health. Midwifery – New Perspectives and Challenges [Working Title]. IntechOpen. Available at: http://dx.doi.org/10.5772/intechopen.110254.

Another key factor contributing to the disparities in women's health issues is the unequal access to healthcare faced by women compared to men. This inequality extends beyond just healthcare services, with women often lacking equal rights and opportunities in decision-making processes related to education, socioeconomic status, income, development, and even within their households. These disparities are rooted in the social gender roles that both men and women are taught and expected to adhere to within society, leading to inequalities based on gender. The concept of social gender encompasses the societal expectations and norms associated with being a man or a woman, which are instilled in individuals from a young age and reinforced through education and socialization.

Women's health is not improving as long as their global social and economic rights are denied. One major barrier to women's health status improvements is their social and political invisibility because the rights to their health and well-being are being violated. The simplest medical ethics axiom—prevention of damage—becomes nearly impossible in certain contexts when the most fundamental ethical standards and human rights are rejected. Specifically, the intentional harm caused by sexual violence during military conflicts keeps women from having the right to be free from physical harm. The psychological and reproductive health of women and their families will be impacted for future generations if women's human rights are eliminated due to war crimes or just cultural norms.

Ensuring the health of mothers and future generations is an ethical obligation that cannot be overstated, yet in many parts of the world, this ideal remains elusive and unattainable. Governments are directly impacted by the correlation between the value of family health status and the global status of abortion and women. Even though governments' disregard for women's safety and health has a negative impact on women's political, economic, and health stability over the long run, abortion is still a top priority in many nations. This creates a significant barrier that the medical field must eventually surmount. Human rights advocacy and education are among the moral duties of a learned profession such as medicine to create a better future. The key to the ethical duty of the learned medical profession and to improving women's health is to highlight the link between the economic and social circumstances of women globally and the health of women and their families.

Two unique health issues that continue to obstruct health promotion are at the core of international medical ethics and link women's cultural roles and status with detrimental medical outcomes. Notable examples are the numerous connections that exist between moral dilemmas, cultural and religious traditions, and women's health rights. Female genital mutilation (FGM) is one example of a culturally affected health issue. Another is the widespread incidence of HIV in women, which is linked to their inability to refuse sexual activity due to cultural expectations, poverty, social status, sexual violence, or cultural submission. Alternatively, they cannot ensure safe sexual activity by insisting on the use of condoms (Benyamini & Todorova, 2017; Değer, 2023).

10.4.2. Hymen Examination or Virginity Testing

The hymen, an elastic membrane with many tiny vessels, covers the vaginal opening to some extent and is typically torn during the first sex. Hymen, which is regarded as a crucial component of femininity and sexuality, has acquired cultural significance by having an impact on people's lives and communities. In certain cultural contexts, a woman's history of sexual activity may disqualify her from consideration for marriage; therefore, if a woman desires to marry and start a family, she may need to hide her past sexual activity. While virginity is no longer considered culturally significant in Western societies, it is still highly valued in Muslim societies in the East. Because of this, virginity tests are frequently used, particularly in Eastern societies.

The virginity test, also known as the hymen examination, is a method used to determine whether a woman has previously engaged in sexual activity through gynecological procedures. The virginity test involves examining the female sexual organ to ascertain whether the subject has engaged in sexual activity. It is also known as the examination of the hymen, two fingers, or per vaginal. The two most popular methods are to measure the size of the entrance or the degree of looseness of the vaginal wall by placing two fingers in the vagina and examining the hymen for size or tears. Both methods are used under the assumption that the subjects have a unique genital appearance from regular sexual activity. The dominant social belief underlying the test is that a woman's virginity is a sign of her moral character and social values, her compliance with marriage, her assessment of sexual assault, her application for a job, or some other context.

Most virginity tests are conducted on single women, typically without consent or in situations where the subjects cannot give consent. An MD, a police officer, or a community leader could be the person inspecting the area. Afghanistan, Bangladesh, Egypt, India, Indonesia, Iran, Jordan, Palestine, South Africa, Sri Lanka, Swaziland, Turkey, and Uganda are among the nations where this practice is reportedly employed. For a variety of regional reasons, the virginity test is administered in different nations. Virginity tests have been administered to schoolgirls in certain Kwazulu Natal, South Africa, and Swaziland communities to discourage premarital sex and lower the HIV prevalence. In India, the test is a component of the evaluation given to rape victims for sexual assault. This exam is now required in Indonesia as part of the application process for women to join the country's police force. Reports of virginity tests are appearing in nations like Canada, Spain, Sweden, and the Netherlands that have no prior history of virginity tests because of growing globalization. Official estimates of the prevalence of virginity tests indicate abortion, even though it is a long-standing custom in some communities. Because of this, accounts of its occurrence appear in a variety of social contexts across national boundaries, although its prevalence is not entirely understood. In certain contexts, routine use of virginity tests has become more widely known due to increased interest in ending sexual violence.

The hymen examination cannot precisely reveal information about vaginal penetration or any other sexual history, according to a systematic review that examined 17 studies on the virginity test. Both people with and without a history of vaginal penetration may have normal results from their hymen examination. It is not guaranteed that an abnormal hymen examination will reveal abnormal hymen properties, such as hymen cutting, tearing, expansion, or scars; these characteristics can be seen in both women with and without a history of sexual activity.

The size of the hymen opening is one hymen characteristic that is frequently looked at in the virginity test. The size of the hymen opening was discovered to be an unreliable indicator of vaginal penetration. The examination technique, the subject's position, their level of cooperation and relaxation, as well as their age, height, and weight, all affect how big or small the hymen opening is. In terms of hymen injury healing, it was discovered that most of these wounds healed quickly and that no prior trauma was visible.

A different method of testing virginity involves sticking two fingers into the vagina to see how loose they are. This examination is not recognized by the medical community as a clinical indicator of prior sexual activity. The vagina is a muscular channel that is dynamic and has a flexible shape and dimension that varies depending on the individual, developmental stage, posture, and hormonal factors like stress and sexual arousal. Nonetheless, there are rumors that in certain nations, like India, the "finger test" is employed to assess the strength of sexual assault evidence.

Limited research has been conducted on the effects of virginity tests on the individuals undergoing the examination. However, based on a review of eight studies, it has been found that virginity tests can lead to physical harm. In one alarming case, five students from Turkey attempted suicide by consuming mouse poison to avoid the virginity test. These tests have also been linked to psychological trauma, including anxiety, depression, loss of self-confidence, and even suicide. Health professionals have noted that violations of privacy and autonomy are negative outcomes of these examinations.

Furthermore, virginity tests can have a negative social impact, resulting in social exclusion, perceived dishonor, discrimination in employment, humiliation, and an increased risk of sexual assault. It has been determined that virginity testing, also known as two fingers, hymen, or vagina head examination, is not a useful clinical tool and can be physically, psychologically, and socially harmful to the individual being tested. From a human rights perspective, virginity tests can be considered a form of sexual assault when performed without consent, as well as a manifestation of gender discrimination and a violation of fundamental rights.

In many countries, virginity tests are often forced on women who claim to be victims of rape or accused of engaging in prostitution and are sometimes used as part of public or social policies to control sexuality, including in hospitals and detention facilities (Benyamini & Todorova, 2017; Değer, 2023).

10.4.3. Hymen Examination in Cases of Sexual Assault

The hymen examination needs to be done in well-lit conditions. When someone is placed in the dorsosacral position, their labiums are gently pulled upward, exposing their vagina, vestibule, and hymen. A chart should be used to display the shape and rupture of the hymen. The following questions should be answered during the hymen examination: 1-What type of hymen? 2-Is there a rupture in the hymen? 3-Is the rupture new or old? 4-How many ruptures are there? 5-Where are the ruptures? 6-Do the ruptures reach the vagina wall? 7-Are there any findings like ecchymosis around the hymen? The clock dial ought to indicate where the ruptures are located. The rate at which hymen heals varies depending on the patient, the quantity and severity of ruptures, local and venereal diseases, and vulva hygiene. The fastest healing time for a single partial rupture, according to the colposcope examination, was nine days. However, the healing process for more intricate ruptures could take up to 24 days. Based on the clock dial, most of the ruptures (62%) occur between 5 and 7. When touched, the ruptured area is red, swollen, painful, and bleeding. The rupture area shrinks after 8 to 10 days, and they typically heal in 7 days. Natural notches on hymens are common and can combine with remnants of tears. They are typically discovered a priori and do not penetrate the vaginal wall. Certain hymens have elastic structures that allow for sexual activity without tearing. Such hymens have an opening as large as 3–3.5 cm. We refer to these as anatomical virgins. These cases occur about 30% of the time. The hymen rupture does not indicate sexual activity without the subject's consent.

Therefore, regardless of the justification, a hymen examination is a violation of human rights. Governments, medical associations, and healthcare professional organizations worldwide—including those without a virginity history—should take the lead in establishing national policies that forbid the use of virginity tests and establish standards for health professionals, public servants, and community leaders. To create more comprehensive and successful educational strategies that involve communities, more research is required to comprehend the regional and cultural origins of the virginity test. Public health experts and medical faculty should revise textbooks, courses, and training programs to remove all recommendations about the virginity test and inform students about the test's lack of scientific support and possible risks.

10.4.4. Female Genital Mutilation/Cutting (FGM/C)

The external genital organs may be removed entirely or partially during FGM/C, or there may be other non-medical injuries to the female genitalia. It is acknowledged as a human rights infringement. There's no known health benefit, but there have been numerous negative outcomes noted. The World Health Organization estimates that FGM/C affects over 200 million women and girls globally. Around 3 million girls are at risk of undergoing FGM/C before turning 15 each year.

While female genital mutilation (FGM) is still practiced in many parts of the world, scholarly research on women's bodies and "clitoris" has increased significantly since the late 1980s, opening the door for contentious discussions. Many national and international regulations aim to outlaw FGM entirely or in part. Girls and women are frequently subjected to FGM in this application, which is said to have a two millennium of history. Examining and addressing legal regulations solely from a health perspective is not the only way to examine the mutilation expressed in various concepts in the literature. Examining this application should consider the reasons, the history of FGM, and both the short- and long-term side effects. This application is one of the most visible and tangible instances of masculine dominance because it is used to restrict women's position in society and regulate their sexuality.

Female genital mutilation was defined as "all the procedures that do not have therapeutic properties or cultural reasons or damage the female genital organs or a partial or full removal of the external genital region" by the World Health Organization, the United Nations Population Fund, and the UN Children Aid Fund in 1997. This definition has been the subject of numerous academic studies. Various concepts, including female genital mutilation, female circumcision, injury, cutting, and even torture, have been employed in literature to explain this practice (Figure 10.1).

Around 30 countries practice FGM/C, primarily in Southeast Asia, the Middle East, and Africa. Strong cultural customs of ethnic origin are followed for a variety of purposes, such as completing a transition ceremony, fostering a sense of ethnic identity, granting social acceptance, protecting virginity, and promoting marriage, loyalty, and religious convictions. Although there is no mention of FGM/C in any major sacred text, like the Bible or the Qur'an, some groups hold that it is a religious requirement. Individuals without medical training, such as midwives and birth officials, perform FGM.

During the application, instruments like knives, scissors, cutting tools, hot objects, and similar ones are used. Most of the time, traditional practitioners handle the application, according to a

2013 UNICEF report. Medical professionals only apply FGM in specific circumstances. In this case, for instance, FGM is exclusively carried out by traditional practitioners in Senegal, Niger, Benin, and the United Republic of Tanzania. Furthermore, since most operations are carried out at home, it is frequently not possible to provide a clean, sterile environment that is appropriate for the procedure.

Female Genital Mutilation or Cutting Classification and Sub classification

Type I: Partial or total removal of the clitoris and/or the prepuce (clitoridectomy)

- Type Ia: Removal of the clitoral hood or prepuce only
- Type Ib: Removal of the clitoris with the prepuce

Type II: Partial or total removal of the clitoris and the labia minora, with or without excision of the labia majora (excision)

- Type IIa: Removal of the labia minora only
- Type IIb: Partial or total removal of the clitoris and the labia minora
- Type IIc: Partial or total removal of the clitoris, the labia minora, and the labia majora

Type III: Narrowing of the vaginal orifice with the creation of a covering seal by cutting and appositioning the labia minora and/or the labia majora, with or without excision of the clitoris (infibulation)

- Type IIIa: Removal and apposition of the labia minora
- Type IIIb: Removal and apposition of the labia majora

Type IV: Unclassified; all other harmful procedures to the female genitalia for nonmedical purposes, for example: pricking, pulling, piercing, incising, scraping, and cauterization

Figure 10.1. *WHO classification of female genital mutilation.*

Source: Bayram, D. V., (2023). Reproductive health and ethical problems in women's health. Midwifery – New Perspectives and Challenges [Working Title]. IntechOpen. Available at: http://dx.doi.org/10.5772/intechopen.110254.

FGM is performed on girls before the age of five and is typically finished by the time the girls reach the age of 15 in half of the aforementioned nations. For instance, it was reported that in Yemen, 85% of girls were exposed to FGM during the first week of their lives. According to survey data from 30 states by 2016, at least 200 million women and children were exposed to FGM, though UNICEF stressed that the precise figure is unknown. It is well known that FGM is pervasive throughout all of Africa, particularly in the Middle East (Iraq, Yemen, and other countries in the region) and Asia (Indonesia). Furthermore, even though the prevalence of FGM varies greatly amongst nations and areas, it is reported that over 40% of cases occur frequently, particularly in Western, Eastern, and North African nations like Mali, Mauritania, Gambia, Guinea, Djibouti, and Sudan. Migration to Europe, North America, Australia, New Zealand, and Japan is known to have resulted in a significant increase in the application rate among female immigrants in these countries. Due to the incomparability of the data currently available in the countries that have experienced migration during the last 30 years, it appears difficult to determine the total number of women and children affected by FGM in these countries and to perform national comparisons. In addition to the national representative data from the application's home countries, some specific data can be obtained thanks to data provided by international research programs. Accordingly, the prevalence of FGM among children in East Africa between the ages of 0 and 14 was 71.4% in 1995 and fell to 8% in 2016. In North Africa, it was 57.7% in 1990 and dropped to 14.1% in 2015. In West Africa, the percentage dropped from 73.6% in 1996 to 25.4% in 2017.

Around 5,13,000 women and girls are thought to be at risk of experiencing the negative effects of FGM/C if they are born to mothers who immigrated from nations that practice the practice or if they are immigrants from these nations living in the United States. Of these women and girls, about half are from Egypt, Ethiopia, or Somalia.

FGM typically affects children between the ages of 4 and 12, and it can lead to several complications, including increased risk of obstetric complications during birth, bleeding, infection, sepsis, infertility, dysmenorrhea, dyspareunia, keloids, cysts, abscesses, as well as psychological effects. Additionally, the application poses a risk to the infant. Type III FGM infibulations should be opened for sexual activity and later in life for childbirth (defibulation). Because of the nearly total closure of the urethra and vagina, infibulation can result in abortion, painful menstruation, and increased urine output. Common complications include painful sexual encounters and urinary incontinence. The psychological and emotional effects of female mutilation are the least well-documented. Three significant psychological effects should be mentioned: "anxiety" brought on by sleeplessness and hallucinations; "response depression" brought on by a delayed healing process; and "psychotic excitement" brought on by divorce and childlessness. The most severe kind of sexual abuse is female genital mutilation (FGM), which is illegal in many nations (Table 10.2).

Table 10.2. *WHO Guidelines on the Management of Health Complications from Female Genital Mutilation*

Risk	Remarks
	Immediate Risks
Hemorrhage	–
Pain	–
Shock	Hemorrhagic, neurogenic, or septic
Genital tissue swelling	Due to inflammatory response or local infection.
Infections	Acute local infections; abscess formation; septicemia; genital and reproductive tract infections; urinary tract infections. The direct association between FGM and HIV remains unclear, although the disruption of genital tissues may increase the risk of HIV transmission.
Urination problems	Acute urine retention; pain passing urine; injury to the urethra.
Wound healing problems	–
Death	Due to severe bleeding or septicemia.
	Obstetric Risks
Cesarean section	–

Postpartum hemorrhage	Postpartum blood loss of 500 ml or more.
Episiotomy	–
Prolonged labor	–
Obstetric tears/ lacerations	–
Instrumental delivery	–
Difficult labor/dystocia	–
Extended maternal hospital stays	–
Stillbirth and early neonatal death	–
Infant resuscitation at delivery	–
Sexual Functioning Risks	
Dyspareunia (pain during sexual intercourse)	There is a higher risk of dyspareunia with type III FGM relative to types I and II.
Decreased sexual satisfaction	–
Reduced sexual desire and arousal	–
Decreased lubrication during sexual intercourse	–
Reduced frequency of orgasm or anorgasmia	–
Psychological Risks	
Post-traumatic stress disorder (PTSD)	–
Anxiety disorders	–
Depression	–
Long-Term-Risks	
Genital tissue damage	With consequent chronic vulvar and clitoral pain
Vaginal discharge	Due to chronic genital tract infections
Vaginal itching	–
Menstrual problems	Dysmenorrhea, irregular menses, and difficulty in passing menstrual blood

Reproductive tract infections	Can cause chronic pelvic pain
Chronic genital infections	Including increased risk of bacterial vaginosis
Urinary tract infections	Often recurrent
Painful urination	Due to obstruction and recurrent urinary tract infections

Source: Bayram, D. V., (2023). Reproductive health and ethical problems in women's health. Midwifery – New Perspectives and Challenges [Working Title]. IntechOpen. Available at: http://dx.doi.org/10.5772/intechopen.110254.

Furthermore, speculum examination may be challenging or impossible in women with Type III FGM/C due to the narrowing of genital scarring or introitus. Treatment options for FGM/C include non-surgical and surgical methods for infertility, genitourinary cysts, and complications related to nerve damage persistent pelvic pain, and sexual dysfunction. Using lubricants, topical lidocaine, and behavioral modifications like refraining from actions that put pressure on the vaginal area are non-surgical interventions for pelvic pain (e.g., cycling). Sexual function has been successfully improved by sex therapy. It is recommended that women who experience Type III FGM/C complications undergo defibulation (i.e., the elimination of the anxiety caused by the constricted vaginal opening).

The current efforts have not yet effectively reduced the number of women and girls who have been exposed to genital mutilation, and they do not meet the health needs of millions of women who are still living with mutilation, despite the growing need for clear guidelines in the treatment and care of women who have undergone genital mutilation to eliminate or abandon the application. International efforts to combat FGM have concentrated on treating pertinent health issues, tending to survivors' needs, and including medical professionals as important stakeholders, mainly to stop the practice. To fulfill this responsibility, the WHO created the 2016 guide on managing FGM-related health complications.

FGM/C is referred to as a type of gender-based violence (GBV) and is a global issue pertaining to gender inequality, public health, and human rights. The 1948 Universal Declaration of Human Rights, the 1966 International Contract on Civil and Political Rights (also known as the Twin Contracts), and the 1966 International Contract on Social and Cultural Rights are also references to FGM because it is a violation of women's and children's human rights. Furthermore, it should be mentioned that two international resource documents are the 1989 Convention on the Rights of the Children and the 1979 Convention on the Prevention of All Discrimination against Women, considering the group exposed to the application. In a ruling, the European Court of Human Rights (ECHR) underlined that subjecting an adult or child to FGM would violate Article 3 of the ECHR.

When examining regional legal regulations, the African Union Organization garnered attention in 1990 regarding the rights and prosperity of children. Under the heading of "eliminating harmful practices" and the medicalization of this procedure, the African Convention on the Rights of the African Humans and People, also known as the Maputo Protocol, specifically forbade FGM in 2005. Furthermore, the African organization declared in 2019 that they were starting a campaign to end women's genital mutilation and that their goal was to eradicate all forms of gender-based violence, including FGM, by the year 2063. As per the Equality Now report from March 2020, out of 92 countries where FGM is practiced, 51 have outlawed it through direct national legislation (refer to Benin, Eritrea, Guinea, Kenya, Italy, etc.) (see Egypt, Djibouti, Ghana, France, Germany, Australia, New Zealand, etc.) and incorporated it into the laws about punishment, child protection, violence against women, and domestic abuse.). Anti-FGM laws are widely enforced by diaspora communities and are specifically implemented in 28 African countries. Additionally, anti-FGM laws exist in other states, including America, Canada, Australia, and New Zealand. Furthermore, it is claimed that the various applications of FGM in different nations represent a significant issue. For instance, the East African Community made transitions between the countries within the other countries, such as Tanzania, where FGM is prohibited from the age of 18 by redrawing the border from Kenya and signing the Women's Genital Mutilation Prohibition Agreement in 2016. Furthermore, the parties are subject to several obligations in this regard under the Istanbul Convention and the Convention on the Prevention of All Discrimination Against Women (CEDAW). Initially, as stated in CEDAW 1st Article 1, "The recognition and use of human rights and fundamental freedoms in political, economic, social, cultural, or other fields based on the equality of women and men" is defined as "distinction against women" under this agreement. This will include any form of discrimination, denial, or limitation that stops, gets rid of, or is motivated by a person's gender. Without a doubt, this definition also covers the application of FGM. Furthermore, in recommendation decision 14, the CEDAW Committee suggested several actions to be taken suitably and efficiently to eradicate the "female mutilation in all of the parties." Similarly, FGM was included in the list of harmful practices that the parties were required to prevent and end for women and girls in the recommendation of Decision 31.

For nations, FGM is a financial burden. According to a study by WHO on the financial implications of treating FGM-related health issues, the current costs for 27 countries for which data are available came to $1.04 billion in a single year (2018). This amount is predicted to rise to $2.03 billion in 30 years (2047) if the prevalence of FGM stays the same, which translates to a 68% increase in inertia costs. But in the following 30 years, these expenses will drop by 60% if nations stop performing FGM.

WHO efforts to eliminate FGM and Medicalization focus on:

1. **Strengthening of Health Sector Intervention:** To develop and implement the guidelines, tools, training, and policy to provide medical care and counseling to girls and women living with FGM and to communicate to prevent implementation.
2. **Evidence Creation:** To produce information about the reasons, results, and costs of the application, including why health service providers do the application, how to leave the application, and how to look at the FGM.
3. **Increasing Advocacy:** Developing publications and advocacy tools for international, regional, and local efforts to terminate the FGM (including tools to predict the potential public health benefits and cost savings of FGM).

FGM/C is therefore a global issue pertaining to human rights and health in the broader framework of GBV. Comprehending the intricate socio-cultural requirements of this practice is imperative, as is formulating policies that best safeguard women and girls from it and present them in the most favorable light. Political will should be demonstrated to support professional education concerning health system reforms as well as the safety and well-being of women and children. Programs for prevention and training can be organized to assist communities in quitting this detrimental habit. Women, educators, school nurses, medical professionals, and security personnel who have been impacted by FGM should all be included in the very disciplined campaign to end FGM. Group education and training should also be a part of this effort. Instead of being an elective, health and well-being education ought to be a part of the core curriculum. Furthermore, it is critical to consider the psychosocial effects of female genital mutilation and identify how medical professionals can support patient care. Examining women's experiences and attitudes regarding FGM is essential, in addition to the effects of intercultural psychology.

10.4.5. Other Aspects

Rapid population growth is a serious problem for nations because of the associated social, economic, environmental, and urbanization issues. It also has an indirect negative impact on "excessive fertility" and directly affects "health."

Population dynamics, a health phenomenon of paramount importance, are influenced by national population policies, individual fertility patterns, the legal status of family planning services, and the availability, acceptability, and accessibility of such services even in cases where they are legal. If risky pregnancies can be avoided through family planning practices, calculations indicate that morbidity and mortality rates for mothers and children will drop by 30% to 40%. Put differently, if family planning services are successfully implemented in developing nations, it may be possible to reduce the number of risky pregnancies and prevent 30–40% of deaths among mothers and infants caused by excessive fertility.

Every year, pregnancy-related complications claim the lives of over 5,00,000 women; only 1% of these deaths take place in developed nations, with the remaining 98% occurring in developing nations. While there have been notable advancements in child health over the past two decades, there hasn't been a commensurate improvement in maternal health. Although family planning services can avert at least one-third of maternal and infant deaths, 300 million couples worldwide still lack access to them. Mother mortality rates in developing nations are 100–200 times greater than those in developed nations. Again, based on available data, unhealthful miscarriages account for 13% of maternal fatalities. According to this data, this cause accounts for at least one out of every 10 mother deaths. Around 25% of people on the planet reside in nations with extremely restrictive abortion regulations. This will unavoidably lead to a rise in the use of illicit and unsafe abortion techniques. Unwanted pregnancies and unsafe abortion practices rank among the major health issues affecting women's health in developing nations. The World Health Organization (WHO) estimates that every year, 46 million women worldwide seek abortions; 19 million of these procedures are carried out in unsafe settings; 68,000 of these women lose their lives; and 53 million of these women suffer from temporary or permanent disabilities.

The World Health Organization defines a non-secure abortion as the ending of an unintended pregnancy by someone lacking the required training and experience, or by someone performing the procedure in a way that does not adhere to basic medical standards. Regretfully, women in developing nations are not as fortunate as those in developed nations. Due to laws that forbid safe abortion or attempts to terminate a pregnancy, women are compelled to apply to illiterate people in most of these nations (56%). The situation is much worse in Africa because of poverty and the Catholic church's prohibitions, as well as in many Central and South American countries that follow them. In these areas, 97–90% of women who wish to terminate their pregnancy are forced to use risky, insecure methods. A Turkish study found that the most common reason for a curettage (88% of cases) was "undesirable pregnancy."

Despite being an essential part of services related to sexual and reproductive health, many women encounter barriers that prevent them from taking advantage of safe curettage procedures. It is estimated that only 35 out of 1,000 women in the 15–44 age range are eligible for curettage services each year. The social, cultural, and legal factors that prevent women from accessing these services are numerous. Though about half of all curettage services provided globally are not safe, access to secure curettage services is regarded as a fundamental human right. An instance of insecure curettage service involves an individual attempting to terminate their pregnancy on their own, a healthcare provider lacking the necessary training and experience, or a failure to follow the proper medical protocols. Another issue is that when women look for curettage services, they run the risk of being stigmatized. The widespread belief that it is immoral and/or socially unacceptable is known as curettage stigmatization. Curette stigmatization is widespread worldwide, but it can differ depending on an individual's age, level of civilization, religion, and social, legal, and cultural context. The woman's curettage decision demonstrates how powerfully society interprets curettage. Curettaging has a detrimental impact on women's social, emotional, financial, and physical well-being. Stigmatization of the curtage can lead to regret, rage, sadness, guilt, and stress. Of the 4,000 women who underwent curettage in a study by Shellenberg and TSUI, 58% of the women required emotional support following the procedure.

The World Health Organization (WHO) releases updated guidelines on abortion care to safeguard women's and girls' health and to lessen the annual number of over 25 million unapproved abortions. Obtaining a safe abortion is a crucial component of health services, according to the WHO. It is possible to fully avoid almost all the deaths and injuries brought on by unsafe abortion practices. Therefore, the WHO advises that women and girls have access to family planning and abortion services whenever they require them. These combined guidelines incorporate over 50 recommendations pertaining to clinical practice, healthcare provision, and legal and policy interventions to support high-quality abortion care, all based on the most recent scientific evidence. The WHO recommends abortion as a straightforward and incredibly safe procedure that can be carried out with the assistance of a person who possesses the required knowledge and skills and in accordance with the length of the pregnancy. Sadly, only half of abortions occur under these circumstances; complications from failed abortions result in millions of women being admitted to hospitals annually and approximately 39,000 deaths. Most of these deaths are more common among people who reside in nations where abortion is legal, such as over 60% of Africa and 30% of Asia. The handbook offers guidance on a variety of basic primary interventions that enhance the standard of abortion care given to women and girls. These include a larger spectrum of health professionals sharing tasks. The availability of medical abortion pills guarantees access to safe abortion services for a greater number of women and guarantees that those in need can obtain the appropriate care information.

As of 2011, there was a legal basis for pregnancy termination for a variety of reasons in all 189 countries worldwide, except just five (the Dominican Republic, Malta, El Salvador, Nicaragua, and Chile). Only in these five nations is a lawful abortion not performed, not even in attempts to save the mother's life. A consistent picture with respect to the level of development is observed when examining the disparities in access to safe abortion services between developed and less developed regions. More than 80% of developed nations justify abortion for social, economic, or medical reasons; other reasons include fetal development issues, women's mental or physical health issues, sexual assault, insects, or the need to preserve women's lives. Only 69% of these nations allow women to access abortion services for any reason. These percentages are 62% and 41%, respectively, in developing nations. Around 48 countries liberalized their abortion laws between 1996 and 2009, including Saudi Arabia, Colombia, Jordan, Portugal, Italy, Australia, Mexico, and Switzerland. In contrast, 14 countries imposed miscarriage restrictions, including Poland, the Dominican Republic, El Salvador, Nicaragua, Argentina, Latvia, Hungary, Hungary Congo, Iraq, Qatar, Japan, Algeria, Belize, and Panama. Brazil, Moldova, Vietnam, and Uruguay enacted new laws to lessen the issue of unsafe abortion practices without resorting to court cases. While there are regrettably some nations where women find it difficult to access safe abortion services due to recent developments in Turkey, overall, there have been improvements in the accessibility of services on a global scale. Positively speaking, these developments can be seen in the fact that nations like Sweden (2007); Denmark (2003); and France (2001) have liberal laws and have never experienced unsafe abortions. These applications resulted in the removal of the residency and citizenship requirements in Denmark and Sweden and an increase in the legal abortion period from 12 to 14 weeks in France. Similarly, Ekvador, who had a very restrictive law regarding the policies of the Catholic Church, implemented a law in 2006 that permits safe abortion services in medical facilities in cases where the woman's health or life is in danger or if the pregnancy resulted from sexual assault. Colombia and Mexico City state liberalized their abortion laws in 2006 and 2007, respectively, making it possible for women to access safe and healthful abortion services. Women deliberately made a significant contribution to this issue, particularly concerning South American legal systems. In conclusion, as of October 2011, 73 countries, or 60% of the world's population, could obtain safe and healthy abortion services only upon request and without a valid reason; five of those nations do not voluntarily grant women the right to an abortion.

But the point that needs to be made clear in this instance is that laws do not always accurately reflect the situation. Notwithstanding liberal legislation, women in many developing and impoverished nations are unable to obtain safe abortion services because of issues with accessing abortion drugs, conservative management attitudes, prejudiced behavior and perceptions of medical professionals, and financial constraints. Legislative limitations highlight a portion of the issue. However, despite legal protections, individuals who support women's safety and willingness to exercise their reproductive rights as well as their human rights must address the challenges that women face in a multifaceted manner. Liberal abortion laws should be passed because they are essential rights, but after that, efforts must be made to guarantee the circumstances under which women can exercise these rights. The legalization of curettage plays a significant role in lessening the stigma associated with the practice as well as the death and morbidity it causes. It is crucial to consider the perspective and mindset of the community where the person living in the stigmatized environment is employed. Six of the studies in Yılmaz and Şahin's systematic review address societal attitudes and opinions. According to the studies, single women's experiences were worse in societies where there was a negative sexual culture. These people are viewed by their families as dishonorable, devoid of integrity, unfaithful, murderous, malevolent, and unfit for marriage. Research has shown that individuals who undergo curettage frequently face heightened stigma. Furthermore, it was found that women who had curettage experienced greater stigma than those who had abortions. There are only societies that permit curettage in abortion cases because it is believed that a woman has no say or judgment during the procedure. Because of this, women who desire to terminate their pregnancy can apply for non-secure pregnancy termination methods to start the abortion procedure. The society's religious perspective plays a significant role in preventing stigma. In the research of Loi et al., 89.9% of the 1,207 participants said that women who undergo curettage have sinned and that, as a result, women who choose not to carry their pregnancies should give birth to their children to atone for their transgressions.

The choice to administer care and curettage is also influenced by the viewpoint of medical professionals. Some participants in Zorddo's work called curettages "a dirty job that no one wants to do," while others claimed that some of them gave women's rights, including the freedom to speak about their bodies. Compared to doctors in Spain, it was discovered that Italian doctors were subjected to higher levels of stigmatization, exclusion, and conscientious discrimination. It was found that doctors in Spain did not stigmatize or object as much as doctors in Italy because only pregnancy terminations for medical reasons occurred in Spanish hospitals. It's said that doctors in Italy are a result of the country's deeply religious culture. In their research conducted in Uruguay (Cárdenas et al., 2018). Once curettage was made legal in Uruguay, the stigma associated with it decreased. Health professionals still referred to curettage as "dirty work, morally questionable practice" even after it was legalized. It was found that fear of stamping and legal threats resulted from the absence of laws that fully protect curettage law and practitioners.

Therefore, abortion has been interpreted differently throughout political history and has been governed by laws, making it a crucial issue for women's health. Women's abortion rights have evolved within the context of political relations. Religion and the state promoted abortion during times of population growth. The same state and religious doctrines responded to this strategy by outlawing abortion during times when the rate of population growth slowed. Women's organizations began during the abortion revolution. Throughout this process, it became clear that as abortion became more commonplace and people had more access to it, so did our understanding of sexual freedom.

Strong costs have been incurred to observe that women's participation in production activities and sexual freedom do not lead to their attainment of freedom. Through sexual emancipation, it has come to light that the female body has been transformed into a tool for sexual exploitation. The development of laws prohibiting abortion is a result of the perception that sexual freedom threatens the institution of the family and social order. The expansion of sexual freedom has given rise to a perilous theory that seeks to institutionally dismantle the family. It has become evident that political interests trump the advancement of women's understanding of freedom when it comes to the right to an abortion (Benyamini & Todorova, 2017; Değer, 2023).

A Closer Look

Microinserts

Microinserts are small, flexible contraceptive devices designed for long-term birth control. These devices, typically made of soft, medical-grade plastic, are inserted into the uterine tubes through a minimally invasive procedure known as hysteroscopy. Once in place, microinserts work by inducing a local inflammatory reaction in the uterine tubes, leading to the formation of scar tissue. This scar tissue gradually blocks the uterine tubes, preventing the sperm from reaching the egg and thereby preventing fertilization. Additionally, the inflammatory response alters the tubal environment, further reducing the chances of pregnancy.

Microinserts offer several advantages over traditional forms of contraception. They are highly effective, with a low failure rate comparable to that of tubal ligation or vasectomy. Moreover, they are reversible, allowing women to regain fertility after removal if they desire to become pregnant in the future. The procedure to insert microinserts is relatively quick and can typically be performed on an outpatient basis, minimizing downtime for the patient. The microinserts provide a convenient and reliable option for women seeking long-term contraception without the need for daily medication or surgery. Their effectiveness, reversibility, and minimally invasive nature make them a popular choice among individuals looking for a hassle-free birth control solution (Benyamini & Todorova, 2017; Değer, 2023).

Summary

- Reproductive health encompasses a wide range of issues related to the reproductive system, including fertility, contraception, pregnancy, childbirth, and sexually transmitted infections (STIs).
- Ethical considerations in reproductive medicine are paramount, as they involve complex decisions that impact individuals, families, and society as a whole.
- Surrogacy is an adoption arrangement, often supported by a legal agreement, whereby a woman agrees to childbirth on behalf of another person(s) who will become the child's parent(s) after birth.
- Health literacy is important for everyone because, at some point in our lives, we all need to be able to find, understand, and use health information and services.
- Gender refers to the socially constructed roles, behavior, activities and attributes that a given society at a given time and place considers appropriate for men and women, and boys and girls and the relationships between them.
- The preceding account showed how women's health and ill-health have been reduced to a matter of their biology, and how disregard for women has permeated throughout medical practice and the health services.

References

1. Aniteye, P., O'Brien, B., & Mayhew, S. H. (2016). Stigmatized by association: Challenges for abortion service providers in Ghana. *BMC Health Services Research, 16*(1), 486. https://doi.org/10.1186/s12913-016-1709-2.
2. Atay, H. (2017). Kürtaj Yasasının Arkeolojisi: Türkiye'de Kürtaj Düzenlemeleri, Edimleri, Kısıtları ve Mücadele Alanları. *Fe Dergi, 9*, 1–16.
3. Ayotte, B. (2000). State-control of female virginity in Turkey: The role of physicians. *Journal of Ambulatory Care Management, 23*(1), 89–91. https://doi.org/10.1097/00004479-200001000-00013.
4. Bayram Değer, V. (2023). Reproductive health and ethical problems in women's health. In *Midwifery–New Perspectives and Challenges [Working Title]*. IntechOpen. http://dx.doi.org/10.5772/intechopen.110254.
5. Behrens, K. (2014). Virginity testing in South Africa: A cultural concession taken too far? *South African Journal of Philosophy, 33*(2), 177–187. https://doi.org/10.1080/02580136.2014.939966.
6. Benyamini, Y., & Todorova, I. (2017). Women's reproductive health in a socio-cultural context. *International Journal of Behavioral Medicine, 24*, 799–802. https://doi.org/10.1007/s12529-017-9667-7.
7. Berenson, A., Chacko, M., Wiemann, C., Mishaw, C., Friedrich, W., & Grady, J. (2002). Use of hymenal measurements in the diagnosis of previous penetration. *Pediatrics, 109*(2), 228–235. https://doi.org/10.1542/peds.109.2.228.

8. Berenson, A., Chacko, M., Wiemann, C., Mishaw, C., Friedrich, W., & Grady, J. (2000). A case-control study of anatomic changes resulting from sexual abuse. *American Journal of Obstetrics and Gynecology, 182*(4), 820–834. https://doi.org/10.1016/S0002-9378(00)70338-0.

9. Berkoff, M. C., Zolotor, A. J., Makoroff, K. L., Thackeray, J. D., Shapiro, R. A., & Runyan, D. K. (2008). Has this prepubertal girl been sexually abused? *Journal of the American Medical Association, 300*(23), 2779–2792. https://doi.org/10.1001/jama.2008.854.

10. Cappa, C., Van Baelen, L., & Leye, E. (2019). The practice of female genital mutilation across the world: Data availability and approaches to measurement. *Global Public Health, 14*(8), 1139–1152. https://doi.org/10.1080/17441692.2018.1459584.

11. Cárdenas, R., Labandera, A., Baum, S. E., Chiribao, F., Leus, I., Avondet, S., et al. (2018). "It's something that Marks you": Abortion stigma after decriminalization in Uruguay. *Reproductive Health, 15*(1), 150. https://doi.org/10.1186/s12978-018-0586-2.

12. Celbis, O., Karaca, M., Özdemir, B., & Isır, A. B. (2004). Cinsel Suçlarda Muayene. *Harran Üniversitesi Tıp Fakültesi Dergisi, 1*(4), 48–52.

13. Çevik, E., Tapucu, A., & Aksoy, Ş. (2003). Toplumsal ve etik bir sorun olarak kızlık zarı incelemesi. *T Klin Tıp Etiği-Hukuku, 11,* 170–177.

14. Clarke, E., & Richens, Y. (2016). Female genital mutilation: An 'old' problem with no place in the modern world. *Acta Obstetricia et Gynecologica Scandinavica, 95*(10), 1193–1195. https://doi.org/10.1111/aogs.13002.

15. Cockrill, K., & Biggs, A. (2018). Can stories reduce abortion stigma? Findings from a longitudinal cohort study. *Culture, Health & Sexuality, 20*(3), 335–350. https://doi.org/10.1080/13691058.2017.1344145.

16. Demirci, Ş., Doğan, K., Deniz, İ. Ç., Doğan, N. Ü., & Günaydın, İ. G. (2008). Sağlam himen morfolojilerinin değerlendirilmesi. *Turkiye Klinikleri Journal of Forensic Medicine, 5*(3), 93–100.

17. Donders, Y. (2011). The right to enjoy the benefits of scientific progress: In search of state obligations in relation to health. *Medicine, Health Care, and Philosophy, 14,* 371–381. https://doi.org/10.1007/s11019-011-9331-1.

18. Esia-Donkoh, K., Darteh, E. K. M., Blemano, H., & Asare, H. (2015). Who cares? Pre and post-abortion experiences among young females in Cape Coast Metropolis, Ghana. *African Journal of Reproductive Health, 19*(2), 43–51.

19. Gelman, A., Rosenfeld, E. A., Nikolajski, C., Freedman, L. R., Steinberg, J. R., & Borrero, S. (2017). Abortion stigma among abortion-income women obtaining abortions in Western Pennsylvania: A qualitative assessment. *Perspectives on Sexual and Reproductive Health, 49*(1), 29–36. https://doi.org/10.1363/psrh.12029.

20. Gökgöl, T. (2012). İsteyerek düşük olgusuna global açıdan bakış: Yasalar ve deneyimler. *Türkiye Halk Sağlığı Dergisi, 10*(Özel Sayı 1), Düşükler.

21. Goldberg, H., Stupp, P., Okoroh, E., Besera, G., Goodman, D., & Danel, I. (2016). Female genital mutilation/cutting in the United States: Updated estimates of women and girls at risk, 2012. *Public Health Reports, 131*(2), 340–347. https://doi.org/10.1177/003335491613100218.

22. Gursoy, E., & Vural, G. (2003). Nurses' and midwives' views on approaches to hymen examination. *Nursing Ethics, 10*(5), 485–496. https://doi.org/10.1191/0969733003ne619oa.

23. Heger, A., Ticson, L., Velasquez, O., & Bernier, R. (2002). Children referred for possible sexual

abuse: Medical findings in 2384 children. *Child Abuse & Neglect, 26*(6–7), 645–659. https://doi.org/10.1016/S0145-2134(02)00354-0.

24. Heppenstall-Heger, A., McConnell, G., Ticson, L., Guerra, L., Lister, J., & Zaragoza, T. (2003). Healing patterns in anogenital injuries: A longitudinal study of injuries associated with sexual abuse, accidental injuries, or genital surgery in the preadolescent child. *Pediatrics, 112*(4), 829–837. https://doi.org/10.1542/peds.112.4.829.
25. Hulme-Chambers, A., Temple-Smith, M., Davidson, A., Coelli, L., Orr, C., & Tomnay, J. E. (2018). Australian women's experiences of a rural medical termination of pregnancy service: A qualitative study. *Sexual & Reproductive Healthcare, 15,* 23–27.
26. Independent Forensic Expert Group Statement on Virginity Testing. (2015). *Journal of Forensic and Legal Medicine, 33,* 121–124. https://doi.org/10.1016/j.jflm.2015.05.012.
27. Kandala, N.-B., Ezejimofor, M. C., Uthman, O. A., & Komba, P. (2018). Secular trends in the prevalence of female genital mutilation/cutting among girls: A systematic analysis. *BMJ Global Health, 3,* e000549. https://doi.org/10.1136/bmjgh-2017-000549.
28. Kavanagh, A., Wielding, S., Cochrane, R., Sim, J., Johnstone, A., & Cameron, S. (2018). 'Abortion' or 'termination of pregnancy'? Views from abortion care providers in Scotland, UK. *BMJ Sexual and Reproductive Health, 44*(2), 122–127. https://doi.org/10.1136/bmjsrh-2017-101794.
29. Kellogg, N., Menard, S., & Santos, A. (2003). Genital anatomy in pregnant adolescents: "Normal" does not mean "nothing happened". *Pediatrics, 113*(1), e67–e69. https://doi.org/10.1542/peds.113.1.e67.
30. Khambati, N. (2014). India's two-finger test after rape violates women and should be eliminated from medical practice. *BMJ, 348,* g3336–g3336. https://doi.org/10.1136/bmj.g3336.
31. Klein, E., Helzner, E., Shayowitz, M., Kohlhoff, S., & Smith-Norowitz, T. A. (2018). Female genital mutilation: Health consequences and complications-a short literature review. *Obstetrics and Gynecology International, 2018,* 7365715. https://doi.org/10.1155/2018/7365715.
32. Leclerc-Madlala, S. (2001). Virginity testing: Managing sexuality in a maturing HIV/AIDS epidemic. *Medical Anthropology Quarterly, 15*(4), 533–552. https://doi.org/10.1525/maq.2001.15.4.533.
33. Leclerc-Madlala, S. (2003). Protecting girlhood? Virginity revivals in the era of AIDS. *Agenda: Empowering Women for Gender Equality, 56,* 16–25.
34. Lloyd, J., Crouch, N. S., Minto, C. L., Liao, L. M., & Creighton, S. M. (2005). Female genital appearance: "Normality" unfolds. *BJOG: An International Journal of Obstetrics and Gynaecology, 112*(5), 643–646. https://doi.org/10.1111/j.1471-0528.2004.00481.x.
35. Loi, U. R., Otieno, B., Oguttu, M., Gemzell Danielsson, K., Klingberg-Allvin, M., Faxelid, E., et al. (2019). Abortion and contraceptive use stigma: A cross-sectional study of attitudes and beliefs in secondary school students in western Kenya. *Sexual and Reproductive Health Matters, 27*(3), 1652028. https://doi.org/10.1080/26410397.2019.1652028.
36. Martin, L. A., Debbink, M., Hassinger, J., Youatt, E., & Harris, L. H. (2014). Abortion providers, stigma, and professional quality of life. *Contraception, 90*(6), 581–587. https://doi.org/10.1016/j.contraception.2014.07.011.
37. Mather, M., & Feldman-Jacobs, C. (2016). Women and girls at risk of female genital mutilation/cutting in the United States. *Population Reference Bureau.*

38. McCann, J., Miyamoto, S., Boyle, C., & Rogers, K. (2007). Healing of hymenal injuries in prepubertal and adolescent girls: A descriptive study. *Pediatrics, 119*(5), e1094–e1106. https://doi.org/10.1542/peds.2006-1591.

39. Mishori, R., Warren, N., & Reingold, R. (2018). Female genital mutilation or cutting. *American Family Physician, 97*(1), 49–52.

40. Mosley, E. A., King, E. J., Schulz, A. J., Harris, L. H., De Wet, N., & Anderson, B. A. (2017). Abortion attitudes among South Africans: Findings from the 2013 social attitudes survey. *Culture, Health & Sexuality, 19*(8), 918–933. https://doi.org/10.1080/13691058.2016.1251046.

41. Narayan, R. K. (2007). *The Essentials of Forensic Medicine and Toxicology* (Vol. 26). Hyderabad: K. Suguna Devi.

42. Olson, R. M., & García-Moreno, C. (2017). Virginity testing: A systematic review. *Reproductive Health, 14*(1), 61. https://doi.org/10.1186/s12978-017-0320-4.

43. Özpınar, S., & Eser, E. (2015). Sağlık hizmeti sunanların güvenli düşük ve tıbbi düşük konusundaki tutum ve algıları; Manisa örneği. *TAF Preventive Medicine Bulletin, 14*(2), 87–92.

44. Padubidri, V., & Daftary, S. (Eds.). (2014). *Shaw's Textbook of Gynecology* (16th ed.). New Delhi: Elsevier Health Sciences APAC.

45. Parikh, C. (2005). *Parikh's Textbook of Medical Jurisprudence and Toxicology* (Vol. 6). New Delhi: CBS Publishers and Distributors.

46. Partoune, A., Dechamps, V., Berrendorf, M., Tezel, M., & Boxho, P. (2020). Les tests de virginité et l'examen hymeneal [Virginity testing and hymen examination]. *Revue Médicale de Liège, 75*(10), 670–675. [Note: Article in French].

47. Pillaim, M. (2008). Genital findings in prepubertal girls: What can be concluded from an examination? *Journal of Pediatric and Adolescent Gynecology, 21*(4), 177–185. https://doi.org/10.1016/j.jpag.2007.10.003.

48. Robatjazi, M., Simbar, M., Nahidi, F., Gharehdaghi, J., Emamhadi, M., Vedadhir, A. A., et al. (2015). Virginity testing beyond a medical examination. *Global Journal of Health Science, 8*(7), 152–164. https://doi.org/10.5539/gjhs.v8n7p152.

49. Sabaratnam, A. (2014). Integrating human rights and women's health: An overview. *The Global Library of Women's Medicine*. Retrieved from: https://www.glowm.com/ (accessed on 24 June 2024).

50. Shalhoub-Kevorkian, N. (2005). Imposition of virginity testing: A lifesaver or a license to kill? *Social Science & Medicine, 60*(6), 1187–1196. https://doi.org/10.1016/j.socscimed.2004.06.006.

51. Shellenberg, K. M., & Tsui, A. O. (2012). Correlates of perceived and internalized stigma among abortion patients in the USA: An exploration by race and Hispanic ethnicity. *International Journal of Gynaecology and Obstetrics, 118*(Suppl. 2), S152–S159. https://doi.org/10.1016/j.ijgo.2012.05.015.

52. Subrahmanyam, B., & Modi, J. (2001). *Modi's Medical Jurisprudence and Toxicology* (Vol. 22). New Delhi: Butterworths India.

53. Süt, H. K., & Küçükkaya, B. (2016). Hemşirelik bölümü'nün himen muayenesi ve himenoplastiye karşı tutum ve bakış açılarının incelenmesi. *Dokuz Eylül Üniversitesi Hemşirelik Fakültesi Elektronik Dergisi, 9*(2), 52–60.

54. The African Union. (2019). The African Union launches a continental initiative to end female genital mutilation and save 50 million girls at risk. Retrieved from: https://au.int/ (accessed on 24 June 2024).

55. The European Court of Human Rights. (2007). Sitting on 8 March 2007. *Third Section Decision as to the Admissibility of Application no. 23944/05 by Emily Collins and Ashley Akaziebie against Sweden.* https://www.refworld.org/jurisprudence/caselaw/echr/2007/en/47485

56. The Foundation for The Global Library of Women's Medicine. (2014). The global library of women's medicine: The educational platform for the international federation of gynecology and obstetrics (FIGO). Retrieved March 27, 2014.

57. United Nations Department of Economic and Social Affairs. (2011). *United Nations World Abortion Policies*. New York, NY: Population Division.

58. Varol, N., Hall, J. J., Black, K., Turkmani, S., & Dawson, A. (2017). Evidence-based policy responses to strengthen health, community, and legislative systems that care for women in Australia with female genital mutilation/cutting. *Reproductive Health, 14*(1), 63. https://doi.org/10.1186/s12978-017-0323-1.

59. World Health Organization. (2016). *WHO Guidelines on the Management of Health Complications from Female Genital Mutilation*. Geneva: World Health Organization.

60. Yılmaz, B., & Şahin, N. (2022). Küretaj ve damgalanma: Bir sistematik derleme. *Turkiye Klinikleri Journal of Medical Ethics, 28*(3), 451–462.

61. Zeren Öztürk, G., Toprak, D., Hurşitoğlu, M., & İpek, Y. (2014). Aile sağlığı merkezine gelen kadın hastaların sezaryen ve küretaj hakkındaki bilgi, tutum, davranışları ve sosyodemografik özelliklerle ilişkisi. *Journal of Clinical Obstetrics & Gynecology, 24*(1), 1–8.

62. Zordo, S. D. (2018). From women's 'irresponsibility' to fetal 'patienthood': Obstetricians-gynecologists' perspectives on abortion and its stigmatization in Italy and Cataluña. *Global Public Health, 13*(6), 711–723. https://doi.org/10.1080/17441692.2017.1320021.

INDEX

P

R

S

Printed and bound by CPI Group (UK) Ltd, Croydon, CR0 4YY
18/09/2026
14965062-0002